Computer Applications in Nursing Education and Practice

Jean M. Arnold, EdD, RN
Associate Professor
Rutgers The State University of New Jersey
College of Nursing

Gayle A. Pearson, DrPH, RN
Director of Continuing Education
Rutgers The State University of New Jersey
College of Nursing

National League for Nursing · New York
Pub. No. 14–2406

To the pioneering nurses who have been in the forefront of integrating computer applications into nursing education and practice, including all of the authors who have made valuable contributions to this book.

The views expressed in this publication represent the views of the authors and do not necessarily reflect the official views of the National League for Nursing.

This book was set in Aster by Better Graphics, Inc. The editor and designer was Nancy Jeffries. Port City Press, Inc. was the printer and binder. The cover was designed by Lauren Stevens.

Printed in the United States of America

Contents

Preface

This unique publication provides descriptions of how nurses are using computer technology to expand nursing knowledge in a variety of clinical and educational settings. Contained within are examples of how nurses created computer applications either using generic or application software.

Rutgers The State University College of Nursing Continuing Education Program has sponsored an Annual National Nursing Computer Conference since 1982. Both the National League for Nursing and the American Nurses Association have co-sponsored this conference. The idea for this book grew out of numerous requests for copies of papers presented at the conference from people who were unable to attend. The writings contained in this book represent refereed presentations at Rutgers and other conferences in 1990 and 1991. The format for the Rutgers College of Nursing Annual National Nursing Computer Conference is to invite keynote speakers and conduct a call for abstracts for presentations, and/or demonstrations. A group of nurses with expertise in computer applications conducts a blind review of submitted abstracts. Generally thirty persons are selected to either present or demonstrate the state of the art of computer applications in nursing. The chapters in this book represent the following categories: practice, administration, education, and research.

A meeting was held at the 1990 Rutgers conference with all of the presenters to discuss the possibility of publishing their papers in a book. All the participants were most enthusiastic about such a publication and emphatically stated that this kind of book was needed. Most persons readily submitted manuscripts.

This textbook is intended for nurses employed in both educational and service institutions, who are involved in nursing informatics. The book could also be used by both graduate and undergraduate nursing students in a variety of computer or administration/management courses.

This publication is the only one in the field at this time in which nurses describe how they developed their computer applications. The inclusion in this book of numerous figures and computer screens provides the reader with a better understanding of the applications described. This feature is not generally found in the literature, but it is a necessary component when describing computer applications. The intent is to share the experiences of nurses who have both developed and used existing computer software for a specific purpose and to prevent reinvention of the wheel.

A unique feature of the book is Section One. It is a resource section which enables nurses to become aware of the information available regarding computer use in the health care delivery system. Section Two provides one of the most comprehensive compilations of papers on bedside computers to date. Section Three includes a collection of papers on a variety of nursing information systems. Section Four contains chapters on administrative aspects of nursing information systems and the chapters in Section Five focus on the use of computers in nursing education. Section Six includes chapters on the development of computer applications for nursing and the concluding section offers a number of research and evaluative studies done within the nursing profession. This book truly illustrates that more nurses are getting involved in using computers and that nursing informatics is a developing specialty within the profession.

We are proud to disseminate the experiences of nurses and others who have made innovative strides in the use of computers throughout the United States.

Jean M. Arnold, EdD, RN
Gayle A. Pearson, DrPH, RN

Contributors

Eula Aiken, PhD, RN, Executive Director, Southern Council on Collegiate Education for Nursing in affiliation with the Southern Regional Education Board, Atlanta, GA.

Jean M. Arnold, EdD, RN, Associate Professor, Rutgers The State University of New Jersey, College of Nursing, Newark, NJ.

Carol A. Bauer, EdD, RN, Assistant Professor, Department of Nursing Education and Services, University of Medicine and Dentistry of New Jersey, Newark, NJ.

Linda Beeber, PhD, RN, Associate Professor, Syracuse University College of Nursing, Syracuse, NY.

Alice J. Belcher, BSN, RN, CCRN, Nursing Information Systems Coordinator, Dover General Hospital and Medical Center, Dover, NJ.

Sharon Oetker Black, PhD, RN, Assistant Professor, Kent State University, School of Nursing, Kent, OH.

Jane Bliss-Holtz, DNSc, RN, Assistant Professor, Rutgers The State University, College of Nursing, Newark, NJ; Assistant Director of Nursing for Research, Newark Beth Israel Medical Center, Newark, NJ.

Rosemarie K. Blume, MA, RN, Associate Professor, County College of Morris, Randolph, NJ.

Frank Brady, MPA, RN, Vice President, Patient Services, Community Health Care of North Jersey, Orange, NJ (formerly Manager of Quality Assurance, VNS Home Care, New York, NY).

Judy L. Luckenbill Brett, PhD, RN, Assistant Vice President, Ancillary Services, Robert Wood Johnson University Hospital, New Brunswick, NJ.

Marcia Brown, BA, Computer Consultant, Lehman College, The City University of New York, Bronx, NY.

Margaret Chalmers, EdD, RN, Director of Health Services, Nursing Care Center at Kimball Farms, Lenox, MA.

Harriet V. Coeling, PhD, RN, Assistant Professor, Kent State University, School of Nursing, Kent, OH.

Barbara Cohen, EdD, RN, Associate Professor, Lehman College, The City University of New York, Bronx, NY.

Lyda Sue Cunningham, MA, RN, Vice President, Nursing Services, Dover General Hospital and Medical Center, Dover, NJ.

Patricia F. Curry, MPA, RN, Nursing Management Consultant, Continuing Education Instructor, Nazareth College, Rochester, NY.

Felicitas A. dela Cruz, DNSc, RN, Associate Professor, Azusa Pacific University, Azusa, CA.

Margaret O'Bryan Doheny, PhD, RN, Assistant Professor, Kent State University, School of Nursing, Kent, OH.

Edward H. Downey, DPA, Chairperson, Department of Public Administration, State University of New York, College at Brockport, Brockport, NY.

Edward E. Duryee, MBA, Director, Financial and Clinical Systems, Memorial Hospital of Burlington County, Mt. Holly, NJ.

Diane M. Eddy, EdD, RN, Assistant Professor, Kent State University, School of Nursing, Kent, OH.

Diane D. Elliott, EdD, RN, Associate Dean, School of Professions and Associate Professor, Department of Nursing, State University of New York, College at Brockport, Brockport, NY.

Christine D. Giamporcaro, BSW, MSEd, Nursing Home Administrator, Oneida City Hospital Extended Care Facility, Oneida, NY.

Greer Glazer, PhD, RN, Associate Professor, Kent State University, School of Nursing, Kent, OH.

Carol Greenberg, BA, CCRN, Assistant Director of Nursing, University Hospital, State University of New York at Stony Brook, Stony Brook, NY.

Robert Guhde, PhD, Associate Professor and Coordinator MIS Emphasis Graduate Program in Public Administration, State University of New York, College at Brockport, Brockport, NY.

Gary D. Hales, PhD, Editor-in-Chief, *Computers in Nursing*, Associate Professor, School of Nursing, University of Alabama, Birmingham, AL.

Mary R. Hassett, PhD, RN, Associate Professor of Nursing, Director of Media Learning Laboratory, Fort Hays State University, Hays, KS.

Patricia M. Haynor, DNSc, RN, Assistant Professor, University of Delaware, College of Nursing, Department of Advanced Nursing Science, Newark, DE.

Janet R. Holloway, MA, RN,C, Associate Professor, Intercollegiate Center for Nursing Education, Spokane, WA.

Gail Hood, BSN, RN, GNP, Director of Nursing, Oneida City Hospital, Extended Care Facility, Oneida, NY.

Carole Hudgings, PhD, RN, former Director, International Nursing Library, Sigma Theta Tau International, Indianapolis, IN.

Angeline M. Jacobs, MS, RN, Professor Emeritus, Azusa Pacific University, Azusa, CA.

Irene Joos, PhD, RN, Assistant Professor and Assistant Director, Learning Resource Center, University of Pittsburgh, School of Nursing, Pittsburgh, PA.

Sally Kilby, RN, MS, Founder, Nursing Information Network, Glendale, CA, and Library Director, American Association of Orthopaedic Medicine, Los Angeles, CA.

Ursel Krumme, MA, RN, Associate Professor, Seattle University, School of Nursing, Seattle, WA.

Claire Lauzon-Vallone, BS, RN,C, Educator Program Manager, Personal Computer Development, Children's Hospital of Pittsburgh, Pittsburgh, PA.

Helen M. Lerner, EdD, RN, Associate Professor, Lehman College, The City University of New York, Bronx, NY.

Gloria H. Lombardi, MA, RN, Associate Professor, County College of Morris, Randolph, NJ.

Sharon J. Majarowitz, MEd, RN, Information Systems Coordinator for Nursing, Memorial Hospital of Burlington County, Mt. Holly, NJ.

Mary N. McAlindon, EdD, CNAA, RN, Administrative Assistant, McLaren Regional Medical Center, Flint, MI.

Maureen McCormac, MS, RN, CCRN, CEN, Director, Nursing Systems, Robert Wood Johnson University Hospital, New Brunswick, NJ.

Katherine McLaughlin, MScN, President, McLaughlin Associates, British Columbia, Canada.

Sharon L. Merritt, EdD, RN, Assistant Professor, Interim Director, Center for Narcolepsy Research, University of Illinois at Chicago, Department of Medical-Surgical Nursing, Chicago, IL.

Kathleen J. Mikan, PhD, RN, FAAN, Professor, University of Alabama School of Nursing, Birmingham, AL.

Emmy R. Miller, PhD, RN, Management Consultant, Superior Consultant Company, Inc., Farmington Hills, MI.

R. Paul Miller, MD, Medical Director, Monroe Community Hospital, Rochester, NY; Assistant Professor of Medicine, The University of Rochester School of Medicine.

Ramona Nelson, PhD, RN, Assistant Professor, University of Pittsburgh, School of Nursing, Pittsburgh, PA.

Lynne Nickle, MS, RN, CS, President, Nickle Associates Inc., Ann Arbor, MI.

Judith S. Ronald, EdD, RN, Associate Professor, Coordinator of Informatics, State University of New York at Buffalo, Buffalo, NY.

Patricia Sayers, MSN, RN, President, Nursing Systems International, Bordentown, NJ.

Ann L. Sedore, PhD, RN, Associate Professor, Syracuse University, College of Nursing, Syracuse, NY.

Elizabeth A. Sheridan, MA, RN, Vice President for Patient Care Services, JFK Medical Center, Edison, NJ.

Roy L. Simpson, RN, Executive Director, Nursing Affairs, HealthQuest/HBO & Company, Atlanta, GA.

Diane J. Skiba, PhD, Director of Informatics, Associate Professor, University of Colorado School of Nursing, Denver, CO.

Arlene Smaldone, MA, RN, Assistant Nursing Director, University Hospital, State University of New York at Stony Brook, Stony Brook, NY.

Susan G. Taylor, PhD, RN, Associate Professor, University of Missouri-Columbia, School of Nursing, Columbia, MO.

Linda Q. Thede, MSN, RN, Director, Learning Resource Center, Assistant Professor, Kent State University, School of Nursing, Kent, OH.

Joan E. Thiele, PhD, RN, Associate Professor of Nursing, Intercollegiate Center for Nursing Education, Spokane, WA.

Brent Thompson, MS, RN, Assistant Professor, University of Delaware, College of Nursing, Newark, DE.

Kathleen Tiedeken, MSN, RN, CNAA, Vice President of Patient Services, Memorial Hospital of Burlington County, Mt. Holly, NJ.

Beatrice B. Turkoski, PhD, RN, Assistant Professor, Kent State University, School of Nursing, Kent, OH.

Jocelyne VanNeste-Kenny, MS, RN, Teaching Assistant, Syracuse University College of Nursing, Syracuse, NY.

Robin W. Wells, MSN, RN, CNA, Director, Test Services, Commission on Graduates of Foreign Nursing Schools, Philadelphia, PA.

Erlinda C. Wheeler, MA, RN, Associate Professor of Nursing, State University of New York, College at Brockport, Brockport, NY.

Mary A. Wyper, PhD, RN, Assistant Professor, Kent State University, School of Nursing, Kent, OH.

Marianne E. Yoder, PhD, RN, Assistant Professor, Northern Arizona University, Department of Nursing, Flagstaff, AZ.

Foreword

Nursing and computers have had a symbiotic relationship since computers were introduced into the health care delivery system twenty years ago. Each has evolved separately, but at the same time, they integrated to form the basis for today's information systems.

During this period, nursing expanded its science, standardized the nursing process, and developed several nursing classification schemes and taxonomies. Also, nursing systems have been developed and implemented in large health care settings. On the other hand, computers have increased their storage, speed, and processing capabilities while getting smaller and less expensive. Because of "chip" and other technological innovations, mainframe computers are being replaced by minicomputers and microcomputers.

Today, nurses are asking "What can computers do for nursing?" My answer is that computerized nursing information systems are available and can support nursing practice, administration, research, and education. Such systems can be used to manage—document, monitor, and communicate—patient care as well as administer nursing services and resources for a health care facility. Also, they can provide educational applications for teaching, testing, and evaluating student, staff and patient education and research applications such as searching the literature, and processing research data.

During these challenging times, technological innovations are revolutionizing the health care delivery system. In nursing, we are expanding our scope of practice as well as our knowledge base. Never before in our nursing history has it been more important for health professionals involved in nursing service, education, and management to be able to communicate with one another and to share necessary information.

With the increase of computers in hospitals and health care agencies, institutions and organizations, we will be required to provide more data in a rapid fashion. Also, we will witness more federal regulation on computer use and access. Federal and state funding for computer demonstration projects has been substantive. Federal regulatory systems will be designed to accommodate the increasing demand for more complex information that impact on patient care, privacy, and security.

With the proliferation of computer applications, the need to disseminate information concerning these innovations has been critical. The rapidly evolving use of computers in all settings where nurses work has created challenges for nursing education. In order to be relevant to nursing practice, nurse educators need to integrate nursing with computers and provide opportunities for students, at all levels, to become knowledgeable in the uses of the technology.

In 1982, as a keynote speaker for the First Annual Computer Conference conducted by Rutgers The State University College of Nursing, I promoted the use of computers as part of nursing practice. The major focus of the conference, initiated by Gayle Pearson, DrPH, RN, and Jean Arnold, EdD, RN, was to educate nurses on existing computer applications. At that time, most nurses had very little knowledge of this new technology.

Since then, the scope and size of the conference has grown, and it is now an annual national event conducted exclusively for nurses. The conferences serve to provide a forum for networking and a sharing of innovations in computer applications in all areas of clinical practice and education among nurses from all areas of the United States. The information gained has been useful for those new to the computer field as well as those who have been involved and have extensive computer experience.

This book, *Computer Applications in Nursing Education and Practice*, is largely a compilation of papers presented at Rutgers The State University College of Nursing's Eighth and Ninth Annual National Nursing Computer Conferences. Since the papers were so provocative, we urged that they be published in order to share the information presented with those who did not attend. This book makes an important contribution to the literature on computer applications in nursing.

The chapters uniquely bring together information for nurses in administrative and staff positions in all clinical settings and will be invaluable for nurse educators in academic or clinical settings. They provide practical knowledge and a discussion of available resources in this field. The papers presented here, highlight why nursing educators have been slow in implementing comprehensive knowledge of information systems within either the undergraduate or graduate curricula. They state that the primary use of computers in nursing schools has been almost exclusively for word processing and literature searches. However, the time has come for computer technology in nursing to be an integral part of every nursing program with a required practicum in their use.

This book bridges the gap between these nursing specialties by bringing together practical information in one volume for all to share. The writings contained here make an important and unique contribution to the literature with information presented not found elsewhere. Also, this book documents where the nursing profession "is" in the "1990s" with regard to computer applications. Today's computerized information systems have just begun to impact on patient care. Nurses need to be prepared in the use of computers in order to meet the demands of the highly technological systems that will continue to expand in the future.

In the next decade, we will witness many revolutionary changes motivated by technological advances that will effect both the quality and quantity of health care. One can envision the patient care unit in a hospital of the future, a computerized environment with robots running errands at the push of a button. What is difficult to comprehend is the role computer illiterate nurses can play in providing adequate health care to patients.

By the turn of the century most health care delivery systems will function with computers and will be managed by computer literate nurses. I believe, that by the turn of the century, "high tech and high touch" will be an integral part of the health care delivery system!

Virginia K. Saba, EdD, RN, FAAN
Chair, American Nurses Association
Council on Computer Applications in Nursing
Associate Professor
Georgetown University School of Nursing
Washington, DC

Section One
Resources for Computer Applications

In the first section the authors recite resources for computer applications. How do I get started using computers? Resources for computer applications are myriad, including periodicals, networking with computer people, membership in computer groups, and travelling the computer circuit. Nelson and Joos provide the reader with a database of resources and strategies for developing a personalized self-education program for learning about the use of computers in nursing.

Hudgings describes The Virginia Henderson International Nursing Library, the first library devoted solely to nursing needs. It is anticipated that this library will be an unparalleled source of information about nurse researchers and their research. The electronic component of the library can be accessed by any individual with a personal computer and communication peripherals.

You can perform a computerized literature search. Learn all about it by reading the chapter by Kilby and McAlindon. Computerized databases, search basics, and a simulated example are included. On-line searches provide you with the most up-to-date information instantaneously.

1

The Virginia Henderson International Nursing Library: Improving Access to Nursing Research Databases

Carole Hudgings

INTRODUCTION

In today's rapidly changing health care environment, professional nurses face a constant challenge of maintaining knowledge of current advances within nursing and other health care disciplines. The explosion of scientific information and recent technological advances have dramatically affected the nature and practice of nursing (Poslusny & McElmurry, 1990). However, nurses frequently find it difficult to keep adequately informed. Although all nurses, and nurse researchers in particular, must function as information specialists, they often have difficulties obtaining information about research in progress and forming networks among other nurse colleagues working in similar content areas. One major factor contributing to inefficiency in the retrieval of relevant information is the lack of a universally accepted classification scheme to organize nursing's knowledge.

Although thousands of nurses conduct and utilize research, no library is devoted to serving as a comprehensive focal point for nursing research. Chapter 1 describes the efforts of the staff of Sigma Theta Tau International to establish an International Nursing Library (INL) to address information needs for nurses worldwide.

SIGMA THETA TAU INTERNATIONAL

Sigma Theta Tau International, the honor society of nursing, was founded in 1922 by six student nurses at Indiana University School of Nursing. These student nurses were interested in starting an organization that would advance the status of nursing as a profession, recognize scholarship, encourage future leaders, and provide a social forum. From those six members in one chapter, the organization has grown tremendously to more than 150,000 members affiliated with 301 chapters in the United States, Canada, Korea and Taiwan. Specific purposes of the organization are to:

- recognize superior achievements in nursing,
- encourage leadership development,
- foster high nursing standards,
- stimulate creative work, and
- strengthen the commitment to the ideals of the profession.

Cognizant of the need to systematically develop programs and services that reflect the needs of members and of the nursing profession, leaders of the Society developed the Ten Year Plan, a strategic planning document that guided the organization's activities during the 1980s. This blueprint for excellence served as a plan to foster expansion and programmatic and financial decisions of the Society (Rose, 1986).

Working within the organization's overall mission (a commitment to improve the health of people worldwide by increasing the scientific base of nursing practice), the Ten Year Plan focuses on three broad goals: knowledge development, knowledge dissemination, and knowledge utilization. Fundamental to the plan is the notion that nursing's knowledge base will be best expanded through a global network of well-prepared nurses. Specific action strategies were identified for these three goals, including one targeted specifically toward the development of the International Nursing Library: to develop an efficient computerized storage and retrieval system for nursing research and nurse researchers (Sigma Theta Tau, 1981). The organization's current strategic planning document (*Actions for the 1990s*) continues the three goals of knowledge development, knowledge dissemination, and knowledge utilization, and adds resource development as a fourth goal (Sigma Theta Tau International, 1989). Emphasis on development of a research resource repository is continued in this plan

which will guide the organization into the twenty-first century.

PLANNING FOR THE VIRGINIA HENDERSON INTERNATIONAL NURSING LIBRARY

Specific work toward the development of the INL began during 1987 (Sigma Theta Tau International, 1987). At this time the *Survey of Interest and Needs for an Electronic Nursing Library and Resource Center* was distributed to members and other nurses at several research conferences. The Survey requested respondents to rank the importance of various services for an ideal information service system and to comment on their current use of library and information technologies. The more than 1,700 nurse respondents identified the following five services as highest priority in an ideal information service system: literature searches, nursing instruments, research funding sources, nursing-related statistical sources, and research in progress. These services were identified as potential services for the INL, and were prioritized into three clusters. The highest priority cluster contained the following: research in progress, profiles of nurse researchers, and a calendar of professional events.

The vision of the INL began to take greater shape as the Society planned services consistent with the organization's emphasis on nursing scholarship and supporting the conduct of nursing research. Three distinct communities emerged as audiences for activities of the INL: nurse researchers, practicing nurses, and the public. INL services are designed to provide communication between and among these three communities. The Library was designed to assist nurse researchers and practicing nurses in the development, dissemination, and utilization of knowledge and to provide the public with information about nursing and nursing research. Rather than duplicating information available through other traditional library resources, the INL is positioned to serve as a unique resource for the nursing research arena by creating on-line nursing databases and by establishing links with existing library networks and other nursing organizations.

The INL expands the traditional concept of library as a repository for printed literary materials by encompassing recent technological advances for information management and communication. Present INL efforts seek to combine traditional library services with state-of-the-art information systems and communications technology to:

- enhance access to nursing information,
- form electronic communication networks among nurse researchers,
- develop selected nursing databases useful to facilitate the conduct and utilization of nursing research,
- provide a classification scheme to organize nursing information, and
- disseminate nursing research findings to the public.

INL PROGRAM IMPLEMENTATION

One component of INL operations includes traditional library services. A small collection of print and nonprint materials (i.e., books, journals, newsletters, audiotapes, and videotapes) provides the first-line resources to respond to requests for diverse information about nursing. In keeping with the scholarship focus of the organization, the emphasis of the current collection of print materials includes nursing research, theory,

and general nursing issues. In addition, interlibrary loans from nearby health science libraries and on-line access to bibliographic databases are used to obtain answers for information requests.

The second component of INL operations is the electronic component. Implementation began in 1989 with acquisition of a host minicomputer to support the development of electronic nursing research databases. (This minicomputer was generously funded by a grant from the Helene Fuld Health Trust.) Additional technological support is provided by search software and personal computer equipment. The host minicomputer stores the electronic databases of the INL, provides an environment for development of databases, and provides access for individuals at remote locations using their personal computers, modems, and communications software. Specific subscription and access information can be obtained by contacting Sigma Theta Tau International in Indianapolis, Indiana.

A powerful and versatile full-text management and retrieval software (BRS/SEARCH Software®) is used as the database management program for storing, searching, and retrieving database information (Hudgings, 1990). Responding to members' identified needs for information about nurse researchers and research in progress, the premiere database of the INL describes nurse researchers and their current projects. This database is an on-line version of the recently published *1990 Directory of Nurse Researchers*. Initially listing 2,500 nurse researchers and their 3,770 research projects, the on-line database of nurse researchers is continually updated and modified to reflect the most recently available information about nursing research.

Currently, searches of the database can be conducted on researcher name and research topics. Demographic information about the researcher and a list of terms describing the research project can be retrieved and printed. Address labels based on researchers' geographic location or subject area can be generated.

Any nurse and nursing student at a setting with INTERNET will be able to access The Virginia Henderson International Library Database. INTERNET is a world-wide electronic network requiring an account number and password. Initial testing of The Virginia Henderson International Library Database was performed at Indiana University School of Nursing in Indianapolis and Capital University in Columbus, Ohio. A user manual will be made available to participating nursing programs.

A wide variety of databases are in the planning stages as future INL services. Projects in the next phase of development include:

- the addition of full-text abstracts for projects in the nurse researcher's database,
- the addition of full-text abstracts of papers presented at nursing research conferences,
- a database of doctoral dissertations including full-text abstracts,
- a database of clinically relevant topics,
- data reflecting international concerns,
- an electronic journal, and
- a calendar of professional events.

Researchers may submit their research abstracts directly to Sigma Theta Tau International Headquarters for inclusion in the database.

CLASSIFICATION OF NURSING RESEARCH

Sigma Theta Tau's classification scheme for nursing research identifies and categorizes terms that describe nursing's research activity, and represents the most extensive classification effort for nursing research today. This classification scheme serves as the infrastructure for the nurse researcher's database and seeks to facilitate networking and collaboration among the worldwide community of nurse researchers (Barnard, 1990).

Currently in its third version, this classification scheme was most recently revised in 1989 to serve as the data collection tool for the *1990 Directory of Nurse Researchers*. This version contains three major sections which identify specific information about the researcher and his or her individual research projects. These sections are:

1. researcher demographics,
2. research project demographics, and
3. keywords for classification of research.

The researcher demographic section contains work and home address, language skills, highest earned education credential, discipline of highest degree, and title of dissertation. The section on research project demographics lists the title of the individual research project and items that describe the conduct of the research in twelve major categories. These descriptors are listed in Table 1.1.

Table 1.1 Sigma Theta Tau International Classification Scheme for Nursing Research (1989) Research Project Demographics (12 categories)

Project Status
Ages of Human Subjects
Categories of Human Subjects
Animal Subject Species
Funding Sources
Nursing Model/Theory Usage
Sites/Location of Data Collection
Type of Research
Design
Data Collection Techniques
Data Analysis Techniques
Type of Project

The section containing keywords for classification of the research project is divided into seven major subsections (see Table 1.2); the first subsection (Clinical Topics) is further subdivided into four divisions of nursing's metaparadigm. A total of 637 discrete keywords describing the topic of the research are listed in this section. These keywords also serve as access points for retrieving relevant information from the electronic nurse researchers database and other planned databases. The classification scheme is intended to be dynamic, and will continue to be modified as the body of nursing knowledge expands. It provides nurses a tool to help structure data and information, thereby assisting with a major crisis facing knowledge workers today (Wurman, 1989).

Table 1.2 Sigma Theta Tau International Classification Scheme for Nursing Research (1989) Keywords for Classification of Research (7 major categories)

Clinical Topics
- Environment
- Health
  — health concepts/constructs
  — health promoting behaviors
  — unhealthy behaviors
- Nursing care activities
  — nursing process
- Person
  — cultural/transcultural focus
  — developmental stages
  — developmental problems
  — developmental processes
  — pathophysiological focus
  — disease/condition/injury
  — response to disease/illness
  — medical interventions
  — physiological systems
  — physiological processes
  — emotions/feelings
  — cognitive responses
  — attributes
  — psychopathological focus
  — social concepts
  — relationships/behaviors
Educational Studies
Health Care Delivery
- Health systems research
- Organizational research
Historical Studies
Methodological Research
Philosophical Perspectives
Professional Issues

SUMMARY

In the current information age, the doubling of information every five years and the increasing specialization of knowledge make it imperative that nurses have access to the latest scientific information to assist in the delivery of high quality care. A variety of technological innovations have increased our access to information during the past two decades. Two of these technological innovations, the developing electronic databases of the INL and the Sigma Theta Tau International classification scheme for nursing research, can enhance nurses' access to information that supports scholarship. Nursing exists within dynamic environments for health care delivery, technological capabilities, and expansion of nursing knowledge. The INL serves as a unique resource for nursing scholarship, reflecting the organization's mission to increase the scientific base of nursing practice.

REFERENCES

Barnard, R. M. (1990). Classification of nursing research. In J. C. McCloskey & H. K. Grace (Eds.), *Current issues in nursing* (pp. 87–93). St. Louis: The C. V. Mosby Company.

Hudgings, C. (1990). Library on-line. *Reflections*, Summer 1990, 19.

Poslusny, S., & McElmurry, B. J. (1990). Developing nursing databases: Critical considerations. *Vard I Norden, 2*(3), 17–23.

Rose, M. (1986). The ten year plan: A blueprint for excellence. *Reflections*, Winter, 6–7.

Sigma Theta Tau. (1981). *Ten year plan*. Indianapolis, IN: Sigma Theta Tau International.

Sigma Theta Tau International. (1987). *International nursing library and resource center strategic plan 1987–1989*. Indianapolis, IN: Sigma Theta Tau International.

Sigma Theta Tau International. (1989). *Actions for the 1990s*. Indianapolis, IN: Sigma Theta Tau International.

Sigma Theta Tau International. (1990). 1990 Directory of Nurse Researchers. Indianapolis, IN: Sigma Theta Tau International.

Wurman, R. S. (1989). *Information anxiety*. New York: Doubleday.

2

Strategies and Resources for Self-Education in Nursing Informatics

Ramona Nelson
Irene Joos

Nursing informatics is a rapidly evolving specialty with enormous potential. This potential will be realized only if there is a sufficient supply of nurses who have a solid knowledge base in informatics. At this point, the number of established educational programs in nursing informatics is limited. However, many nurses have successfully educated themselves using a variety of formal and informal resources. This chapter presents a database of these learning resources and a systematic approach to using the database in developing a program of education. The resources in the database include formal educational programs, as well as informal educational opportunities such as journals, organizations and conferences. The first step in using these sources is the establishment of goals and a plan for achieving them.

SETTING GOALS

The data, information, and knowledge incorporated in the field of nursing informatics originates from a variety of disciplines. To even the experienced computer user this knowledge base can appear overwhelming and disorganized. Figure 2.1 presents a model for organizing the knowledge base of nursing informatics.

In this model the knowledge base is divided into three interrelated areas: the health care system, nursing, and computer and information science. Nursing is further divided into the four traditional roles: research, administration, nursing practice, and education. Although the model consists of everything known and is constantly growing as new information is discovered, two factors can focus the learner. First, there is a baseline of information needed by all nurses: information about the health care system, computer and information science, and nursing, including the speciality of nursing informatics. Second, there is the information needed by nurses interested in the specialization of informatics. In both cases, the information needed is strongly influenced by the nursing role being emphasized.

For example, nurses interested in education and/or research will have a different set

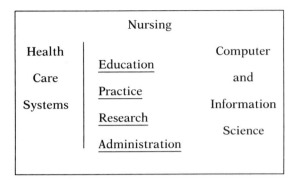

Figure 2.1 A systematic approach to organizing topics in nursing informatics.

of goals and learning needs from nurses interested in practice and/or administration. This is true whether we are talking about the core of information necessary for all nurses or about nurses interested in informatics specialization. One must identify the purpose of the learning before exploring specific content.

Three professional organizations provide four resources that can be used with the model in Figure 2.1 to answer the question: "What should I be learning?" The most comprehensive approach to this question is detailed in *Preparing Nurses for Using Information Systems: Recommended Informatics Competencies* by the Nursing Informatics Task Force on Nursing Education: Working Group Eight. Working Group Eight is the Nursing Informatics Interest Group of the International Medical Informatics Association (Peterson & Gerdin-Jelger (Eds.), 1988). The first paragraph explains the purpose of their report.

The purpose of the Working Group Eight Task Force on Education was to define broad competency statements about nursing informatics for the practicing nurse, the nurse administrator, the nurse educator, the nurse teacher, and the nurse researcher. The competencies were to be "useful for guiding these nurses' preparation

for using informatics competencies in performing their nursing role." (Peterson & Gerdin-Jelger (Eds.), 1988, p. 4)

Working Group Eight identified nursing informatics-related role functions for each of the nursing roles. Three levels of competency are presented for each of these role functions. These levels of competency are user, developer or modifier, and expert or innovator. Examples of these role functions and related competencies are found in Table 2.1, which presents one role function for each of the nursing roles. The role functions are then followed by a competency example for each of the three levels.

While Working Group Eight considers each of the four nursing roles, *Computers in Nursing Education* is targeted specifically to the nurse educator (American Nurses Association [ANA], 1987). This brief, but informative reference assists faculty in identifying what they need to know about computers. Each chapter presents key questions regarding the chapter topic and then responds in outline fashion to the proposed question. For example, Chapter 3, Preparing Faculty to Use Computers in the Curriculum, focuses on what faculty should know about computer use in nursing practice and in the curriculum. One of the questions from this chapter is "How can faculty prepare for their role with computers?" (p. 11).

Guidelines for Basic Computer Education in Nursing (Ronald & Skiba, 1987, p. iv) was written "to help nursing educators prepare students to use the computer as a tool for an information-intensive profession." This book addresses faculty developing basic or introductory courses in nursing informatics. Chapter 3 contains a well-organized and an easy-to-follow topical outline of appropriate content. While this book is targeted to faculty, any nurse can use it to identify the computer/information science content for his or her own program of study. The content

Table 2.1 Nursing Informatics: Role Functions and Related Competencies*

	EDUCATOR	ADMINISTRATOR	PRACTICING NURSE	RESEARCHER
ROLE FUNCTION	Teaches with computer-based instructional materials.	Assures ethical standards and data protection.	Documents nursing practice.	Manages and manipulates data.
USER	Prepares over-heads using graphic soft-ware.	Familiar with ethical standards.	Able to use the documentation system in the health care setting.	Uses statistical packages and other related research software programs.
DEVELOPER/ MODIFIER	Critiques general software for potential use to support preparation of instructional materials.	Monitors that ethical standards are upheld.	Analyzes the documentation system.	Modifies software programs to support data manipulation functions.
INNOVATOR/ EXPERT	Designs, develops and implements hardware and software systems for instructional support activities.	Participates in the development of ethical standards.	Participates in the design of documentation systems.	Develops innovative techniques for data collection or analysis in nursing research.

* Reprinted by permission from Peterson, H.E., & Gerdin-Jelger, U. (Eds.). (1988).

focuses on what nurses need to know about computer or information science in the context of nursing.

The fourth reference targets nursing administrators and clinical nurses. *Computer Design Criteria for Systems that Support the Nursing Process* is published by the American Nurses Association (1988). The document was developed by the Task Force on Computer Design Criteria for Systems that Support the Nursing Process, which is a committee of the ANA's Council on Computer Applications in Nursing. The previous references provide guidance on content one should be learning in the field of nursing informatics. This reference, however, describes "for both practicing nurses and computer system vendors the criteria for computer applications to support and document the nursing process" (p. 1). This document concludes by summarizing five impediments to better use of automated systems. One of the major impediments is a lack of nursing perspective.

What is needed are more nurses who have in-depth education in both nursing and information systems technology, so that systems will be designed from both a sound technological basis and a nursing viewpoint. (p. 34)

In summary, all four references identify general goals and directions for a program of study, however, with certain limits. Each cautions the reader on the changing nature of nursing informatics. The developers of each of these documents are important nursing leaders representing key professional organizations. As one plans a program of education, it is important to remain current. The viewpoints of these leaders and organizations can be expected to change! Keep up with your professional organizations. The publications from these organizations will continue to provide guidance.

EVALUATING INFORMAL EDUCATIONAL OPPORTUNITIES

Organizations, journals and conferences provide a wide range of informal learning opportunities. Choosing the specific learning activity involves evaluating many opportunities in terms of your identified goals.

Organizations

One of the most effective techniques for learning current issues and information is active involvement with others who have similar interests. Organizations offer this opportunity. There are a large number of organizations to choose from. These can be grouped into six basic types.

1. Special interest groups (SIG). Each professional health organization represents a group of health care professions, and the pertinent SIG represents the use of information systems within that group. Both the American Nurses Association (ANA) and the National League for Nursing (NLN) support councils related to nursing informatics. Other health profession groups of interest to nurses include the American Hospital Association (AHA); Healthcare Information and Management System Society (HIMSS); the Healthcare Financial Management Association (HFMA); the Interdisciplinary Association for Advancement of Rehabilitation and Assistive Technology; and the American Medical Record Association (AMRA).

2. Information science and computer organizations. While professional health organizations have been forming special interest groups in informatics, professional information science and computer groups have been developing special interest groups related to health care. The information science and computer groups tend to be large organizations with several SIGs and local chapters. Many of the SIGs are themselves large organizations and do not require membership in the parent organization. Three of the major organizations in this classification are the Association for Computing Machinery (ACM), the American Federation of Information Processing Societies (AFIPS), and the American Society for Information Science (ASIS).

3. Health computing organizations. Each of these organizations was established by individuals involved with issues and problems of health care computing. Each organization represents a different issue or interest within the broad context of health care computing. The largest and most broadly representative group is the American Medical Informatics Association (AMIA). It includes several SIGs, with one for people interested in nursing information systems. Other health computing groups include Computer Use in Social Service Network (CUSSN); Healthcare Information Systems Sharing Group (HISSG); Health Level Seven (HL7), and the Soci-

ety for Clinical Data Management Systems (SCDMS).

4. Information science specialty organizations. As the field of information science grew, a number of other specialty groups besides health care computing developed. The focus of these organizations is of interest to select groups of individuals involved in health care computing. For example, the American Association of Artificial Intelligence (AAAI) focuses on artificial intelligence in all areas including health care. The Association for Development of Computer-based Instructional Systems (ADCIS) focuses on educational applications. Membership includes educators and vendors. Nurses may join the SIG in health education. Currently, a tentative agreement exists between ACM and ADCIS that could eventually lead to ADCIS becoming a SIG within ACM. Three other organizations in this group are Health Science Communications Association (HeSCA), the Institute of Electrical & Electronic Engineers (IEEE), and Education Communication (EDUCOM).

5. User groups. User groups consist of individuals working with a specific language, software, and/or vendor. For example, the Massachusetts General Hospital Utility Multi-Programming System, (MUMPS®) user group is concerned with the development and the use of the language MUMPS. Finding specific user groups is best done through the appropriate vendor. These groups, helpful to vendors, are therefore frequently supported by them.

6. Local groups. While the groups discussed so far may have local or regional chapters, they are national or international organizations. The final group of organizations operate locally only. Two

examples are the Tri-State Nursing Computer Network located in Pittsburgh and Capital Area Roundtable on Informatics in Nursing (CARING, also referred to as the Rounders) located in Washington, DC. Both groups were started by nurses working with information systems. If such a group exists in your area, you can usually find the group by talking with other nurses involved with computers.

Selecting an Organization. Certainly anyone interested in learning about nursing informatics should become active in at least one of the related organizations. The choice is based on one's goals. There are a number of ways to obtain information for deciding on the appropriate organization. First send a letter to the organization asking for information. The flyers and applications provide cost, focus of membership, benefits, and other related information. Many of the organizations support one or more publications. Reviewing the publications as well as attending an organization-sponsored conference will provide more specific information. Finally, talk with members, especially those who are nurses. An alphabetical listing of organizations can be found in Appendix A.

Journals and Newsletters

In any field journals and newsletters provide the latest published information. Currency is especially important for nurses working in the fast-changing field of informatics. Considering the value of the content, most journals and newsletters are an inexpensive resource available to the readers on their own time schedule.

Types and Focus. Appendix B provides an extensive list of current journals and newsletters. These can be classified into four basic types: 1) journals focused on the computer/vendor business, 2) official publications of computer-related professional organizations, 3) research in computer applications, and 4) nursing computer applications. Any one journal or newsletter may apply to more than one grouping. Newsletters are further divided into two types: 1) newsletters conveying organizational news from a specific organization and 2) those containing the very latest information on a specific topic.

1. Computer/vendor business. Journals focused on the computer/vendor business provide a good source of concise information on who the vendors are, what systems they offer, who is buying what system, and what are the success stories. *HealthCare Informatics* and *Computers in Healthcare* are two of the most widely read journals profiling hospital information systems. Their Canadian counterpart is *Healthcare Computing & Communications: Canada*. Each year *Computers in Healthcare* publishes a market directory of the health systems vendors. A more critical analysis of the vendors is usually found in newsletters. Because of the research costs involved, these newsletters are expensive.

2. Professional organizations. Journals which serve as official publications of professional organizations focus on the current events, issues, and developments related to the stated purpose of the organization. Many of these journals are provided to the members of the organization as part of their dues. Newsletters from large professional organizations usually involve a SIG. *Input/Output* from the American Nurses Association ANA Council on Computer Applications in Nursing is a good example. There may be one or two brief articles on computers in nursing with a

significant portion of the newsletter reporting current events in the SIG.

3. Research developments. Many research journals are also official publications of professional organizations. For example, *Computers and Biomedical Research* is an official publication of the American Medical Informatics Association (AMIA). Some research journals as well as journals representing various specialties require the reader to have a specialized background in the terminology and the basic concepts of the field. For example, the journal *Computerized Medical Imaging and Graphics* assumes a background in radiology.

4. Nursing computer applications. Currently, one journal and one newsletter focus on the specialty of nursing. Articles published in the journal *Computers in Nursing* cover all areas of nursing: administration, practice, research, and education. For nurses interested in informatics this journal is a "must read." Included in the subscription is a yearly directory of computer-assisted software. The newsletter *Nurse Educators Microworld* is targeted to nursing educators. It contains the latest information on new releases of software, current developments, conferences, and discounts. The newsletter itself is offered to nursing faculty at half price.

Prices. Journals and newsletters range in price from free to under $400. The average price is between $30 and $40. Free journals are of two types. These are either free with membership in a professional organization or are free to a select group of individuals. For example, *T.H.E. Journal* provided a free one-year subscription to qualified individuals in educational institutions and training departments in the USA and Canada. The most expensive publications are newsletters which critique the vendors. For example, *Na-*

tional Report on Computers & Health is published 25 times per year.

Selecting Journals. Which journal to subscribe to depends on your background, needs, goals, time and finances. Select two or three which will help you achieve your goals or do your job and then read them. For example, if you are a nurse educator, involved in using and developing Computer Assisted Instruction (CAI) and Interactive Videodisc (IVD), you probably want to read *Nurse Educators Microworld, Computers in Nursing, Journal of Educational Technology Systems,* and *Journal of Computer Based Instruction.* If you are a nurse educator, preparing to teach about clinical applications or a nurse analyst in a clinical setting, you probably want to consider *Computers in Healthcare* and *National Report on Computers & Health.* If you are a nurse managing a learning resources center or computer lab, you want to consider those listed above for the educator plus generic computer publications. *PC Today* is a good choice for the beginner. For the more advanced user, *PC Computing* or *Byte* are helpful.

Conferences

Conferences provide an opportunity to hear the latest information directly from experts in the field. Larger conferences also have extensive vendor exhibits offering a first hand look at commercial products. Conferences vary greatly in size, focus, and location. They can be classified into four types: 1) nonhealth-related, 2) health-related, 3) educational, and 4) nursing. Like journals, this classification scheme is imprecise, with any one conference fitting into more than one area.

1. Nonhealth-related conferences. These conferences focus on developments occurring in both hardware and software.

They are vendor sponsored (eg, Software Publishing Co., IBM, or Hewlett-Packard) or large trade shows (eg, PC Expo or Portable Computing & Communication Networks). Vendor-sponsored conferences last one-half to one day. They function as a marketing tool for the vendors, providing them with an opportunity to demonstrate their latest product. As a result, there is little or no cost involved. Trade shows represent many vendors with extensive exhibits and tutorials. This type of conference usually lasts three days with registration between $300 and $800.

2. Health-related conferences. These conferences focus on automation and information processing in practice, education and research settings. Many are sponsored by organizations, journals, and/or institutes and occur at set intervals. Important examples include, SCAMC (Symposium on Computer Applications in Medical Care), MEDINFO (Medical Informatics), and Computers in Healthcare Conference and Exposition. These are large conferences with multiple workshops that meet the needs of different types of health care personnel.

3. Education-related conferences. With these conferences the focus is on the use of automation and information processing in different educational settings. Many include health education or nursing special interest groups such as the ADCIS (Association for the Development of Computer-based Instructional Systems) conference held every fall. The special interest groups, interactive video and health education, are among its sponsored tracts. Other good conference choices are AECT (Association for Educational Communications and Technology) and EDUCOM. Educa-

tional conferences tend to be priced between $170 and $230 depending on professional membership and early registration.

4. Nursing conferences. These conferences are designed for nurses in education, practice, administration, and/or research settings. The Nursing Informatics Conference is an international conference held every three years and is sponsored by IMIA Working Group Eight. At the national level, the Council on Nursing Informatics of the National League for Nursing sponsors a biennial conference. Proceedings from these conferences are published. Nursing conferences have also been sponsored by universities. One of the most noted is the Annual National Nursing Computer Conference at Rutgers, The State University of New Jersey. This conference is held every spring and is sponsored by the Continuing Education Program within the College of Nursing. Periodically, the National Institutes of Health (NIH) also sponsors a computer and nursing conference.

Locating Conference Schedules. Besides word of mouth there are two basic strategies used in locating conferences: reading about upcoming conferences in journals or other publications or receiving directional information from conference sponsors. Published announcements can be found in advertisements, in the "calendars and bulletins" of a journal or newsletter, and on electronic networks.

The information can be obtained directly by being on a mailing list. Call conference sponsors to be placed on a mailing list. Because conference sponsors buy mailing lists from each other, organizations, journals and even vendors, being on one mailing list can provide one with a consistent source of free new information.

CHOOSING A FORMAL EDUCATIONAL PROGRAM

There are a number of formal educational options that can be utilized in developing expertise. These options vary from undergraduate to postdoctoral opportunities in a variety of disciplines. These programs are divided into four groups: 1) nonhealth-related, 2) health-related, 3) medical informatics, and 4) nursing informatics.

Nonhealth-Related

Nonhealth-related programs include those in computer science, information science and specialty tracts within graduate programs. Computer science and information science are offered as both graduate and undergraduate degrees. Computer science degrees focus on the technical aspects involved in the effective use of the computer. These programs require a strong math background. Typical courses include Information Structures, Assembly Language, Compiler Design, and Scientific Computation. A directory of programs is published biannually by the Association for Computing Machinery (ACM).

Programs related to information science focus on the development of information systems through a process of needs analysis, design, implementation, and evaluation. Prerequisites are more general than those required for computer science degrees. Typical courses include Information Technology, Data Structures, Systems Analysis, and Human Information Processing. A representative list of programs in information science can be obtained from two sources. Many programs in information science are related to programs in library science. These programs are included in the list of programs accredited by the American Library Association. The second source, the Ameri-

Table 2.2   Published Directories of Computer/Information Science-Related Educational Programs

PROGRAMS	DIRECTORY	ADDRESS
Computer Science	*Administrative Directory of College & University Computer Science/Data Processing Programs and Computer Facilities.* (1988). New York: ACM Press. Order No. 212880	ACM Order Department, P. O. Box 64145, Baltimore, MD 21264
Information Science	*Graduate Library Education Programs Accredited by the American Library Association under Standards for Accreditation,* 1972 (October, 1988).	Accredited List American Library Association/COA, 50 East Huron Street, Chicago, IL 60611 Single copy free with SASE
	Programs Related to Information Science: A Representative List	American Society for Information Science, 1424 16th Street NW, Suite 404, Washington, DC 20036 Single copy free with SASE

can Society for Information Science provides a representative list of programs in information science (a list of published directories is in Table 2.2).

Finally, a number of different graduate programs include a track related to the management of information. The focus of each of these programs is the graduate specialty. The information track is developed in terms of the specialty. For example, in a graduate business program (e.g., MBA), an information track focuses on the management of business information systems.

Health-Related Programs

Health-related informatics programs occur as track within health related specialties. Some typical schools and programs include Public Health, Hospital Administration, Pharmacy, and Medical Records. The focus of these programs is the preparation of practitioners for the specific specialty. The information track emphasizes the use of informatics concepts and computers in that specialty. Besides the core courses for the specialty, students are required to complete a set number of credits in the information track. Typical courses include Introduction to Application Software, Information Systems in Health Care, and Data Management and Analysis.

Programs in Medical Informatics/Information

Programs in medical informatics/information vary from undergraduate to post-doctoral. Undergraduate programs exist at the University of Victoria in Victoria, BC, Canada and at the Rochester Institute of Technology in New York. Both of these programs involve cooperative education and lead to a baccalaureate degree. The goal of these programs is to produce a specialist who can meet the information system needs of health care providers.

Graduate programs in medical informatics in this country have been supported by the National Library of Medicine. The goal is to provide individuals qualified to address issues in the use of computers, automated information systems in health care, health professions education and biomedical research. Institutional training grants and individual postdoctoral fellowships support these goals: Institutional training grants are available to students accepted as doctoral candidates at participating institutions. Applicants for individual postdoctoral fellowships must arrange for an appointment to an appropriate institution and acceptance by a sponsor. Further information on this program can be obtained from:

Biomedical Information Support
  Branch
Extramural Programs
National Library of Medicine
8600 Rockville Pike
Bethesda, MD 20894
Telephone (301) 496-4221

Although many of these graduate programs are located in Schools of Medicine, the applicant need not be a physician. The students demonstrate a varied background in the health and/or information science fields. A list of medical informatics programs was recently published in *MD Computing* (Ball & Douglas, 1990).

Nursing Informatics

A variety of opportunities exist for learning content specific to nursing informatics. These include a summer institute, undergraduate courses, as well as formal graduate and postdoctoral programs. The increased importance of nursing informatics can be seen in the number of basic nursing programs that now offer related courses. Many schools permit nurses, especially their own alumni, to enroll in these courses. Because

these courses are geared to the undergraduate, they are at an introductory level.

Currently only the University of Maryland and the University of Utah offer graduate programs in nursing informatics. Both of these institutions also offer summer programs. Since 1988, the University of Utah has offered a summer postdoctoral program. This program lasts about four weeks and provides postdoctoral credits. However, graduate study in nursing informatics need not be limited to these two schools of nursing. Another approach is to identify institutions that are doing research in this area. Many times they offer an opportunity to study or work with experts in the field. Some examples include University of California at San Francisco, Georgetown University, University of Texas at Austin and Case Western Reserve.

CONCLUSION

This chapter provides a database for learning nursing informatics, along with references which can be used to develop individual learning goals. However, these resources and references alone will not provide expertise in nursing informatics. The reader will also need time, money, and patience. In most fields, it takes about seven years to move from novice to expert status. One does not learn this type of content quickly. Be patient; give yourself time. It takes a long time to feel like you are really learning the content. For bright people this slow initial learning curve is a difficult experience. Be kind to the learner as you plan a program of self-education. Furthermore, education is never free. We expect to pay for education when it is provided in a degree granting institution; but a program of self-education also costs money. Plan your budget just as carefully as you plan your learning goals. Without money there are no resources to achieve your goals. Without goals there are no reasons for spending the money.

REFERENCES

American Nurses Association. (1987). *Computers in nursing education*. (NE-13, 2.5M, 1/87). Kansas City, MO: American Nurses Association.

American Nurses Association. (1988). *Computer design criteria for systems that support the nursing process*. (NS-30, 2.5M, 6/88). Kansas City, MO: American Nurses Association.

Ball, M. J., & Douglas, J. V. (1990). Informatics programs in the United States and abroad. *MD Computing, 7*(3), 172–175.

Peterson, H. E., & Gerdin-Jelger, U. (Eds.). (1988). *Preparing nurses for using information systems: Recommended informatics competencies*. New York: National League for Nursing.

Ronald, J. S., & Skiba, D. J. (1987). *Guidelines for basic computer education in nursing*. New York: National League for Nursing.

Appendix A Organizations

AAAI
American Association for Artificial Intelligence
Menlo Park, CA 94025-3496

ACM
Association for Computing Machinery
New York, NY 10036

ADCIS
Association for the Development of Computer-based Instructional Systems
Columbus, OH 43210

AFIPS
American Federation of Information Processing Societies
Reston, VA 22091

ALA
American Library Association COA
Chicago, Illinois 60611

AMIA
American Medical Informatics Association
Rockville, MD 02852

AMRA
American Medical Record Association
Chicago, IL 60611

ANA/CCAN
American Nurses Assoc. Council on Computer Applications in Nursing
Washington, DC 20024-2571

ASIS
American Society for Information Science
Washington, DC 20036

CUSSN
Computer Use in Social Services Network
Arlington, TX 76019-0129

HFMA
Healthcare Financial Management Association
Westchester, IL 60154

HIMSS
AHA Healthcare Information & Management Systems Society
Chicago, IL 60611

HISSG
Healthcare Information Systems Sharing Group
Roswell, GA 30075

HL7
Health Level Seven
Chicago, IL 60666-9998

HeSCA
Health Sciences Communications Association
St. Louis, MO 63112

IEEE
The Institute of Electrical and Electronic Engineers
Piscataway, NJ 08855-1331

IHC
Interactive Healthcare Consortium
Alexandria, VA 22312

MRI
Medical Records Institute
Newton, MA 02160

NLN/CNI
National League for Nursing Council on Nursing Informatics
New York, NY 10014

RESNA
Interdisc Assoc for the Advan of Rehab & Assistive Technology
Washington, DC 20036

SALT
The Society for Applied Learning Technology
Warrenton, VA 22186

SCDMS
The Society for Clinical Data Management Systems
Covina, CA 91723-1906

Appendix B Journals and Newsletters

AI Expert
Miller Freeman Publishers
Boulder, CO 80321-1241

AI Magazine
American Association for Artificial Intelligence
Menlo Park, CA 94025-3496

AI Today
Yellowstone Information Services
Elkview, WV 25071

AI Trends
The Relayer Group
Scottsdale, AZ 85254

AI Week: The Artificial Intelligence Newsletter
AI Week
Atlanta, GA 30339

Assistive Technology
Demes Publications
Washington, DC 20036

Closing the Gap
Henderson, MN 56044

Communications of the ACM
Association for Computing Machinery
New York, NY 10001

Computational Medicine Technical Committee Newsletter
Dr. Margaret Peterson
New York, NY 10021

Computer
IEEE Computer Society
Los Alamitos, CA 90720-1264

Computer News for Physicians
BMI/McGraw-Hill
Minneapolis, MN 55435

Computer Talk: Directory of Medical Computer Systems
Computer Talk Associates, Inc.
Blue Bell, PA 19422

Computer Use in Social Service Network Newsletter
Computer Use in Social Services Network
Arlington, TX 76019

Computerized Medical Imaging and Graphics
Pergamon Press, Inc.
Elmsford, NY 10523

Computers and Biomedical Research
Academic Press Inc.
San Diego, CA 92101

Computers and Medicine
Medical Group News, Inc.
Glencoe, IL 60022

Computers in Biology and Medicine
Maxwell Macmillan Pergamon
Elmsford, NY 10523

Computers in Healthcare
Cardiff Publishing Company
Duluth, MN 55802

Computers in Human Services
The Haworth Press, Inc.
Binghamton, NY 13904-1580

Computers in Nursing
J.B. Lippincott Co.
Hagerstown, MD 21740

Expert Systems Strategies
Cutter Information Corporation
Arlington, MA 02174

Expert Systems: The International Journal of Knowledge Engineering
Learned Information, Inc.
Medford, NJ 08055-8707

HealthCare Informatics
Health Data Analysis, Inc.
Evergreen, CO 80439

Healthcare Computing & Communication: Canada
Health Data Analysis, Inc.
Edmonton, Alberta
CANADA T5P4P4

Healthcare Financial Management
Health Financial Management Association
Westchester, IL 60154-9817

IEEE Expert
IEEE Computer Society
Los Alamitos, CA 90720-9970

Input/Output
ANA Council on Computer Applications in Nursing
Kansas City, MO 64108

Interactive Healthcare Newsletter
Stewart Publishing Co.
Alexandria, VA 22312

International Journal of Clinical Monitoring & Computing
Kluwer Academic Pubs. Group
Hingham, MA 02018-0358

Journal of Clinical Computing
Buffalo, NY 14214

Journal of Computer Based Instruction
ADCIS Headquarters
Columbus, OH 43210-1116

Journal of Educational Computing Research
Baywood Publishing Company, Inc.
Amityville, NY 11701

Journal of Educational Technology Systems
Baywood Publishing Company, Inc.
Amityville, NY 11701

Appendix B   continued

Journal of Medical Systems
Plenum Publishing Corp.
New York, NY 10013
Knowledge in Society
Transaction Publications
New Brunswick, NJ 08903
M.D. Computing
Springer-Verlag
Secaucus, NJ 07096-9813
Methods of Information in Medicine
FK Schattauer Verlag
Lenzhalde 3, Germany
Micropsych Network
Methodist College Press
Johnson, VT 05656
National Report on Computers and Health
United Communications Group
Bethesda, MD 20814-3382

Nurse Educators Microworld
Saratoga, CA 95070-9998
PC AI
Phoenix, AZ 85023-9978
Patient Accounts
Healthcare Financial Management Assoc.
Westchester, IL 60154
Physicians and Computers
Bannockburn, IL 60015
RESNA News
Washington, DC 20036
Spang Robinson Report on Artificial Intelligence
John Wiley & Sons, Inc.
Ridgefield, NJ 07657-9876
Using Personal Computers in Nonprofit Agencies
Center for Community Future
Berkeley, CA 94705

3

Searching the Literature Yourself: Why, How, and What to Search*

Sally A. Kilby
Mary N. McAlindon

WHY SEARCH

Information is the basis of power, for the person who "knows" has an advantage over those who do not "know." The process of "knowing" includes reading what others have said and done so that we can build upon their knowledge. In *Powershift* Toffler (1990) describes the 1990s as a new era for informatics, the process of gaining power through the data–information–knowledge triad.

Blum (1986) defines data as discrete entities that are described without interpretation, information as data that have been interpreted, and knowledge as information that has been synthesized so that interrelationships are identified. An excellent source of data and information is the printed word that has become available electronically. Access to this electronic databank and information can be obtained through a literature search, which you can accomplish by yourself!

An electronic literature search is a process whereby you identify in specific terms what information you need, choose the database most likely to contain it, access the database through a computer, and examine the literature related to your topic.

There are two ways to search the literature. The first is through professional searchers, generally librarians who have been trained in computerized searching and who are knowledgeable about a variety of databases. They are able to choose the most appropriate database for your search and know the techniques and shortcuts that can save time and money and ensure maximum retrieval. Disadvantages of this method may include a lengthy turn-around time between your request and the search results, and the possibility of not obtaining the results that you expected.

The second method of searching the literature is to do it yourself. The advantages of this method are that you can:

* The authors thank Penny Coppernoll-Blach, DIALOG Customer Services, Biomedicine, and other representatives of DIALOG Information Services, who reviewed this manuscript and offered numerous valuable suggestions.

- Run literature searches at almost any time of day or night—at *your* convenience.

- Search from a computer terminal located in the library or in your home or office (depending on the system being searched).

- Conduct an on-the-spot search to respond to questions that need immediate answers.

- Modify a strategy during the search if you are not finding the information you need. As a result, searches may be more on-target.

- Browse through the databases and build your knowledge each time you search. Literature searches are a direct form of continuing education—to assist you with keeping up with trends and familiarizing yourself with a new area.

- Take advantage of a wonderful opportunity for serendipitous discovery of data related to your topic.

- Quickly identify pertinent literature as it is indexed (one database, MEDLINE®, is updated weekly).

- Easily and efficiently create and update tailor-made bibliographies.

- Experience a feeling of power as you realize that you have access to a vast amount of information from your computer.

There are limitations to doing your own searching: the do-it-yourself search may not be for everyone. Although the basics of searching are not difficult to master, an ongoing investment of time and money will be necessary. Databases are constructed differently, with different subject heading lists and searching features. You must also learn the commands of the specific search software you are using. Software and database features are regularly updated, requiring you to stay abreast of these enhancements in order to capitalize on your investment.

Generally speaking, your searching will not be as efficient as that of a professional searcher (in terms of time and search productivity), so this must be taken into account in looking at the overall benefits. Direct searching may or may not save you time, depending partially on how well you have prepared your search strategy, and on your ability to use a computer. In addition, some programs for non-librarians do not offer the more sophisticated and powerful features that are available on software designed for professional searchers.

Cost may be an issue, since direct literature searching may not be part of a nursing department's budget. In addition, special arrangements must be made with libraries or other services to obtain copies of articles cited in the search. Lastly, there will always be areas of literature that you can't reach. As Conway and Messerle (1990) have stated, "you don't know what you don't know."

Many health care professionals choose direct searching for some topics and call on a professional librarian for others. A good compromise might be to do the simple, straightforward searches yourself, and let the professional librarian do the complicated, exhaustive ones.

You'll find it's easy enough to find a few good citations on a topic, but more difficult to make sure you have retrieved all of the relevant ones. You can easily identify hundreds (sometimes thousands) of articles on a general topic; you may want an on-line searcher to pinpoint exactly the type of article you are seeking or to find data when your search turns up very little.

By doing the simple searches, you will learn the process and have immediate access to some of the literature. You will have clarified your search terms, and you'll be better able to explain what you need.

HOW TO SEARCH

Discuss your needs with your institution's library or learning resource center director; there may be a variety of free programs already available. You may even be able to "dial-up" the library's system from a microcomputer in your office or home. Even if an on-site system is not available, the librarian will be able to advise you about the hardware and software needed to set up an efficient searching system.

Electronic Options

You or a librarian can conduct electronic searches in the following ways:

On-line. With a microcomputer and a modem, you are connected to distant "vendors" of databases such as BRS Information Technologies™, PaperChase®, the National Library of Medicine (NLM), and DIALOG Information Services.* All offer user-friendly programs for nonlibrarians (see Appendix A). You contract directly with the vendor, with a "gateway service," and/or with the producer of "front-end" or interface software. The user is generally charged hourly database rates, a fee to print citations, and telecommunications fees. Some institutions contract with vendors to provide services to all affiliated personnel. Setting up an on-line system for direct searching is described in detail in the section entitled, "The ABCs of Going Online with DIALOG's Knowledge Index" (see page 28).

CD-ROM. CD-ROM means compact disc, read only memory. This refers to small com-

pact discs, similar to audio discs, that can store massive amounts of material. Information on these laser discs is "read" by a compact disc drive ($500–$1200) connected to a microcomputer.

Subscriptions to databases may run $1,000 per year and include periodic updates. Dozens of databases in the health care field are now available on CD-ROM, including MEDLINE, NURSING & ALLIED HEALTH (CINAHL), ERIC, PSYCHOLOGICAL ABSTRACTS® (known as PsycLIT®), and HEALTH PLANNING AND ADMINISTRATION®. Because of cost, CD-ROM is still a technology for your department or library. However, some CD-ROM systems offer dial-up access from off-site computers. Appendix B lists three CD-ROM vendors.

Local Mounting. Database tapes can be leased and mounted on main frame computers of colleges, universities, or other large organizations. Searching is made available via terminals throughout the campus—generally at no cost to the individual or the specific department.

WHAT TO SEARCH

Databases are produced by the government, by non-profit organizations, and by for-profit private companies. Figure 3.1 illustrates "the information path"—the database production process. As mentioned previously, databases are available via on-line and through CD-ROM vendors or institutions that have arrangements with vendors and producers. Database vendors provide access for a fee and take responsibility for the search software, billing, and customer service.

Databases used in nursing are primarily bibliographic. That is, they include citation information (e.g., author names, title of the

---

* DIALOG is a trademark of Dialog Information Services, Inc. Registered, U.S. Patent and Trademark Office.

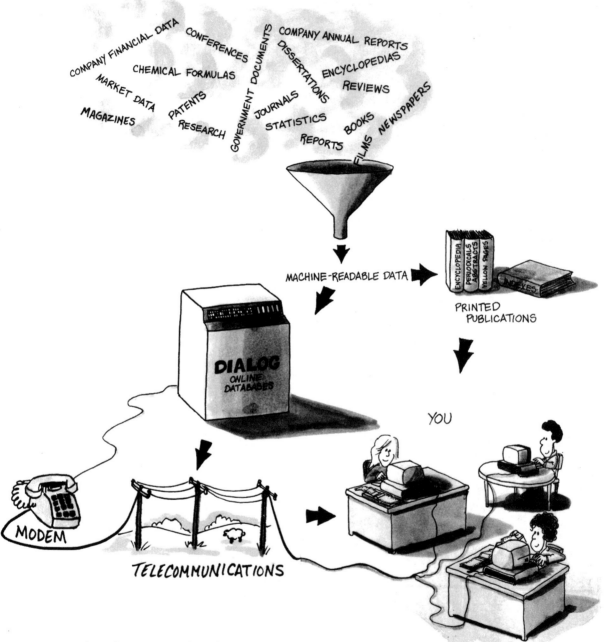

Figure 3.1 The information path is the process by which information about articles and other materials is made available to searchers in print and on-line formats. DIALOG Information Services, Inc., is one of the world's major database vendors, providing access to more than 400 databases. Reprinted with permission, Dialog Information Services, Palo Alto, CA.

article, journal name) and perhaps an abstract. Journal literature is the focus of most databases, although some databases also index books, audiovisuals, software, dissertations, and other materials. A few contain the full text of journals or books (e.g., BRS's Comprehensive Core Medical Library) or synthesized information on a topic (e.g., Physician Data Query—or PDQ—for cancer).

Databases of interest to nurses are listed in Table 3.1.

Information about an article or other publication is contained in one complete record. Each record is comprised of "fields"—the title, journal name, publication date, and so forth. Indexing terms (i.e., subject headings, descriptors) or abstracts may be added to the record.

Table 3.1 Computerized Databases of Interest to Nursing

Database	Description
MEDLINE®	Comprehensive coverage of English-language and foreign biomedical literature since 1966. Produced by the National Library of Medicine, the database includes all nursing journals indexed in the *International Nursing Index*. On-line database is inexpensive to search and widely available. Uses Medical Subject Headings (MeSH), a broad-based, controlled vocabulary, for indexing content.
NURSING & ALLIED HEALTH (CINAHL)	Database focuses on nursing and allied health. Covers English-language journals from 1983–present (print version coverage from 1956 to present). Coverage of nursing journals in English approximately the same as MEDLINE. However, subject heading list, features, and content are more specific to nursing. Indexes nonjournal literature, including dissertations.
EDUCATIONAL RESOURCES INFORMATION CENTER (ERIC)	Largest education database in the world; indexes research documents, journal articles, technical reports, program descriptions and evaluations, and curricular materials.
HEALTH PLANNING AND ADMINISTRATION (HEALTH)®	Focuses on health care planning, organization, financing, management, manpower, and related subjects. Some overlap with MEDLINE. Uses MeSH for indexing.
HEALTH AND PSYCHOSOCIAL INSTRUMENTS FILE	Contains information on national and international instruments in nursing and health care, psychosocial sciences, and organizational behavior/human resources. Includes questionnaires, interview schedules, observation checklists/manuals, index measures, coding schemes, scenarios/vignettes, and rating scales. Developed by nursing research/psychology professor Evelyn Perloff, with initial funding from NIH Division of Nursing, National Center for Nursing Research. Available only on BRS.
Physician Data Query (PDQ)	Contains comprehensive information on more than 80 types of cancer. Includes up-to-date information on prognosis, staging, standard and investigational treatments, protocols, patient information and resources.
PsycINFO®, PsycLIT® (PSYCHOLOGICAL ABSTRACTS®)	Covers worldwide literature in psychology and such related disciplines as psychiatry, sociology, anthropology, education, linguistics, and pharmacology. Journal articles, technical reports, and dissertations included.

HOW TO: THE ABCs OF GOING ONLINE WITH DIALOG'S KNOWLEDGE INDEX®

Equipment

Hardware. To do an on-line search, you need a microcomputer and a modem connected to a telephone line. The computer can be equipped with a floppy or hard disk drive, and must have a free connection (port) for the modem attachment (the word modem means *mo*dulate/*dem*odulate). The modem digitizes signals between computers over telephone lines. Modems transmit data at between 300–9600 bits per second (BPS), or baud rate, and many searchers find 1,200–2,400 baud modems practical.

The Hayes Company marketed the first desktop computer-intelligent modem that was capable of automatic dialing and answering, and established the communications protocols that became the standard in this country (*Communications*, 1988). Modems can be purchased for under $200 from computer dealers, by mail through advertisements in computer magazines, and quite often from universities at discounted prices. Both stand-alone and internal models are available.

Software. You will also need a telecommunications software program. PROCOMM PLUS®, Crosstalk®, and Smartcom® are popular programs for IBM/compatibles; Micro-Phone™ and White Knight™ are popular Macintosh programs. The producers of these software programs provide manuals and help lines for users. It is also extremely helpful to find a colleague or computer resource person who can answer your questions and show you the shortcuts of using the software.

Choosing an On-line Vendor

When choosing a vendor, remember that some vendors offer many databases; others offer only a few. The major vendors with user-friendly programs are DIALOG Information Services and BRS Information Technologies, a division of Maxwell Online. DIALOG is the largest, with more than 400 databases. BRS is second with more than 100 databases (McAlindon, personal communication, May 17, 21, 1991). EasyNet®, CompuServe®, and other gateways provide access to these and other vendors.

Both DIALOG and BRS offer after-hours services that are less expensive. Knowledge Index is the "after 6 P.M." DIALOG service; After Dark is the BRS service. To give you an idea about the financial arrangements, Knowledge Index (KI) has an initial subscription fee of $35, which includes a user manual with quarterly updates, a subscription to the newsletter, *Knowledge Index News*, and two hours of free connect time worth $48. The 100 databases accessible through KI are available from 6:00 P.M. through 5:00 A.M. Monday through Thursday, and from 6:00 P.M. Friday through 5:00 A.M. Monday local time. Personal search assistance is available by calling a toll-free number during these hours. Connect-time and telecommunications charges run $.40/minute, and telephone access is available through Tymnet®, SprintNet® (formerly Telenet®), and Dialnet®. (International customers are billed for local telecommunications.) There are no monthly minimum fees (M. McAlindon, personal communication, May 17, 21, 1991).

Users can access many diverse databases through a vendor using the same commands; this makes searching relatively easy, regardless of the database you choose. Vendors provide materials that describe the individual databases.

When choosing a vendor, consider responsive customer service, a user-friendly manual, and whether or not the vendor provides access to all the databases that you need. Many vendors offer demonstration disks. Be sure to ask about the initial subscription fee, manuals, ongoing fees, minimum use requirements, and other costs such as connect time and access costs.

You are ready to search after your computer and modem are set up and connected, you have paid your fees to a vendor, and you have received a password and reviewed the manual.

Developing a Search Strategy

First, you must choose the database most likely to contain the information you need. Read the vendor's user manual for the subject areas covered by each database. The medicine section of *Knowledge Index User's Manual* (1991) lists eight databases. The manual explains the subject areas, scope, and origin of each database. The manual also includes a sample citation, instructions about how to display results, and a search example.

You will want to purchase the thesaurus for each database you frequently search. MEDLINE, Cumulative Index to Nursing and Allied Health Literature (CINAHL), Educational Resources Information Center (ERIC), PsycINFO (PSYCHOLOGICAL ABSTRACTS), and other databases publish their own thesauri (subject heading lists, controlled vocabularies). Database producers also publish very detailed guides for searchers.

Searching Basics. All searching programs include instructional manuals, on-line help screens, and customer service assistance to help you learn each system's unique features. However, the basics of searching remain the same. What follows are a few overall concepts that will insure more effective searching, whether it is conducted by yourself or a librarian:

- Think through the topic you are researching. What are the concepts you are investigating? Write several questions about the issue. Talk to a colleague to further clarify the topic. This way you can identify the major concepts to be searched. Major databases use "controlled vocabularies" of subject headings to index materials. Finding the term or terms (keywords) that are used by that database to index the content you are interested in will improve searching effectiveness substantially.

- When thinking about concepts, it is helpful to know that most databases provide easy ways to retrieve data on frequently requested aspects of a topic (e.g., trends, drug therapy, adverse effects). In addition, you can limit your search to publications, that focus, for example, on specific age groups, research studies, reviews, or other areas.

- Electronic searching is extremely powerful, enabling you to retrieve data that meet a number of criteria simultaneously. The most frequently used function in electronic searching is "boolean combination" of keywords in order to retrieve only the materials that discuss the appropriate combination of concepts. This is known as "anding." For example, you can ask for references that focus on certification within the specialty of critical care nursing. When the concepts "critical care nursing" and "certification" are "anded," the searcher is asking for all articles that discuss critical care nursing *and* certification. While there may be hundreds of articles on each of these topics, a much smaller number will address both topics in a substantive way.

When you are ready to develop a search strategy, write out the first search statements. This will save you time, money, and confusion when you access the database. Write down all the commands that are needed to search, the terms used to display the data, the commands needed to order documents on-line, and the logoff commands so that you can exit the database quickly.

Log on to the vendor and set your computer to save incoming data to either disk or printer. Saving the data to disk is quicker and you will have it for reference.

A search for articles about "on-line searching" using the database vendor Knowledge Index® and the NURSING & ALLIED HEALTH (CINAHL) database might look like this:

?*Begin* Medi14 [CINAHL in Knowledge Index]*

---

* Notes in brackets do not appear on screen.

?*Find* on-line literature searching
?*Type* s1/1/all [type set 1, long form that includes abstracts, all abstracts]
?*Logoff*

"Begin," "Find," "Type," and "Logoff" are database commands that are used with all databases on Knowledge Index®. Citations found on the search are shown in Figures 3.2 and 3.3. The search was done for only $2.41.

In this example, we are asking the program to find all articles with the words "on-line," "literature," and "searching" either in the title of the citation, the abstract, or the thesaurus terminology. This is a quick way to find some materials; you will find that you

```
begin medi14

Date:       04jun91

Now in MEDICINE (MEDI) Section (MEDI14) Database NURSING & ALLIED
HEALTH (CINAHL) 83-91/MAY
(C. CINAHL CORP. 1991)

?find online literature searching
          462  ONLINE
         2374  LITERATURE
          950  SEARCHING

     S1       2  ONLINE LITERATURE SEARCHING

?type s1/1/all

 1/L/1
0001956
  Selective  use  of  online  literature  searching  by  a  drug
information service
  Knodel LC; Bierschenk NF
 American Journal of Hospital Pharmacy, 1983 Feb; 40(2): 257-9 (4
ref)
  SERLINE Serial ID: A24270000
  Descriptors:  * Reference Databases, Health--Utilization ; *
Computerized Literature Searching--Utilization ; * Libraries,
Pharmaceutical

 1/L/2
0001955

Use and cost analysis of online literature searching in a univer-
sity-based drug information center
  Schneiweiss F
 American Journal of Hospital Pharmacy, 1983 Feb; 40(2): 254-6
(21 ref)
  SERLINE Serial ID: A24270000

  Descriptors:   *  Computerized   Literature  Searching--Econom-
ics  ;  * Computerized   Literature   Searching--Utilization
;   *  Libraries, Pharmaceutical ; * Reference Databases,
Health--Utilization
```

Figure 3.2 Results of literature search using on-line literature searching.

will use the information from this search to identify established thesaurus terms (descriptors on the printout) that indexers attach to articles on this topic. If we ran the search again, using the term "computerized literature searching" (a thesaurus term), the number of terms retrieved would be much higher.

Ordering Documents

There are several ways of obtaining the sources you need once you have the bibliographic information. The easiest and least expensive method is to go to the library, locate the journal, book, or document, and take notes on what you need. If the publica-

```
?keep s1/1,2
        S0        2   S1/1,2

?order ki
Order RB001
0122323
   Online searching in the small college library -- ten years
Order RB001 confirmed

Order RB002
0120215
   Communications software for online searching on a PC
Order RB002 confirmed
Your order will be charged to your credit card.  Type HELP
RATES for current charges.  Please direct questions to
Dynamic Information, Burlingame, CA at 415/259-5000.  Type  ORDER
CANCEL + Order Number (e.g.,ORDER CANCEL RC012)
to cancel your order.

?order list
 Order    Vendor  File   Requested     Transmitted     Notes

 RB001      KI      218   04jun91  12:04
 RB002      KI      218   04jun91  12:04

?Help rates

HELP RATES

*KNOWLEDGE INDEX - $24 per hour
Access to KNOWLEDGE INDEX is based on the amount of time you  are
connected  to  the KNOWLEDGE INDEX system. There are  no  minimum
fees or monthly handling charges.
                    ---
*KNOWLEDGE INDEX allows you to purchase the full text of docu-
ments and articles while online. Charges will be made directly to
your credit card.  Full instructions for document ordering appear
in your User's Workbook.

   -Copies of articles:
      $7.50 (North America)
      $9.50 (outside North America)
      plus $.35 per page photocopied

   -Copies of documents:
      $10.00 (North America)
      $12.00  (outside  No. America)
plus  actual cost of document (phone calls,  purchase,  shipping,
and other related costs)

   -Copies of NTIS documents:
      $10.00 (North America)
      $15.00 (outside North America)
      plus North American NTIS price
   -Rush orders:
      $7.50 surcharge
?logoff
Menu system v. 5.53  ends.
        04jun91 12:06:11
User401095 Session B20.4
     $2.41     0.103 Hrs FileKI
     $2.41   Estimated total session cost    0.103 Hrs.
Logoff: level 26.04.03 B  12:06:12
```

Figure 3.3 Ordering documents on-line.

tion is not available, the library can order it for you from another library.

You may also order on-line through your vendor or from an information service. Most services will send the requested documents and bill your credit card. Be prepared to give the journal name, title of article, and the author's name.

Orders placed through DIALOG's Knowledge Index® or another program are transmitted electronically to a document supplier, who locates the articles and mails them. The commands to do this are "Keep," "Order," and "List." Write these commands as part of your search strategy so that you will not have to look them up while on-line:

> ?*Keep* s1/1–2 [Keep set 1, articles 1–2]
> ?*Order* ki [Order through Knowledge Index]
> ?*Order* List [List the order numbers, vendor, file, dates requested]
> ?*Help Rates* [The cost of articles, on-line time]

Figure 3.3 illustrates the ordering function. The cost for this order was $10 per article, with the documents arriving in 10 days.

Note: Information on prices, vendors, search features, and system requirements were current at the time of manuscript submission. June, 1991.

On-line searching is worthwhile for nurses in education and practice. In addition to gaining information for research projects, clinical instruction, and speeches and seminars, you can also find the cost of a new car, make airline reservations, and move money from one bank account to another. In addition, you will be the person who has access to information, the person who "knows," the person with the power.

REFERENCES

Blum, B. (Ed.). (1986). *Clinical information systems*. New York: Springer Verlag.

Communications. (1988). Alexandria: Time-Life.

Conway, S., & Messerle, J. (1990). Searching MEDLINE: Finding the needles in the medical haystack. *Group Practice Journal 39* (3), 26–34.

DIALOG Information Services. (1991). *Knowledge Index User's Manual*. Palo Alto: DIALOG Information Services.

Toffler, A. (1990). *Powershift*. New York: Bantam Books.

Appendix A—User-Friendly On-line Searching Services For Health Care Professionals

Name	Description
BRS Colleague	Offers some 40 databases in the biomedical field, including MEDLINE, NURSING & ALLIED HEALTH (CINAHL), and HAPI (HEALTH AND PSYCHO-SOCIAL INSTRUMENTS file). Cost: one-time registration fee plus monthly usage fees. Discounts available. BRS Colleague Student Program provides access at a 50% reduction in cost. BRS After Dark for non-prime time searching.
DIALOG Menus℠	Provides access to 300 popular databases. Hourly database rates apply. Knowledge Index® for non-prime time searching. Classroom Instruction Program available for a flat $15/hour fee.
EasyNet®	Telebase Systems' gateway providing access to 13 database vendors. Also available through CompuServe® and many other gateways.
Grateful Med®	Front-end program for searching MEDLINE and other NLM databases ($29.95, which includes communications software). For a few dollars per search, you can conduct simple searches. Loansome Doc is a new service for ordering article copies.
PaperChase®	User-friendly interface for searching MEDLINE and HEALTH PLANNING AND ADMINISTRATION (also available via CompuServe gateway).
Pro-Search™	Front-end system for searching BRS and DIALOG databases from Personal Bibliographic Software, Inc. Use company's Biblio-Links® and Pro-Cite® to organize references and create bibliographies according to standardized styles.

Vendors

BRS Information Technologies: McLean, VA 22102
DIALOG Information Services: Palo Alto, CA 94304
National Library of Medicine: Bethesda, MD 20894
PaperChase: Boston, MA 02115
Personal Bibliographic Software, Inc. (PBS): Ann Arbor, MI 48106
Telebase Systems: Wayne, PA 19087

Appendix B—Vendors of CD-ROM Databases

Although a number of CD-ROM vendors offer a range of health care databases, the following three vendors provide access to *both* MEDLINE and NURSING & ALLIED HEALTH (CINAHL), the primary databases used in nursing. Additional databases are available from these vendors.

Cambridge Scientific Abstracts
Bethesda, MD 20814

CD Plus
New York, NY 10001

SilverPlatter Information, Inc.
Sausalito, CA 94965

Section Two
Bedside Computers in Nursing Practice

Hales describes the potential benefits of bedside computers based on previous research. The historical perspectives, current, and future trends of bedside computers are also addressed in this chapter. Bauer describes the impact of the state of New Jersey Nursing Incentive Reimbursement Awards on the implementation of bedside computers in hospitals. Three types of computer systems are described with reference to examples in following chapters. The next three chapters are nurses' accounts of the methods they used to innovate nursing care with bedside computers. Belcher and Cunningham describe how nurses selected and implemented a critical care bedside computer system that provides point of care documentation. Miller and Sheridan describe why and how a bedside nursing information system should be implemented with a new nursing care pattern; in this situation, the case management model. The experience of working with two vendors to implement a nursing information system is described by three authors in the final chapter of this section. The effects of the bedside computers on joint practice, quality assurance, and nursing education are also addressed.

4

Bedside Data Acquisition:
Past, Present, Future

Gary D. Hales

INTRODUCTION

Although investigating the current uses and reasons for non-use of bedside terminals and predicting their failures and successes based on critical evaluation criteria are clearly vital to examining this technology in healthcare, taking an historical perspective is just as important. Discussing the development of bedside terminals allows us to see both the parallel development of bedside systems and hospital/healthcare information systems and the essential need for primary user input in design and implementation. By remembering the past and realizing the present, we may promote a better future.

HISTORICAL PERSPECTIVES

The development and use of a portable EPSON hand-held unit and one of the original portable lap top computers, the Radio Shack Model 100 with a monumental 32K of RAM reflected the desire for computer hardware and software developers to meet a need they saw existing in health care. It is not surprising that the impetus for computer use directly by health care givers might have sprung more from the desire of computer companies to produce a viable product than from users who might have been more comfortable with procedures already in use.

Andrews and Gardner (1988) found that "Although using [these] portable computers for charting was shown to be a feasible method for entering data, [respiratory] therapists using the portable computers preferred using ward terminals for entry." Given the limitations of this technology, this finding is not surprising. The portable computer had very limited functions, was not designed with this particular use in mind, and was not constructed for ease of data entry in a situation wherein the therapist moved from patient to patient. Andrews and Gardner do note that the goal at Latter Day Saints (LDS) hospital, where the study was conducted, is to have bedside terminals at all beds by the early 1990s. Lastly, small hand-held computers manufactured by Radio

Shack again were shown at some conventions with software for collection of health data. These devices resembled large rulers and had a very limited screen output and limited memory capacity.

The use of bedside terminals began, in the most basic sense, with the introduction of physiological monitoring devices in the early 1970s. These systems included the PROMIS system, introduced at Latter Day Saints Hospital in Salt Lake, the Technicon system, which premiered at El Camino Hospital, and the TDS Help system. These systems do not meet the operational definition of bedside terminals systems (i.e., interactive data collection and retrieval devices), however, these early attempts preceded the development of such systems. Another physiological monitoring system, of less repute than the above, was the Unibed system described by Prakash, Meij, and Zeelenberg (1982). Essentially this was a microcomputer-based system, significant because of the type of computer used.

The first bedside terminal was the PNUT or Portable Nursing Unit Terminal shown in figure 4.1. This revolutionary device was hand held, contained a temperature probe, and held simple patient information. The unit was designed to be carried by the nurse from patient to patient, information entered at the bedside, then uploaded from a base unit at the nursing station via an RS 232 connection to minicomputer. This base station was to be designed for two way communication. Information would be loaded from the PNUT to the base unit, and downloaded from the base unit to the PNUT. Due to the limited memory available at that time, two-way communication was necessary in order to have current information on a number of patients available to the nurse. This writer assumes that the eventual scheme called for connection to a Hospital Information System (HIS). The absence of this device in today's market attests to its failings, not the

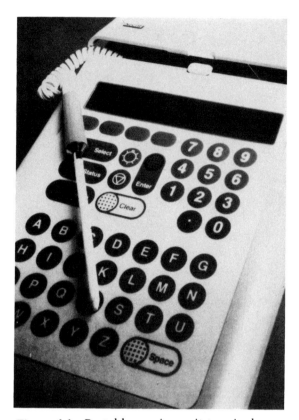

Figure 4.1 Portable nursing unit terminal.

least of which was the screen size. Another problem would have been that the device was hand-held. The unit, by NCR, was announced and shown at several meetings, pilot tested, and never, to the writer's knowledge, used commercially.

None of these early devices survived, but all contributed to the history of bedside terminals. These early attempts exemplify the usually unsatisfactory technique of fitting existing devices to new technology. If one combines the portability of the PNUT with the screen display of the Hewlett-Packard system, the result is very close to the early version of the Clinicom unit, discussed on the following page.

Much more pedestrian in design, but still being used, are the MEDTAKE and ULTICARE systems. The MEDTAKE system used a much more conventional design, terminal, and keyboard. The small footprint of this unit (15″ × 18″) made it an unobtrusive addition to the patient's room environment. The downscaled design was complemented by a reduced key set; Pesec (1988) reports that this reduced set incorporated a "handful of function keys labeled with common patient care activities . . . plus a numeric keypad." He also states "MEDTAKE was designed to automate the patient charting process and record the activities directly at the bedside." This type of input would not promote free text entry use of the terminals for physician orders, nursing care plans, or other text intensive functions. The customized bedside system (manufactured by MICRO) communicated using twisted-pair cable with a PC/XT (or clone) at the nursing station and thence to MICRO Healthsystem's DEC-based hospital information system. The connection to the HIS is an important chronological advance.

Another development was the ULTICARE system design which differed from the MEDTAKE unit in the use of a complete keyboard. This allowed free input not dictated by preconceived opinions regarding what healthcare workers needed and did not need.

The CRITIKON system, VitalNet shown in Figure 4.2, has the advantage of a smaller keyboard set and a display screen that may be wall mounted. In this unit you have the advantages of the small size of the unit plus the availability of screen input using a light pen.

Another system to appear in the middle eighties was the Clinicom system. The early design for the Clinicom unit, now under revision, resembles the even earlier PNUT. The Clinicom system used a 30-oz hand-held unit to collect patient data. The unit maintains

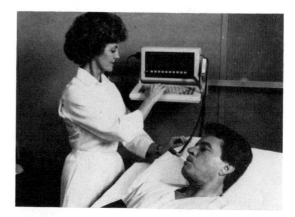

Figure 4.2 The Critikon System, VitalNet.

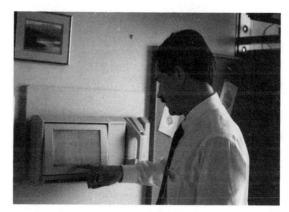

Figure 4.3 The Clinicom System.

continual communication with a base unit via a special radio frequency. The system can detect potential treatment conflict since information entered into the portable unit can be immediately compared to information available to the base unit. The newest configuration of this system includes a touch screen monitor shown in Figure 4.3. Touch screen technology is also used in the CRS system of bedside terminals.

The UBITEX system exemplifies multiple input modes. It utilizes large and small keypads and a mouse [Figure 4.4].

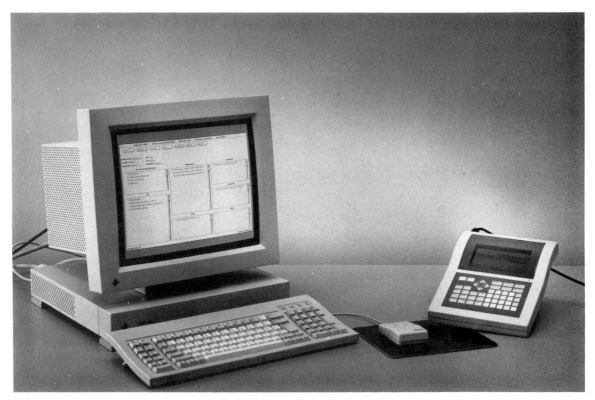

Figure 4.4 The Ubitex System.

Hewlett-Packard has also been investigating the use of bedside terminals for some time. They currently offer the Carevue 9000. Marquette Electronics and the 3M company have also added to the history of bedside systems through the use of different input/output (I/O) devices, touch pad, and track ball respectively. Finally, during the year 1990, Big Blue entered the fray with the 7690 computer. The IBM system features a rather unique design in which the bedside computer, based on the PS2, is mounted on a wall rack. The screen and keyboard fold out for use, leaving little to clutter the work space. Output is displayed through an adjustable back lit screen that can be seen in the dark and adjusted for viewers of different heights. Data is input by means of bar code reader, keyboard, or touch screen. This use of multiple input mechanisms, seen on other systems too, is an ergonomic design that permits the nurse to be flexible in the use of the system. The IBM unit can also be connected to networks, communication systems, and HISs. The Spectrum Healthcare Systems bedside unit uses the IBM unit as its hardware base shown in Figure 4.5.

Two devices that presage developments in the years to come are the INTELLICARE system and a computer image projection device. Figure 4.6 depicts the Sunquest information Systems' INTELLiCARE that processes continuous speech rather than single utterances. The nurse in the photograph has

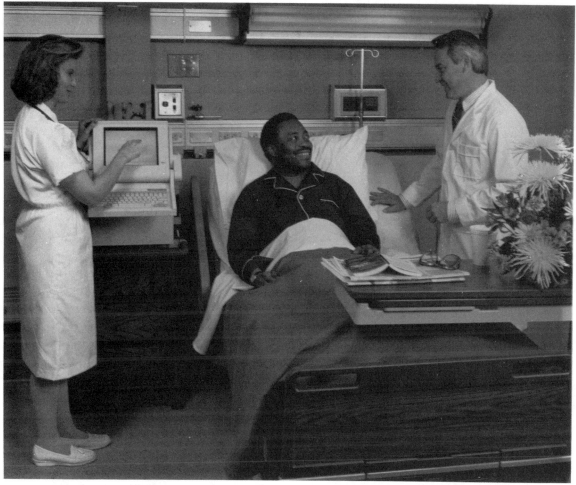

Figure 4.5 The IBM System. Photo courtesy of International Business Machines Corporation.

generated the display on the screen by saying "Make a graph displaying heart rate, temperature, and systolic pulmonary artery pressure." The INTELLiCARE system is a clinical information system for an intensive care unit.

In summary, Table 4.1 lists the major bedside software and hardware companies as of May, 1991. The information in the table is taken from an extensive survey of hardware and software bedside systems (*The Buyer's*

Guide to Bedside Computer Systems, 1991). This book also contains the KPMG-Peat Marwick study cited below as well as a study conducted at St. Joseph's Hospital in Milwaukee, Wisconsin. The whole computer industry moves so fast, that the list may be partially out of date by the time this book is printed. Some of the above cited vendors also produce hardware products unique to their systems; others use hardware from well-known hardware companies. Since this

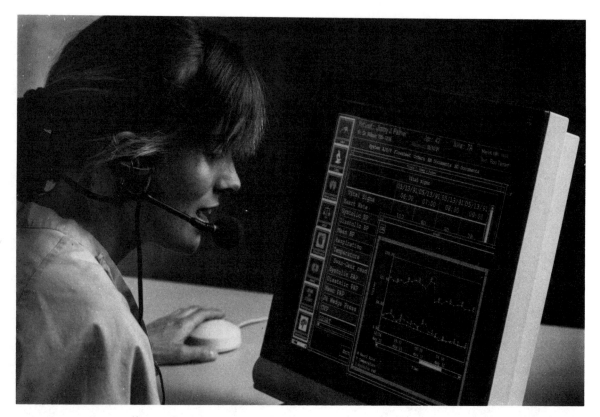

Figure 4.6   The Intellicare System.

situation remains very fluid as of the printing of this text, it is suggested the reader contact the company to determine the current hardware platform.

INPUT AND OUTPUT DEVICES

All of the typical input/output devices (i.e., key boards, touch screens, light pens, bar code readers) are being used in healthcare. However, only one of these devices, the IN-TELLICARE Sunquest system cited above, includes the most exciting I/O and the mechanism that will be *the* way data will be entered in the year 2000 at the latest: speech.

At the 1989 SCAMC (Symposium on Computer Applications in Medical Care) meeting, there was a panel discussion on automated speech recognition presented by a number of physicians and one hospital administrator. While all of the conference speakers recognized the current limitations of speech systems, voice independence or "speaker adaptive" speech recognition, they also saw the tremendous potential for this incipient technology.

Most speech recognition systems must be trained. That is, the speaker must input his or her voice commands a number of times so the computer can later recognize them. The speech thus recognized is not free flowing speech such as we use in our person-to-person communications but rather clipped phrases. Even with that limitation, the speakers reported very positive results in laboratory and emergency room settings.

Table 4.1   Companies Offering Bedside Software (May 1991)*

Company	Software
ACT/PC (608) 273-8860	ARGUS 2000
Clinicom (303) 443-9660	Clinicare
Clinicomp (714) 248-4015	CIS
Clinical Resource Systems (512) 478-1792	EmSTAT
Datacare (800) 999-3040	Decision Series Total
Daughters of Charity (214) 641-0385	Bedcom-1
Emtek (800) 832-8006	System 2000
First Technology (817) 232-3013	EMERGISOFT
Healthquest (404) 804-2932	Clinipac
Health Data Sciences (714) 888-3282	Ulticare
Hewlett-Packard (617) 890-6300	Carevye 9000
JR Systems (203) 966-7401	Nursing Information Systems
Micro Healthsystems (201) 731-9552	Medtake
Nursing Systems International (609) 499-3916	NIS
Phamis (206) 622-9558	Lastword
Puritan Bennett (619) 438-4138	Clinivision
Quantitative Medicine (301) 263-1301	Quantitative Sentinel
Second Foundation (802) 862-3052	ProTouch
SMS (215) 251-3164	Invision and Unity
SpaceLabs (206) 882-3700	PC Chartmaster
Sunquest (802) 885-7700	Caregiver and Intellicare
TDS Healthcare Systems (404) 847-5424	7000 Series
3M Health Information Systems (801) 265-4400	HELP
Trinity Computing Systems (800) 243-3952 NICU (800) 231-2445 ICU	NICU & ICU Link
Ubitex Corporation (204) 942-2992	Nursing Information System

* Information taken from *The Buyer's Guide to Bedside Computer Systems*, 1991.

The ideal use of such a system—person-to-computer, computer-to-person vocal contact—is not that far off. First, we will see speaker adaptive systems that will print their responses on a screen. This will shortly be followed by voice-generated responses. From there, it is impossible to predict.

RESEARCH IN BEDSIDE SYSTEM USE

A number of authors have investigated the applications and advantages of bedside terminals. Pesec (1988) suggests that these systems save time because the nurse does not have to return to the nursing station to check the chart for instructions or previous recordings that are now available at the bedside. While Pesec makes these statements in regard to the MedTake unit, these benefits are common to other systems of this kind.

Another very important consideration is IEEE Project 1073, the Medical Information Bus (MIB) committee. Paganelli (1989) describes the importance of a standardized method of connecting devices from various manufacturers such that data can be shared. An excellent analogy of the potential chaos of non-compatible bedside devices is provided by the example of kitchen appliances. She wrote "Imagine that you are remodeling your kitchen and considering the electrical wiring requirements. Your appliances are from several manufacturers: you have a MAYTAG range and a General Electric Toaster oven. . . . the range has a three-pronged plug and the toaster oven has a five-pronged plug.'' The potential for confusion and expense is clear. The IEEE project is designed to address this problem before it becomes a reality in hospital settings. A study done by KPMG-Peat Marwick for the TDS Healthcare Systems Healthcare 4000 models seems to reflect the findings of others in this area.

The TDS Health Care System survey of their model 4000, conducted by KPMG-Peat Marwick found that use of bedside terminals had a variety of benefits. These include:

1. reduction of medication errors by 34 percent,
2. reduction of patient use of nurse call systems by 26%,
3. increase in discharge teaching documentation and patient recall by 14 percent,
4. a stationary device was preferred over a portable device,
5. a light pen was the most efficient mechanism for data entry,
6. total productivity was increased by 80 to 120 minutes per nurse/shift/day,
7. nurses were excited and adapted quickly to use,
8. patients and families were indifferent, considering devices just another piece of equipment,
9. from a cost–benefit point of view, current intensive care use is more effective, and
10. full-function software (e.g., order entry/results reporting, care planning, assessments, patient accounts, intake and output, vital signs) were needed if the system was to maximize its potential.

Further support for successful implementation and positive outcome of bedside devices are reported by Levo, Averbuch, Halpern, and Jordan (1987), Seiver, Kohatsu, and Rowles (1987), Drazen and Huske (1988), McKinney (1988), and Cerne (1988).

The following list of potential benefits of bedside terminals is a synthesis of benefits described in three studies (Soontit, 1987; KPMG-Peat Marwick, 1988; Hughes, 1988; Halford, Burkes, & Pryor, 1989; Herring & Rochman, 1990).

1. increased nurse productivity,
2. increased nursing hours for direct patient care,
3. accessibility of patient data at bedside,
4. decreased unit clerk's work hours,
5. decreased overtime costs,
6. improved accuracy and legibility of data,
7. immediate availability of patient charts,
8. increased patient compliance,
9. improved contents of nursing notes,
10. efficient retrieval of data,
11. more timely response to patient needs,
12. positive patient identification,
13. improved nursing morale,
14. improved standardization and quality of charting, and
15. more time available for patient education.

SUMMARY AND CONCLUSIONS

Evaluation Considerations in Bedside Terminals

The following were deemed important considerations in evaluating bedside terminals (Paganelli, 1990). These considerations are recommended to any group planning to implement a bedside system.

1. Create a "vision" of the system you wish to implement; understand the "flow of data."
2. Does the system do a better job of manipulating and presenting data than the present manual system?
3. Can the system be modified and reconfigured without the vendor's help?
4. Does the vendor support the MIB?
5. What has the vendor done to address potential down-time problems?
6. Is the display conducive to use (e.g., color, fonts)?
7. How easy is terminal/workstation mounting?
8. Considering training purposes, is the system intuitive?
9. Is there a database component for research? (also cited by Zielstorff, McHugh, & Clinton, 1988)

The Impact of the User

After examining the literature, talking to experts, developers, and users, it seems that systems have evolved in response to recently past and current informatics needs. The user seems to have had input in "focus groups" and in responding to studies. Yet, there remains some doubt as to what forces have actually driven the development of these systems. There are a very limited number of systems currently in use, probably under 100 across the whole country.

In general the design and development of bedside systems have followed patterns of traditional data collection within the hospital. There is nothing immediately inap-

propriate or adverse in this; in fact, it is to be expected. One hopes, however, that this situation will not continue. Preferably, users, especially nurses, will make a concerted effort to make their needs known and encourage development of innovative uses of this technology. At this point, the driving force has been traditional data collection methodologies, leading us to use a potentially revolutionary technology to do things in the old ways. The vendors and a small number of users they have consulted would appear to be the decision makers in system development. One cannot fault this process totally since those who forced themselves and their opinions on others deserve to have their positions considered. On the other hand, there are a lot of people who have not contributed, whose experience is needed in development, and who should become actively involved in the process. Hospital information systems developed without the input of the most significant user group—nurses. This should not be the case in bedside terminals.

The impact of the user, then, has been present, but nursing input has been insufficiently influential. Zielstorff et al. (1988) makes a generic comment about systems that support nursing, but is applicable to bedside terminals specifically:

> *Nurses may be able to profit from the explanations of available technologies, benefits, impediments, and selection and evaluation considerations. Ultimately, the intent is to bridge the communications gap that sometimes exists between computer experts and nursing experts in order to improve the quality and usefulness of automated systems that promote more efficient and effective nursing care." (p. 35)*

In closing, the following quote from the KPMG-Peat Marwick (1988) study cited earlier clearly states the problem and suggests a potential solution.

If bedside terminals are to be successfully utilized the concept must complement the mission and goals of the institution. Additionally, use of bedside terminals must reinforce the philosophy and practice of nursing. (p. 2)

REFERENCES

Andrews, R. D., & Gardner, R. M. (1988). Portable computers used for respiratory care charting. *International Journal of Clinical Monitoring and Computing, 5*, 45–51.

Ball, P. A., Candy, D. C. A., Puntis, J. W. L., & McNeish, A. S. (1985). Portable bedside microcomputer system for management of parenteral nutrition in all groups. *Archives of Disease in Childhood, 60*, 435–439.

Cerne, F. (1988). Bedside terminals have nurses' support: study. *Hospitals*, June 20, 85.

Cerne, F. (1989). Study finds bedside terminals prove their worth. *Hospitals*, February 5, 72.

Drazen, E. L., & Huske, M. S. (1988). Bedside patient care systems. *Spectrum*, September 1988, *2*, 39–43.

Halford, G., Burkes, M., & Pryor, T. A. (1989). Measuring the impact of bedside terminals. *Nursing Management, 20* (7), 41–45.

Herring, D., & Rochman, R. (1990). A closer look at bedside terminals. *Nursing Management, 21*, (7), pp 54–61.

Hughes, S. (1988). Bedside terminals: Clinicom. *M.D. Computing, 5*, 22–28.

Janssen, J. H. A., Ackermans, J., Folkert, T., Verstraelen, B., de Zwann, C., Bar, F., & Brugada, P. (1984). Bedside digital subtraction angiography in critical care medicine. *Critical Care Medicine, 12*, 1067–1070.

Khoor, S., Kekes, E., Fugedi, K., Tote, J., & Berentey, E. (1988). Expert system on microcomputer: A bedside analysis of mechanocardiograms. *Acta Cardiologica, 43*, 273–276.

Koska, M. T. (1988). Bedside terminals. *Hospitals*, June 5, 100.

KPMG-Peat Marwick (1988) for TDS Corporation. *TDS Healthcare systems corporation bedside terminal study*. Author: Atlanta, GA.

Levo, Y., Averbuch, M., Halpern, Z., & Jordan, P. (1987). Computer-aided information system to support direct patient care: The application of a hand-held data collector in a department of medicine. *International Journal of Biomedical Computing, 20*, 175–179.

Lynn, L. A., & Sunderrajan, E. V. (1986). Bedside respiratory analysis by pocket computer. *Critical Care Medicine, 14*, 62–64.

National Report on Computers & Health. (1991). *The Buyer's guide to bedside computer systems*. Rockville, MD: Source.

Nolan-Avila, L. S., Paganelli, B. E., & Norden-Paul, R. E. (1988). The medical information bus: An automated method for capturing patient data at the bedside. *Computers in Nursing, 6*, 115–121.

McKinney, P. (1988). Can point-of-care terminals ease the threat? *Computers in Healthcare (Nursing Edition)*, April.

Paganelli, B. E. (1989). Criteria for the selection of a bedside information system for acute care units. *Computers in Nursing, 7*, 214–221.

Pesec, J. (1988). Bedside terminals: Medtake. *M.D. Computing, 5*, 16–21.

Prakash, O., Meij, S., & Zeelenberg, C. (1982). Computer-based patient monitoring. *Critical Care Medicine, 10*, 811–822.

Replogle, K. J. (1986). A computer at every bedside: Issues and obstacles. *Critical Care Nurse, 6*, 14–21.

Schank, M. J., & Doney, L. D. (1987). General-purpose microcomputer software: New tools for nursing professionals. *Nursing Management, 18*, 26–28.

Seiver, A., Kohatsu, S., & Rowles, D. (1987). Bedside computers in the surgical intensive care unit. *Angiology*, March, 248–252.

Solingen, S., & Shabot, M. M. (1988). A 32 key keyboard for the HP PDMS. *International Journal of Clinical Monitoring and Computing, 5,* 31–34.

Soontit, E. (1987). Installing the first operational bedside nursing computer system. *Nursing Management, 18,* 23–25.

Stead, W. S. (1983). Evolution of technology brings computers to the bedside. *Kidney International, 24,* 436–437.

van Bemmel, J. H. (1987). Computer assisted care in nursing—Computation at the bedside. *Computers in Nursing, 5,* 132–139.

Zielstorff, R. D., McHugh, M. L., & Clinton, J. (1988). *Computer design criteria: For systems that support Nursing.* Kansas City: American Nurses Association.

5

Information Management in Nursing Care: One State's Approach

Carol A. Bauer

INTRODUCTION

Information management is a necessity for nurses who wish to maintain high standards in their work because the nursing profession and health care in general have changed phenomenally. The information nurses must be able to access in order to practice has expanded dramatically. Monumental advances in science and medicine during the past decade demand that nurses meet the challenge created by our rapidly proliferating information society. Moreover, nurses must continually insure safe, effective, and competent care. The need for information access is also influenced by the complexity of nursing practice and the diversity of its patient population. The evolution of new and complex nursing roles has put an additional strain on existing nursing resources. More than ever, professional nurses must provide information for other health professionals, quality assurance programs, third party payers, accrediting bodies, and others in the public arena in response to consumer demand for accountability and cost containment.

Critical to the professional role of nurses is the changing delivery system and clinical practice. In order to derive personal and professional satisfaction from nursing, nurses must incorporate information technology into their practice.

BACKGROUND

In response to escalating health care costs, an increasing population of uninsured, and the overlapping organizational structure of health care services, New Jersey, in 1978, created a mandatory reimbursement system that included all payors and all hospitals (Siegel, Weiss, & Lynch, 1991). This rate setting system implemented the state's public policies of high quality of care, access to safe care, promotion of financial solvency of acute care hospitals, and cost containment (Merlino & Parker, 1978). Known as the DRG system, it was later adopted by the federal Medicare program. A unique feature of the legislation was the establishment of the Hospital Rate Setting Commission which determined the reimbursement rates for all payors and hospitals in New Jersey. This was later to be a mechanism for channeling funds to hospitals struggling to recruit and retain nurses during the nursing shortage.

New Jersey was hard hit by the nursing shortage of the 1980's. The shortage was felt first in the state's acute care hospitals. In October, 1987, the governor of New Jersey convened the Nursing Shortage Study Commission whose task was to assess the adequacy of the supply of current and future registered nurses and ancillary nursing personnel and to insure that the supply was proportional to the demand for the health care requirements of the citizens of New Jersey (New Jersey State Nursing Shortage Study Commission, 1988).

After six months of intensive study, the Commission presented the governor with immediate and future-focused recommendations to remedy the nursing shortage. Computerized clinical and management systems were proposed to improve the work environment. Nursing education was urged to prepare graduates who were computer literate and ready to operate computer-based information systems found in the health care environment. The New Jersey State Nursing Shortage Study Commission also addressed the creation of a separate incentive fund to enable New Jersey health care institutions and agencies to develop professional practice models that foster nursing recruitment and retention. A competitive grant funding process was put forth to operationalize this recommendation.

The Nursing Advisory Committee, created by the New Jersey Commissioner of Health, was a direct outcome of the recommendations of the New Jersey State Nursing Shortage Study Commission. This Committee, comprised of nurses in service and education, doctors, hospital administrators, and insurance industry representatives, embellished the recommendation of the Nursing Shortage Commission with further innovations in nursing practice models and environments. In 1989, the Nursing Incentive Reimbursement Awards (NIRA) program came from temporary adjustments in the reimbursement rates for those acute care hospitals whose proposals were selected for implementation. The NIRA program criteria for funding were modeled after the Robert Wood Johnson-Pew Foundations grant program which used these criteria: 1) innovative projects, 2) impact on the nursing shortage, 3) the hospital's commitment, and 4) ability to replicate the proposal.

The nurses of New Jersey now had funding to address the causes of nursing attrition: image, decision-making, and time management. The purpose of the NIRA program was to improve the nurses' work environment and increase recruitment and retention of nurses (New Jersey State Department of Health, 1989). The proposals were reviewed by an expert panel chaired by Dr. Lucille Joel, President of the American Nurses Association. Proposals were selected on the basis of having the most impact on the nursing shortage, the commitment of the hospital, and the ability of the proposal to be replicated in other units or hospitals. A cross-section of hospitals in the state were chosen according to size, type, and location within the state. A total of $20 million was allocated for the program over a two year period.

COMPUTER APPLICATIONS

Of the 23 proposals awarded funding for the first year of the program, 1990, 15 were for the implementation of new bedside or unit-based computer systems. Fifteen hospitals were to be the prime initiators of nursing information management in New Jersey.

Less than 50 hospitals nationwide had bedside computer systems in 1989 (Drazen, 1990). This was an uncharted area into which these 15 hospitals took the lead to introduce the latest information technology. Many problems and pitfalls were experienced by these pioneers.

Colleagueship among the project directors was facilitated through regularly scheduled meetings sponsored by the New Jersey Department of Health, whereby project directors of all funded hospitals reported on the status of each project. Bonding of the project directors created an informal network for consultation and support.

The initial period was used to select a system compatible with the particular institution. Most of the major vendors competed in this selection process. The desired features of a nursing documentation system were used as selection criteria. These included reduced charting time, elimination of duplication, increased accuracy, and compliance with quality assurance criteria and improved legibility. Charting consumes a significant percent of nurses' time, a limited and costly resource in today's health economy.

Three types of computer systems are currently on the market: stand alone systems for general acute care, stand alone systems for critical care, and interfaced hospital information systems with a nursing application. The majority of hospitals chose a stand alone system for general acute care, thereby impacting on the greatest number of hospital beds. These systems enable the nurses to enter vital signs, intake and output, routine care, medications, assessments, and care plans. As these are stand alone systems, the data entered and maintained by nursing remains separate from the hospital information system and is accessed at a separate terminal. Interfaces can be developed to enable the nursing system to have the maximum impact on patient data management.

Only one of the 15 hospitals chose a stand alone critical care system. This stand alone computer system, as well as two other computer projects cited, is described in detail elsewhere in this publication (see Belcher and Cunningham, Chap. 6). Stand alone computer systems are less popular as they are limited to a select group of patients and interfaces must be written for these systems in order to transfer the data to the hospital information system. The software is designed to manage information. Information management software programs are designed around flowcharting and graphics displays which manage the immense amount of data collected and monitored in the critical care setting. The selling point of this software is that it services a patient population requiring expensive labor and capital outlays. Therefore, stand alone computer systems represent a significant, but highly specialized market.

In contrast, an interfaced hospital information system includes a nursing application with two-way interface between bedside computers and the hospital information system (see Miller & Sheridan, Chap. 7). Assessment, care plans, and documentation are available for each type of bedside computer. An example is provided in this text (Tiedeken, Majarowitz, & Duryee, Chap. 8). A major advantage is the accessibility of information at the nurses' station for patient care and all clinical services. Multiple users may access the system at the bedside or any other system terminal. These systems are the most costly and the anticipated dollar savings may not be readily apparent as there is a delayed payback for computer technology. Evaluation is more difficult because of the comprehensiveness of the system and the effects on delivery of care.

SYSTEM IMPLEMENTATION: PROBLEMS AND CHALLENGES

Once the 7.1 million dollars were awarded for 1990, the real challenge began. Computer technology is a highly complex and specialized field. Implementing the systems demanded the expertise and cooperation of multiple hospital departments whose priority was not the installation of bedside computers for nursing. Articulating the schedules of the vendors and the plant engineering staff who had to provide wiring, carpentry, and other structural alterations required keen administrative coordination. In some cases, this work was not anticipated or budgeted in the original proposal. Delays at any step of the process led to serious time lags and cost overruns.

Most hospitals had to make structural adjustments to accommodate the computer terminals in patient rooms. Already overcrowded with equipment, hospital architecture was not designed for bedside computers. In some hospitals, less than ideal placements of terminals resulted in nurses being distanced from the patient's bedside contrary to the intent of the system.

Education of nursing staff in order to make the system operational also required coordination of staffing schedules and readiness of equipment. Equipment did not always arrive according to delivery dates, this resulted in the nurses being ready to "go live" before the computers were operational. False starts led to disinterest and diminished cognitive and manual skills.

IMPACT ON NURSING

Although not a panacea for the nursing shortage, computers are here to stay and are rapidly becoming an essential part of patient care technology. Some hospitals view computerization as a way of projecting a high tech image to assist with recruitment and retention of nurses. Nurses, once they have overcome their "computerphobia," do not wish to return to paper and pencil documentation, illegible charting and incomplete patient data.

Nursing's need for computerization will only grow, during the second year of the NIRA program 16 more hospitals received funding for bedside or unit-based systems (Dunston, 1990). These awards will expand existing computer technology or introduce computer systems into the hospital nursing environment.

Nursing information systems have become a significant portion of the technology market. Vendors now realize the economic potential in designing and manufacturing systems which are user-friendly and meet nursing specifications. Computers are now used in hospitals, home health care agencies, cancer centers, clinics, and learning resource centers where the nurses indicated the systems benefited both their patients and themselves, saving time, and improving patient care (Thomas, 1991).

This state's experience with computer technology will have a nationwide impact on nursing documentation and delivery of care. The opportunity to obtain funds for expensive technology, usually out of reach for most hospital-based nursing departments will have a broad and lasting effect. The establishment of nursing databases, accurate, legible documentation, and readily accessible patient information will enable nurses to improve clinical decision making. Nursing research will have access to large data banks to validate nursing interventions. These outcomes will ultimately enhance the quality of care to the public.

REFERENCES

Drazen, E. (1990). *Bedside computer systems overview, bringing computers to the hospital bedside: An emerging technology.* New York: Springer Publishing Company.

Dunston, F. J. (1990). *1991 Nursing incentive reimbursement awards.* Trenton, NJ: State of New Jersey, Department of Health.

Merlino, J. P., & Parker, B. T. (1978). An act

concerning the provision and payment for medical services and establishing a hospital rate setting commission and amending and supplementing P. L. 1971, c. 136 and P. L. 1938, c. 366. *State of New Jersey, Senate, No. 446.*

New Jersey State Department of Health (1989). *Nursing incentive reimbursement awards program, requests for proposals.* Trenton, NJ: New Jersey Department of Health.

New Jersey State Nursing Shortage Study Commission (1988). *Nursing Shortage Study Commission Report to the Governor.* Trenton, NJ: State of New Jersey, Department of Health.

Siegel, B., Weiss, A., & Lynch, D. (1991). Setting New Jersey hospital rates: A regulatory system under stress. *University of Puget Sound Law Review, 14*(3), 601–631.

Thomas, M. (1991). Computers free nurses for care. *The American Nurse,* July-August, 1.

6

Implementation of Bedside Computers in Critical Care

Alice J. Belcher
Lyda Sue Cunningham

INTRODUCTION

"I don't have time to learn how to use a computer, much less take time to use it. I have patients to take care of!" "I hate computers, I never intend to touch one!" "What, me use a computer, you must be kidding!"

These were some of the responses from several of the critical care nurses in a 360-bed voluntary community hospital prior to the implementation of a bedside computerization project. The nursing administration had just announced receipt of a grant from the New Jersey State Department of Health (NJDOH) through its Nursing Incentive Reimbursement Award Program. Funds were made available to 23 New Jersey hospitals to create innovative methods to decrease the effects of the persistent nurse shortage. Large sums of hospital monies were being expended for overtime salary costs and agency nurse fees in order to keep nursing units functioning. The critical care staff nurses had known about the grant application and its intended purpose to procure

funds to install bedside computers, but no one thought it would become a reality. Much to everyone's astonishment, funding became available to carry out the bedside computerization plan. This scenario is just one of the ways that computerization impacts nursing in the 1990s. Because the effects of the nursing shortage were most acute in the critical care unit, it was felt that installation of bedside computers in that area would best accomplish the goals and objectives of the project. From a literature review and interviews with critical care managers in successfully computerized hospitals, it was felt that the following objectives/goals could be accomplished:

- Improve recruitment and retention of nurses
- Open closed critical care beds
- Enhance the ICU/CCU high-tech image of the hospital
- Decrease nonnursing tasks
- Reduce unplanned overtime

- Reduce agency nurse costs
- Improve job satisfaction of nurses
- Enhance documentation of care

The account that follows reveals how a clinical information system (CIS) was successfully implemented in a critical care unit. Initial results of research studies that measure the impact of this project will also be discussed.

STAGES OF IMPLEMENTATION

Selection Process

The hardware and software products of three different vendors were reviewed. The product had to include:

1. Software developed specifically for critical care use
2. Ease of use by noncomputer literate staff
3. Ability to configure the software to individual hospital needs
4. Ability to configure future changes on site
5. An open architecture to allow for interfacing with the hospital information system and other foreign devices

Other *desired* product qualities include the following:

- multisectioned flowsheet
- auto physiocalculation
- drug calculator
- patient care plans
- medex and kardex
- narrative charting
- graphing/trending
- admission/assessment screen
- audit tool
- multilevel security
- quality assurance tools
- acuity/classification
- severity of illness
- database export
- printed reports
- trackball or penlight
- modem interface to physician offices
- work lists of nursing tasks
- reference library

Before making a final vendor selection, two on-site visits were made to other hospitals using critical care bedside information systems. Staff nurses willingly shared their opinions regarding the improved quality of documentation and the overall impact on their ability to deliver patient care. Management shared useful insights and suggestions for a successful project implementation.

Vendor Selection

The vendor chosen was Hewlett-Packard (H-P). Their CareVue 9000 bedside computer system is designed specifically for critical care and is totally configurable to individual hospital needs. While all of the above applications were not immediately available, it was felt that this stable and innovative company would develop them shortly. Additional factors influencing the decision included the product appearance, ease of use, and speed of data entry using the trackball for the noncomputer-literate user. The hospital also had a long history of satisfaction with service and products from this company for other equipment.

Change Process

To begin the unfreezing phase of Kurt Lewin's change process (Sullivan & Decker,

1988), the task force asked the vendor to demonstrate the system for the nursing and medical staff. The purpose of the hands-on demonstration was to convince nurses and doctors that the computer system could enhance their practice, decrease nonnursing tasks, and thus allow more time for patient care and hopefully decrease patient length of stay. It was anticipated the system would enhance the high-tech image of the hospital, improving recruitment and retention, and decrease overtime and agency nurse expense. The nursing and medical staff generally adopted an "I'll believe it when I see it" attitude, but they did maintain open minds and volunteered for committees related to the project.

Setting Expectations

Then the real work began! A manager assumed primary responsibility for the project. A time line was developed (see Table 6.1). The hospital implementation team consisted mostly of directors of departments who would be directly impacted by this new system (medical records, biomedical, information systems, risk management, nursing administration, and medical staff).

The hospital team was introduced to the Hewlett-Packard implementation team at a kick-off meeting, where the responsibilities and expectations of each person, department, and team were outlined. As a result, a general commitment to the success of this venture was generated, expectations outlined, and a lasting partnership was envisioned between the vendor and the hospital.

Designing the Software

Twelve members of the nursing staff volunteered to work on the configuration

committee. An H-P clinical specialist conducted a one-day training session. Many meetings were held to design and build the menus and code tables for the flowsheet and drug calculator. That initial work required two months. The first version of the software was loaded by the H-P Company and the configuration committee began reviewing the flow of menus and making changes. The members held many impromptu meetings with their peers to gain a consensus about controversial issues concerning charting on the flowsheet. Staff interaction during the designing phase was very important in the change process. Nurses began to realize that they would have to chart in a more organized and complete manner when using the computer. The discussions and decision-making processes also helped them to recognize the value of this change in their work habits and encouraged ownership of the system.

Meanwhile, other details had to be solved: (1) what small room could function as a system control room (with controlled humidity and temperature, and dedicated power and telephone lines); (2) would the workstations be permanently mounted or placed on a mobile cart in the patient rooms; (3) where in the patient rooms would the workstation be placed—which side of the bed; (4) who would pull the cable for the system; and (5) was the hospital carpenter available to build shelves and platforms?

Training

Nine of the nursing staff volunteered to be trainers. Hewlett-Packard provided a two-day intensive "Train-The-Trainer" course at the local H-P facility. Trainers learned (1) how to use the system expertly; (2) how adults learn; and (3) how to teach adults. During the next six weeks, the nine nurses set up classes and trained 80 other nurses

Table 6.1   Sample Time Line Chart

Task Name	Resources	Duratn (Days)	Start Date	End Date	Status	Mar 5	12	19	26	Apr 2
Summary of PLAN-1		162	8-Jan-98	24-Aug-98		!!!!!!!!!!!!!!!!!!!!!!!!!!!!!				
1.02 Kickoff Meeting	AB, JH, NH	1	8-Jan-98	8-Jan-98		.	. !	.	.	
1.03 Detailed Impl. Plan	JH, AB, NH	1	12-Feb-98	12-Feb-98		.	. !	.	.	
1.01 Ship Loaner Hardware	NH, LC, DD, MS	3	14-Mar-98	16-Mar-98	R	.	. XXX-	.	.	
1.05 Prepare Site	LC, DD, MS	10	15-Mar-98	28-Mar-98	R	.	. XXXXXXXXXX------			
1.04 Train Hospital Impl. Team	JH	0.5	20-Mar-98	20-Mar-98	C p	.	. !	.X	.	
1.06 Configuration Training	JH	1	21-Mar-98	22-Mar-98	C ps	.	. !	. XX	.	
1.10 Dev. Rules of System Use	AB, Hosp, JH	10	13-Aug-98	24-Aug-98	CR	.	. !	.	.	
1.07 Design Displays	AB, Hosp, JH	40	23-Mar-98	18-May-98	CR ps	.	. !	.	XXXXXXXXXX	
1.08 Develop Reports	AB, Hosp, JH	40	23-Mar-98	18-May-98	CR ps	.	. !	.	XXXXXXXXXX	
1.09 Build Application Config	HP, JH, AB	20	23-May-98	21-Jun-98	C s	.	. !	.	.	
1.11 Load Application Config.	LC, DD, JH	0.5	3-Jul-98	3-Jul-98	C s	.	. !	.	.	
1.12 Review Application Config	AB, Hosp, JH	20	5-Jul-98	1-Aug-98	C	.	. !	.	.	
1.14 Educate Hosp. Instructors	JH, HP	4	7-Aug-98	10-Aug-98	CR	.	. !	.	.	
1.13 Develop Conversion Plan	AB, JH, NH	5	7-Aug-98	13-Aug-98	R	.	. !	.	.	
1.15 Educate System Manager	LC, DD, JH	1	13-Aug-98	13-Aug-98		.	. !	.	.	
Summary of INSTALL		40	11-Jun-98	6-Aug-98	C	.	. !	.	.	
2.02 Manufacture Software	HP	5	21-Jun-98	28-Jun-98	C p	.	. !	.	.	
2.01 Ship Hardware	MS, JH	10	11-Jun-98	22-Jun-98	C	.	. !	.	.	
2.03 Install/Test Hardware	MS, LC, DD, JH	5	25-Jun-98	29-Jun-98		.	. !	.	.	
2.04 Install/Test OPSYS Softw.	LC, DD, JH	1	2-Jul-98	2-Jul-98		.	. !	.	.	
2.05 Copy Application Config.	LC, DD, JH	1	2-Aug-98	2-Aug-98	C	.	. !	.	.	
2.06 Conduct System Test	LC, DD, MS, JH	1	3-Aug-98	3-Aug-98	C	.	. !	.	.	
2.07 Freeze Application Config	AB, JH, Hosp, LC, DD	1	6-Aug-98	6-Aug-98	C	.	. !	.	.	
Summary of CONVERT		38	7-Aug-98	28-Sep-98	C	.	. !	.	.	
3.02 Training/Double Charting	AB, Hosp, JH	20	27-Aug-98	24-Sep-98	CR	.	. !	.	.	
Milestone (Clinical Use)		0	27-Aug-98	27-Aug-98	C	.	. !	.	.	
3.04 Dev. Sys.Accept. Criteria	JH, AB, Hosp, NH, HP	7	7-Aug-98	15-Aug-98	R	.	. !	.	.	
3.03 Finalize Conversion Plan	AB, Hosp, JH, HP	2	14-Aug-98	15-Aug-98	R	.	. !	.	.	
3.01 Instruct End Users	AB, Hosp, JH	15	27-Aug-98	17-Sep-98	R	.	. !	.	.	
3.05 Convert to CV 9000 - Beta	AB, Hosp, JH, HP	2	25-Sep-98	26-Sep-98	C	.	. !	.	.	
3.06 Meet Sys.Accept. Criteria	AB, Hosp, JH, NH, HP	1	27-Sep-98	27-Sep-98	C	.	. !	.	.	
3.07 Transition to Support	JH, HP, NH	1	28-Sep-98	28-Sep-98	C	.	. !	.	.	
Milestone (End of Phase I)		0	28-Sep-98	28-Sep-98	C	.	. !	.	.	

```
XXXXX Detail Task        ##### Summary Task    M  Milestone
xxXXX (Started)          ==### (Started)       >>> Conflict
XXX-- (Slack)            ##--  (Slack)         ..XXX Resource delay
------------------ Scale: 1 day per character -------------------
```

and 45 physicians. Each nursing staff member required an average of eight hours of training. A few utilized an optional four-hour practice session. Each nurse was required to enter practice patient data into the computer flowsheet. Upon successful completion of the exercise, each nurse was issued a confidential password. The physicians were taught only how to enter the flowsheet to review their patients' information.

All trainers were trained to be system operators (first-line trouble shooters who could, for example, bring up a workstation that might be accidentally unplugged, load paper into the printers, clear paper jams, and so forth). Three people were trained to be system managers (using different software tools to manage the overall system and interact with the regional control center) as knowledge of computer programming is not necessary to carry out these tasks.

Policies and procedures were developed to aid the nursing staff in use of the system. Double charting was carried out for one week (computer as well as the handwritten 24-hour flowsheet) to ensure that no major flaws had occurred in the configuration.

Conversion (Paper to Computer)

"Go-Live Day" occurred ten months after the start of the project. It was treated as a celebration for the nursing staff and their patients, with decorations and food for the staff. A one-to-one patient–nurse staffing ratio was planned to ensure a trouble-free transition. There were H-P clinical specialists in the intensive Care Unit 24 hours a day for the first three days. A trainer was scheduled on each shift for the next two weeks, which provided the nurses with immediate help with any problem or question that might arise. The patients were delighted to be part of the initial computerized record system.

The conversion to the computer system was smooth and efficient. Benefits that have been measured and observed to date are believed to be the result of following the installation and implementation plans explicitly, with an emphasis on completion of each detail, thus avoiding pitfalls and errors that could have led to costly delays and failure.

PROBLEMS

Of course there were problems. Nevertheless, they were people problems, not hardware or software problems. The project director and implementation team were aware from the beginning that installation of this new charting method required both work and cultural habit changes for the nursing staff. The opening statements from this article reflect the resistant attitudes that had to be overcome. Consequently the nursing staff were involved from the beginning in the entire project, to initiate the unfreezing and move them through the other phases of the change process (Sullivan & Decker, 1988). Their work in configuring the entire system resulted in enhanced organization and time management skills, and they had a greater vested interest in the success of the system along with acceptance of ownership. Work habits had to change as the staff learned to enter data at the point-of-care rather than waiting several hours to transcribe a large amount of data from their scribbled notes and memory. Still, the cultural habit change took longer to occur. Several weeks after "going live" the nursing staff moved their workstations to the doorways of patient rooms and from that vantage point they could communicate with their peers while entering data. This practice continues the socialization process that nursing has carried out for years while charting at the nurses station. However, that practice decreases the time-saving aspect of bedside charting since the information is not entered at the point-of-care immediately after delivery of patient care.

While the staff have accepted and are utilizing the bedside computer system beneficially, there are only a few applications in place at present. Thus, the staff has not realized the full value of computerization on their practice. Only after the care plans, medication administration record, work lists, classification and acuity tools, and laboratory and x-ray results are put into place (see list p. 54) will the full significance and impact of this product be known. Only at that point will there be full acceptance and utilization of the bedside computer as a significant change in nursing practice and patient care. At that time the change process can be considered completed and refrozen (Sullivan & Decker, 1988).

BENEFITS

Nine months after the bedside computer system was initiated the following benefits were tangible:

1. The documentation became more comprehensive, accurate, and timely. Charting became much more complete and organized because each nurse was reminded, by row labels on the computer screen, of information she or he should chart and patient care she or he should complete. Costly errors of duplication and omission were thus eliminated. (This function will be enhanced in the future as patient care plans are created in the computer and the resultant work lists are generated.) Moreover, all printed information was much easier to read because it was presented in a consistent and orderly manner.

2. All vital signs on the bedside monitor are automatically linked into the computer, yielding increased accuracy in recording. Ventilators, IV pumps, and blood gas machines will soon be interfaced to capture that data automatically. (See Figure 6.1.)

3. End-of-shift overtime for charting-related activities has disappeared. Overtime expense has decreased by 67 percent. Use of agency nurses has decreased by 58 percent. System "uptime" is 99.98 percent.

4. Confidentiality and access to the patient's chart have improved as only users with a valid password can gain access to the patient record.

Other, more subtle changes have been observed. The census and acuity have been routinely higher on the computerized unit than on the noncomputerized unit—even though patients are assigned randomly. It appears that the nurses are placing the sickest patients on the computerized unit. Additionally, when, in July 1991, the nursing staff took their annual hospital critical care exam to requalify for their career ladder placement, their scores averaged higher than those taken previously. We believe the computers may have focused their thinking processes on clinical information. Finally, easily viewed information on the flowsheet has encouraged a more consultative approach to patient care by the primary nurse with her charge nurse and/or the physician.

EVALUATION

To enable the nursing profession to grow through its own efforts, nurses must conduct and publish their own research regarding all new innovations in nursing care rather than be regulated by other agencies and vendors. Therefore, studies were conducted to measure the impact of this bedside computerization project in the critical care units of this medium-sized (360-bed), nonteaching, voluntary community hospital. That involved comparing the computerized intensive care unit with the noncomputerized coronary care unit. The studies were conducted three months before the project began, six months after "going live," and will be conducted again at 18 months or when all applications are in place.

Areas studied included: (1) nursing work satisfaction, (2) patient satisfaction with care, (3) physician satisfaction with nursing care, (4) overtime expense and agency fees,

Figure 6.1 flowsheet

	91Aug27 07:00AM	08:00AM	09:00AM	10:00AM	11:00AM	12:00PM	01:00PM	02:00PM	03:00PM	04:00PM	05:00PM
Vital signs											
Temperature		36.8				36.7				36.9	
Temp Site		R				R				R	
Alarms		On	On			On				On	
Heart Rate		85	87	92		88	89	91	92	92	90
Respiration		15	14	20		12	17	17	18	16	20
Basic Rhythm		Afib/c		Afib/c		Afib/c				NSR	
Secondary Rhythm											
PVC										Freq	Trigem
Morphology										Unifoc	
PAC											
Cuff BP S/D		113/ 64	109/ 61	115/ 63		107/ 56	102/ 54	95/ 51	99/ 52	100/ 53	97/ 53
Position		Lying	Lying			Lying			Lying	Lying	Lying
Hemodynamy											
PAP S/D		45/ 24	47/ 18	43/ 16		35/ 13			18/ 12	25/ 10	26/ 14
PA Mean			29						14	15	
PA Wedge		18									
Right Atrial		10									
Cardiac Output Aver.		3.76									
IV drips											
Amrinone mcg/min		300	300	300		300	300		300	300	300
Dobutamine mcg/min		400	400	400		400	400		400	400	400
Dopamine mcg/min		200	200	150		100	50		0	50	100
Lidocaine mg/min		1	1	1		1	1		1	1	1
D1/2NS 1000		10	10	10		10	10		10	10	10
100 D5W 50											
100D5W 50KCL						10	10		10	10	10
50 D5W 60 KCL											
Pulmonary Vent/Resp											
Oxygen Delivery						[1]	NC		NC	NC	
O2 Concentration							6l		6l	6L	
Ventilator		Serv900	Serv900			Serv900					
FIO2		40	40			40					
Tidal Volume		750	750			750					
Ventilator Mode		SIMV	SIMV			SIMV					
Vent/Set/Pt Rate		12/ 14	12/ 14			12/ 14					
PRESSURE SUPPORT		10	10								
Intake/Outputs Totals											
D5W+Lido		14	7	7		14	7		14	14	
D5W.45		20	10	10		20	10		20	20	
D5W+Dopa		22	11	11		22	6		3	6	
D5W+Dobuta		24	12	12		24	12		24	24	
NS .45%+Inocar		14	7 [1]	7		14	7		14	14	
D5W+KCL						10	10		20	20	
D5W+KCL											
IV Meds Fluids/cc's											
Urine Foley		210	120	[2] 160		1260	1000		525	740	160
IV Fluids In Total	0 384	94 478	47 525	47 572	0 572	104 676	52 728	0 728	95 823	98 921	0 921
PO/NG Intake Total											
Urine Out Total	0 346	210 556	120 676	160 836	0 836	1.32.1L	1.03.1L		03096	5253621	7404361
Stool Total											
Total IN	0 384	94 478	47 525	47 572	0 572	104 676	52 728	0 728	95 823	98 921	0 921
Total OUT	0 346	210 556	120 676	160 836	0 836	1.32.1L	1.03.1L		03096	5253621	7404361
Net Body Balance	+ 38	-79	-152	-265	-265	-1421	-2369	-2369	-2799	-3441	-3601

Figure 6.1 Sample vital sign section of flowsheet.

Table 6.2 Nurse Satisfaction Surveys

Item	Preinstall		Postinstall	
	Standard Deviation	**Weighted Control**	**Standard Deviation**	**Weighted Control**
Pay	1.125	3.6	1.126	3.90
Autonomy	0.823	3.4	0.852	3.39
Task Requirements	0.979	2.8	1.018	2.88
Organizational Req.	0.951	2.8	0.918	2.46
Interaction	0.947	3.0	0.911	3.11
Professional Status	0.583	3.3	0.520	3.08

Source: Knickman et al., 1991.

(5) quality of patient records, and (6) recruitment and retention data.

Nurse satisfaction was measured with the Stamps and Piedmont "Index of Work Satisfaction" tool, (Slavitt, Stamps, Piedmont, & Haase, 1979). The initial and first follow-up standard deviations with weighted components of the nursing staff satisfaction surveys (evaluated by New York University Research Department) are reported in Table 6.2.

Preinstallation work sampling studies revealed that the nursing staff spent an average of 37.71 percent of their total time on nonpatient care tasks, with 19.3 percent of that time spent on charting-related activities. This compares to an average of 30 to 40 percent of total time as reported in the literature.

Patient satisfaction was measured with the modified Risser "Patient Satisfaction" instrument (Hinshaw & Atwood, 1982). Patients were chosen at random from a population that had been admitted at least 24 hours prior to administration of the instrument and deemed able to communicate effectively by their primary nurse. Results of that survey indicated that 100 percent of patients interviewed had a high degree of satisfaction with nursing care.

Physician satisfaction with nursing care was measured with an instrument developed by the hospital and tested for validity and reliability (Lynn, 1989). That survey revealed that 92 percent of the physicians thought that patient care was excellent, and 57 percent were inclined to agree that the chart forms and vital sign sheets were easy to read. It showed a consensus for the need to improve the ease of use of the medical record.

Vendor and independent studies are beginning to validate the reduction of costs of operation as a result of these bedside computer systems. Since funding is the major deterrent to computerizing nursing, studies must corroborate that entering more complete, accurate, and timely patient data from the point-of-care can contribute to a more accurate revenue collection for hospitals. When that has been proven beyond a doubt, funding will be available for the computerization of nursing functions. The most comprehensive tool for measuring savings achieved by the use of bedside terminals has been developed by Ken Kahl (1990, 1991). Further research studies for the bedside computer project will be completed after all of the applications are in place.

CONCLUSION

The installation of an information system is a complex and expensive process for any hospital, thus it pays to do it right from the start. Without careful planning, commitment from top hospital administration, a sound partnership with the vendor, and involvement of the end users, the investment is jeopardized.

This summary of strategies and suggestions for implementing a bedside computer system can be utilized in any nursing care setting, in any size hospital. It is meant to be a helpful guide for others to achieve success in this challenge of the decade, by implementing nursing information systems in order to allow a new and more efficient level of quality patient care.

REFERENCES

Hinshaw, A. S., & Atwood, J. R., 1982. A patient satisfaction instrument: precision by replication. *Nursing Research, 31,* 170–175.

Kahl, K. (1990). Bedside automation. In *Proceedings of the 1990 Annual HIMSS Conference* (pp. 71–94). New Orleans, LA: American Hospital Association.

Kahl, K. (1991). Bedside automation: Measuring the savings achieved by use of bedside terminals. In *Proceedings of the 1991 Annual HIMSS Conference* (pp. 89–92). San Francisco, CA: AHA.

Knickman, J., Kovner, C., Hendrickson, G., Whittier, D., & Graf, H. (1991). *An evaluation of the New Jersey nursing incentive reimbursement award program: An interim report.* New York: Health Research Program of New York University.

Lynn, M. R. (1989). Instrument reliability and validity: How much needs to be published? *Heart & Lung, 18,* 421–423.

Slavitt, D., Stamps, P., Piedmont, E., & Haase, A. (1979). Measuring nurses' job satisfaction. *Hospital and Health Services Administration,* Summer, 62–76.

Sullivan, E., & Decker, P. J. (1988). Managing and initiating change. *Effective Management in Nursing, 2,* 98–100.

7

Integrating a Bedside Nursing Information System into a Professional Nursing Practice Model

*Emmy R. Miller**
Elizabeth A. Sheridan

Do computers improve the quality of nursing care and increase nursing productivity? Is it necessary to place computer support at the bedside to achieve those goals? We believe that the answer to both questions is a qualified "Yes." The qualification is that effective utilization of a bedside nursing information system is contingent upon a nursing care delivery system that is designed to capitalize on operational changes in the ways in which nurses deliver care to patients. At JFK Medical Center, we found that the combination of a professionally based nursing care delivery system and a bedside nursing information system resulted in an increase in the direct patient care time of registered nurses, a decrease in time spent in documentation and clerical activities, and an improvement in the quality of nursing documentation.

PROJECT BACKGROUND

A key challenge facing nurse executives today is the task of redesigning nursing services and systems so that the quality of clinical services match their cost and reimbursement systems (O'Malley, Loveridge, & Cummings, 1989). To meet this challenge, nurses in administrative and clinical positions must work together to design and implement effective nursing care delivery systems that are quality focused and consumer driven. Such systems must deal with the day-to-day operational issues of providing patient care services, utilize nursing personnel effectively and appropriately, and manage the huge volumes of clinical, administrative, and regulatory information required in today's health care environment.

One approach to improving the effectiveness of patient care delivery systems is the use of automation. On average, medical/surgical nurses spend 34 percent of their time handling information (Jydstrup & Gross, 1966). It has been suggested that the use of computers to assist in that activity has resulted in improvements in both the quality

---

* At the time this project was conducted, Dr. Miller was a consultant with Ernst & Young.

of care and nursing productivity. Yet, only 7 percent of those health care organizations with automated systems used those systems for nursing care planning, and only 4 percent documented nursing care in their systems (Summers, Ratliff, Becker, & Resler, 1989).

Despite the low utilization of automation to support nursing, nursing informatics is a reality for nurses in the 1990s. The combination of a constrained economic environment and a nursing shortage have focused attention on the potential of information systems for nursing. The Secretary's Commission on the Nursing Shortage (1988) and the Commonwealth Fund Paper (Roberts, Minnick, Ginzberg, & Curran, 1989) recommended the use of automated information systems to support nurses and help them use their time more efficiently.

In New Jersey, we have begun to address the challenge of incorporating automation into nursing care delivery systems. The Department of Health's Nursing Incentives Reimbursement Award (NIRA) Program, which sponsors innovative programs to improve nursing and patient care, enhance nurses' job satisfaction, and increase patient satisfaction granted two $500,000 awards to JFK Medical Center to implement their Four-Point Plan for Nursing (see Figure 7.1). One purpose of the Four-Point Plan is to strengthen the role of the professional nurse in both clinical and administrative decision-making. Another important purpose is to improve the working environment so as to enhance job satisfaction and nurse retention, as well as reinforce nurse commitment to quality patient care.

At JFK Medical Center, there was a commitment to innovation in professional practice accompanied by the belief that a systems approach was the most effective way to introduce the components of the Four-Point Plan. A fundamental principle of our plan was to place nurses at the bedside and keep them there! The use of automation

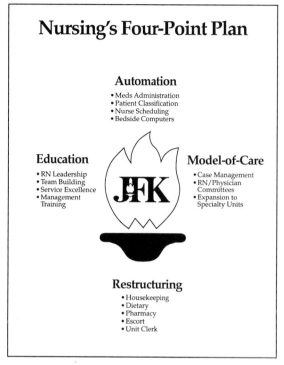

Figure 7.1 Nursing's four-point plan.

to assist with information management activities and restructuring the care delivery systems were key strategies to enact this objective. In addition, these strategies would provide the professional nurse with the authority, accountability, and autonomy to manage the care of patients.

The project described in this chapter focuses on two parts of our Four-Point Plan: The Model of Nursing Care Delivery and the Bedside Nursing Information System. Prior to implementation of our Four-Point Plan, nurses at JFK Medical Center were familiar with a number of computer-supported functions that had been provided by the hospital information system since 1987. These functions included admission, transfer, discharge, order communication and results reporting, and nursing care planning. In fact, JFK Medical Center was one of the first nursing departments in New Jersey to implement a computerized nursing system.

About JFK Medical Center

JFK Medical Center is the flagship of the JFK Health Systems, Inc., located in Edison, New Jersey. It is a 509-bed multihospital complex, composed of the Anthony M. Yelencsics Community Hospital and the Johnson Rehabilitation Institute. JFK Health Systems, Inc. is the largest health care network in New Jersey. It provides acute, rehabilitative, and outpatient/ambulatory services to the community. In addition, JFK Health Systems provides long-term care in its three not-for-profit nursing, convalescent, and rehabilitation centers.

Our award-winning Four-Point Plan for Nursing capitalizes on a number of strengths of the organization. There is a strong supportive relationship between JFK Medical Center and its corporate parent, JFK Health Systems, Inc., and this support has been critical, both in the grant application process and the implementation of the project. Equally strong has been the support from the Medical Center's Board of Trustees. Finally, the Information Systems Department has provided a great deal of assistance and encouragement on both technical and implementation issues.

DESCRIPTION OF THE PROJECT

The project was based upon the belief that successful use of a bedside nursing information system was contingent on the design of the nursing care delivery system. The availability of a bedside nursing information system moves a number of important functions away from central areas, such as the nursing station, to the point of care—the bedside.

Documentation of care activities, recording of patient data, and nursing care planning can be performed more quickly and effectively at the bedside; furthermore, the availability of patient information at the point of care can enhance clinical decision making, and quality of care can be improved (Hughes, 1988; Wiederhold & Perreault, 1990).

Some of the benefits associated with moving these clinical information management activities to the point of care include improved accuracy and quality of clinical information, increased compliance with documentation standards, more timely recording of patient data, and decreased nursing time spent in documentation (Johnson, Burkes, Sitting, Hinson, & Pryor, 1987; Halford, Pryor, & Burkes, 1987). To realize these benefits, however, nurses must change their usual patterns and routines of delivering patient care. For example, typically nurses perform the bulk of their documentation activities at the end of their shift of work. This pattern often results in poor data quality because nurses must recall and summarize the patient data to be recorded. Nurses frequently work overtime as well. The successful utilization of a bedside nursing information system requires that nurses enter their observations, care activities, and care planning information at the time care is delivered, rather than at the end of the shift.

The project described here contains two distinct but interrelated components. The first is the installation of a bedside nursing information system. The second component is the redesign of the nursing care delivery systems to accomplish three goals:

1. Establish the accountability of the registered nurse to provide direct nursing care and to manage the care of patients through collaboration, coordination, and supervision of other members of the health care team;

2. Support direct patient care through appropriate utilization of licensed practical nurses (LPNs) and nursing assistants, as well as adequate clerical and support services; and

3. Incorporate a bedside nursing information system to support nursing documentation, care planning, and the management of patient care.

These goals reflected our key assumption: that new nursing practice patterns must be designed to take advantage of the benefits of bedside automation, rather than simply adding bedside documentation to existing practices.

Approach to the Nursing Care Delivery System

The nursing care delivery system, also referred to as the model of nursing care, defines how a group of nurses organize and provide care activities for a group of patients. This system includes roles and responsibilities, nurse–patient assignment patterns, communication activities such as shift report and patient care conferences, work flows, and nursing unit routines. There are five recognized models of nursing care delivery: functional nursing, team nursing, total patient care (TPC), primary nursing, and case management. Each model has specific attributes and characteristics in a defined combination, however, in the clinical practice setting, many nursing units may incorporate characteristics from more than one model into their nursing care delivery system, with one model usually predominating (Rocchiccioli & Colley, 1989).

The predominant nursing care delivery system used prior to the initiation of this project was total patient care (TPC). Under this system, each RN and LPN was responsible for providing all aspects of direct care and documentation for a group of assigned patients. Nursing assistants provided selected aspects of physical care, such as bathing and feeding. Care activities were coordinated and directed by a charge registered nurse, who did not assume a patient assignment but was responsible for medical order processing, communicating with physicians and other health care providers, and generally coordinating the activities of the nursing unit. Clerical and computer support was provided by the nursing unit secretary (NUS).

Case management was selected as the nursing care delivery system that best met the professional practice goals of the project. This is a relatively new model of nursing care that is designed to organize patient care through an episode of illness so that specific clinical and financial outcomes are achieved within an allotted time frame (Togno-Armanasco, Olivas, & Harter, 1989). Nursing case management has also been suggested to hold promise for enhancing the professional autonomy of nurses within institutional settings (Prescott, Phillips, Ryan, & Thompson, 1991).

Case management is often superimposed on another patient care delivery system, such as primary nursing. A similar approach was used for this project. A nursing case management model was developed with two distinct levels. Level I was concerned with designing and implementing systems to ensure the delivery of professional nursing care to patients and to promote smooth operations of the nursing unit. Level II included the implementation of the nurse case manager role, development of case management plans (critical paths), and monitoring of utilization and financial data. To date, Level I has been successfully implemented, and planning for Level II is in progress. The remainder of this chapter will focus on the activities and results of Level I of the nursing case management model.

The Design Process for Nursing Case Management

We used a values-driven, participative process to design Level I of the nursing case management model. The project team was composed of nurse managers and staff nurses from the pilot nursing units, representatives from Nursing Service, and a consultant. This group was charged with developing the nursing case management model, as well as an implementation plan for the introduction of the new model on two pilot medical/surgical nursing units.

A number of educational and team-building sessions were conducted for the project team. This group also reviewed the current operations and nursing care delivery systems of the pilot nursing units. The purpose of these activities was to define a shared philosophy and vision of nursing practice, as well as establish a foundation for the design of the case management model. The result of these sessions was a philosophy statement that was used to guide model design activities.

With a philosophy statement to guide the thinking of the project team, the following steps were accomplished:

1. Specific roles were designated within the model, including the professional registered nurse (RN), the licensed practical nurse (LPN), the nursing assistant, and the nursing unit secretary (NUS).

2. The scope and responsibilities of the charge nurse role were substantially reduced and renamed "shift coordinator"; furthermore, this role was no longer exempt from a patient care assignment. The reduced scope of the shift coordinator role made it possible for an RN acting as a clinical leader to assume these responsibilities.

3. Major responsibility for professional nursing care and supervision of other nursing staff was located in a new RN role, the clinical leader, who assumed responsibility for a group of patients for one shift; continuity of patient care was maintained by consistent assignment of the Clinical Leaders.

4. Nurse–patient assignments were organized to use staff members most effectively, yet provide professional nursing (i.e., RN) supervision and coordination of care.

5. Shift report was organized to expedite clinical information exchange and to minimize redundant reporting and copying of information.

6. Unit work-flow expectations were delineated on a shift-by-shift basis.

The documentation resulting from these activities constituted Level I of the nursing case management model and provided a basis for planning its implementation.

An important consideration in each of these steps was the incorporation of the bedside nursing information system. The new model included a number of operational guidelines that reflected specific modifications in practice patterns or routines to utilize the bedside nursing information system effectively. These operational guidelines addressed such issues as the need to document care activities as they were performed instead of at the end of the shift, establishment of specific times for documentation of care activities such as patient assessment, and changing nurses' perceptions of care planning from a "paper work" activity to a dynamic process for managing and coordinating patient care.

Implementation of the New Patient Care Delivery System

The implementation of the new patient care delivery system occurred in two phases.

In the first phase, we instituted the new model of nursing care delivery without the support of the bedside nursing information system. This phase lasted two months, and it enabled the nursing staff to adopt the operational components of the new delivery system without the additional stress of the bedside nursing information system. In the second phase, the addition of the bedside nursing information system actually facilitated the functioning of the new patient care delivery systems.

Strategies for implementation of the new nursing care delivery system (Phase I) included the following activities:

- team building and role clarification sessions for all nursing staff members on the pilot units, emphasizing teamwork, collaboration, and the value of each role in the model;

- preparation of written guidelines and operational routines for the new nursing care delivery system;

- educational sessions addressing professional practice issues, physical assessment, nursing diagnoses, nursing care planning, and specialty care issues pertinent to the unit's patient population; and

- identification of key staff members on the pilot units to serve as resource personnel during the implementation process.

Using these strategies resulted in the successful implementation of the new nursing care delivery system. We then turned our attention to the installation of the bedside nursing information system.

Addition of the Bedside Nursing Information System

Activities such as cabling and installation of the bedside hardware occurred during the implementation of the new nursing care delivery system. In addition, training sessions for the nursing staff commenced after the new patient care delivery system had been in place for one month. At this point, we were concerned that the bedside nursing information system installation would distract staff from the new nursing care delivery system, and that they would revert to old practice patterns and routines. Establishing the new patient care delivery system was a more abstract undertaking than the more concrete system installation, which offered tangible, immediate requirements and rewards.

During the staff training and actual system implementation, system issues did require the majority of time and attention of both the project team members and the pilot units' nursing staff. Despite this shift in focus, the new nursing care delivery system continued to operate smoothly. The operational guidelines were followed, and responsibilities specifically concerned with documentation and patient assessment were highlighted during system implementation. As one staff nurse said, "The model is really easier, now that we have the computer!" This smooth transition was due to considerable efforts by the project team members to monitor staff performance, reinforce new behaviors, and address problems promptly.

RESULTS OF THE PROJECT

We conducted a study of our new patient care delivery system and bedside nursing information system. The project was implemented on two pilot nursing units (4 South and 4 West), while two similar medical/surgical units (3 West and 3 Central) were used as control units, thus we used a nonequivalent control group design. The full results of this study will be published elsewhere; however, we will present some of our experiences here.

The results of our project indicated that the purported benefits of a bedside nursing information system can be obtained when the bedside system is part of an effective patient care delivery system. When we examined the nursing staff's perception of their nursing care delivery system using an instrument designed for that purpose (Miller, 1989), we found that the nursing staff on the pilot nursing units had made substantial changes. The pilot units showed a definite shift away from their baseline model, total patient care; furthermore, these nursing units indicated that aspects from primary/case management and team nursing were predominant in their nursing care delivery system. These changes were consistent with the goals of the new nursing care delivery system of expanded accountability for

RNs and enhanced teamwork among all nursing staff.

In addition, the time nurses spent in various activities was measured using the standard industrial engineering technique of work sampling. Results from the work sampling data prior to project implementation revealed that nurses on the pilot and control units spent between 33 percent to 37 percent of their time in direct nursing care. Nursing staff using the new model on the two pilot units were spending 40 percent and 42 percent, respectively, in direct patient care, representing increases of 6% and 9% per nursing unit (see Figure 7.2). The percentages of time spent in direct and indirect care did not vary at all for one control unit (3 West), and *slight variation* was seen for the other (3 Central). These findings indicate that increased time

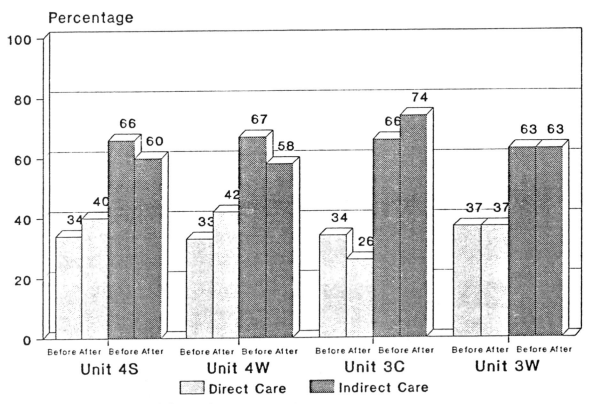

Figure 7.2 Comparison of observed nursing care time.

for direct patient care can be attributed to the changes introduced with the project described here.

The types of activities that occupied nurses' time also changed. Prior to this project, indirect care activities and nonproductivity occupied the majority of nursing staff's time. For RNs, clerical activities and computer order entry were very time consuming. After implementation of the model, computer order entry and clerical activities were no longer predominant indirect care activities for RNs. These indirect care activities were replaced by professional activities, conferring with and supervising nursing staff and performing direct care activities such as treatment, medication administration, communication, teaching, and support activities.

The time spent in documentation was also examined through work sampling. Our baseline work sampling data revealed that prior to implementation of the model registered nurses and LPNs spent, on average, over 80 minutes per shift in documentation activities. After implementation, RNs on the pilot units decreased documentation time by more than 20 minutes per registered nurse. An even larger decrease was seen among the licensed practical nurses group, with charting time decreasing by 36 and 44 minutes on the two pilot units.

In addition, an audit tool was used to examine the quality of nursing documentation. This audit tool consisted of 18 items, designed by the project team, to examine the flow of information in the patient record, based upon the steps of the nursing process. The baseline audit of documentation quality showed that compliance with the 18 indicators averaged 38 percent and 45 percent on the two control units, while the pilot units were slightly higher at 50 percent and 52 percent. After the implementation of the new nursing care delivery system and the bedside nursing information system, the quality of their documentation improved. Compliance with the documentation audit criteria in-

creased by 25 percent and 27 percent respectively on the two pilot units, while the control units' compliance remained stable.

CONCLUSION

A number of benefits of bedside information systems have been proposed, including decreased charting time, improved quality of documentation, and more time spent in direct patient care by the nursing staff. A number of studies of bedside system implementation, however, have failed to demonstrate such results. For example, Bradshaw, Sitting, Gardner, Pryor, & Budd (1988) found an increase in charting time and a decrease in direct patient care time in their study of a bedside system in an intensive care unit.

Our results indicate that obtaining the benefits of a bedside information system can be accomplished. Often, the implementation of a bedside nursing information system is viewed only as a means to decrease the time nurses spend in certain activities, with minimal attention paid to the issues of quality of care and larger operational concerns. This project is unique in that the focus was not on time savings, per se, but rather on how nurses' time could best be used. We believe that the success of our project was due to the successful integration of a bedside nursing information system into a nursing care delivery system that supports professional nursing practice, increases the time that nurses spend with patients, and enhances the quality of information in the patient record.

REFERENCES

Bradshaw, K. E., Sitting, D. F., Gardner, R. M., Pryor, T. A., & Budd, M. (1988). Improving efficiency and quality in a computerized ICU. In *Proceedings of the Twelfth*

Annual Symposium on Computer Applications in Medical Care, (pp. 763–767). Washington, DC: IEEE Computer Society Press.

Halford, G., Pryor, T. A., & Burkes, M. (1987). Measuring the impact of bedside systems. In *Proceedings of the Eleventh Annual Symposium on Computer Applications in Medical Care*, (pp. 359–362). Washington, DC: IEEE Computer Society Press.

Hughes, S. (1988). Bedside information systems: State of the art. In M. J. Ball, K. J. Hannah, U. G. Jelger, & H. Peterson (Eds.), *Nursing Informatics: Where caring and technology meet* (pp. 138–145). New York: Springer-Verlag.

Johnson, D. S., Burkes, M., Sitting, D., Hinson, D., & Pryor, T. A. (1987). Evaluation of the effects of computerized nurse charting. In *Proceedings of the Eleventh Annual Symposium on Computer Applications in Medical Care*, (pp. 363–366). Washington, DC: IEEE Computer Society Press.

Jydstrup, R. A., & Gross, M. J. (1966). Cost of information handling in hospitals. *Health Services Research, 1*(3), 235–245.

Miller, E. R. (1989). *Classifying nursing care delivery systems used on nursing units: The Model Assessment Tool (MAT)*. Unpublished manuscript.

O'Malley, J., Loveridge, C. E., & Cummings, S. H. (1989). The new nursing organization. *Nursing Management, 20*(2), 29–32.

Prescott, P. A., Phillips, C. Y., Ryan, J. W., & Thompson, K. O. (1991). Changing how nurses spend their time. *IMAGE: The Journal of Nursing Scholarship, 23*(1), 23–28.

Ricchiccioli, J., & Colley, B. (1989). Models of nursing practice: The basis of diagnosis-based nursing practice. In E. R. Miller (Ed.), *How to make nursing diagnosis work: Administrative and clinical strategies* (pp. 119–138). Norwalk: Appleton & Lange.

Roberts, M., Minnick, A., Ginzberg, E., & Curran, C. (1989). *A commonwealth fund paper: What to do about the nursing shortage*. New York: Commonwealth Fund.

Summers, S., Ratliff, C., Becker, A., & Resler, M. (1989). Computerized nursing diagnosis and documentation of nursing care in inpatient health care agencies. In R. M. Carroll-Johnson (Ed.), *Classification of Nursing Diagnoses: Proceedings of the Eighth National Conference* (pp. 270–274). Philadelphia: J. B. Lippincott.

Togno-Armanasco, V. D., Olivas, G., & Harter, S. (1989). Developing an integrated nursing case management model. *Nursing Management, 20*(10), 26–29.

U.S. Department of Health and Human Services. (1988). *Secretary's Commission of Nursing* (Final Report, Vol. I). Washington, DC.

Wiederhold, G., & Perreault, L. E. (1990). Hospital information systems. In E. H. Shortliffe & L. E. Perreault (Eds.), *Medical informatics: Computer applications in health care* (pp. 219–243). Reading, MA: Addison-Wesley.

8

The Development of a Nursing Information System in Collaboration with Two Vendors

Kathleen Tiedeken
Sharon J. Majarowitz
Edward E. Duryee

BACKGROUND

Memorial Hospital of Burlington County (MHBC), part of the Memorial Health Alliance, is a 402-bed nonprofit community hospital located in Mt. Holly, New Jersey. The hospital offers a full range of medical services and is affiliated with tertiary centers for additional specialized care. The corporate organization includes a nursing home, visiting nursing service, and a foundation.

The medical staff is relatively young and loyal to the institution. There is a family practice residency program affiliated with the University of Medicine and Dentistry/New Jersey Medical School in New Jersey. Medical staff leadership is provided by appointed, voluntary chiefs of departments and elected, voluntary officers. Collaboration between the physicians and the nursing staff has always been excellent, with each appreciating the skills of the other.

The nursing department practices a modified team nursing delivery system which utilizes four levels of caregivers: courier,

nursing assistant, licensed practical nurse (LPN) and registered nurse (RN). Since 1983, the HBO & Company* hospital information system, has been used at the nursing stations for order entry, reporting results from radiology and laboratory, and for some interface with the pharmacy.

IMPACT OF NURSING SHORTAGE ON NEW JERSEY AND MHBC

In 1989 New Jersey experienced a high vacancy rate especially for RNs in hospital-based practice; the vacancy rate sometimes approached 18 percent. Many nurses left hospitals to work in temporary staffing agencies which offered high pay and maximum flexibility. Additionally nearby states offered much higher salaries and better benefits packages. MHBC competed with about 15 hospitals within a 20-mile radius in New

---

* HBO & Company should not be confused with the cable television company of the same name.

Jersey alone, as well as with many Philadelphia hospitals. To further compound recruitment efforts, the supply of nurses had dwindled due to low student enrollment in nursing programs.

In 1988 the nursing department had developed a business plan which targeted many areas that needed to change in order to recruit and retain qualified staff. These included flexible hours including the 24/40 weekend option, the three-day work week of 12 hour shifts or 36/40, and later in 1990, a four-day work week of nine-hour shifts in the surgery department. Other endeavors included scholarships for students enrolled in nursing programs or other allied health fields, increased tuition reimbursement, a creation of our own internal pool (Mega Pool) dedicated to offering salaries competitive with agencies, and contracting with only a few agencies to offer care when needed under our requirements. In addition to this, in a rather bold move, salaries were significantly increased for certain shifts and certain units within the medical/surgical and critical divisions that had sustained high vacancy levels. These actions resulted in a drop in RN vacancy rate that went from a high of 18 percent in 1988 to a vacancy rate of approximately 7 percent in 1989. This enabled the nursing organization to be in a stable position to accept the challenge of competing for a research grant.

ENACTMENT OF NURSING INCENTIVE REIMBURSEMENT AWARD PROGRAM

The New Jersey State Department of Health, in response to concerns by many constituencies within the state, reconstituted the Nursing Advisory Committee to the Commissioner of Health. It was this group which recommended the Nursing Incentive Reimbursement Award (NIRA) Program. The main objective of the NIRA grant was to recruit and retain professional nursing staff. Since MHBC had already included the use of bedside computers in their five-year plan, we had already started to explore some products in the industry. This preparation and the existing position of a nursing informatic specialist encouraged MHBC to submit a grant based on bedside technology. This person then also became the Project Coordinator.

The focus of the MHBC grant was to integrate, within the first year, a bedside nursing system with the existing hospital information system on two nursing units. The grant specified the need for design and consultation with vendors as well as development of a program at Burlington County College to provide a learning experience for nursing students to use computers in nursing before graduation. The same hardware and software used by the nurses at MHBC were donated to the college for this purpose. A video was produced showing the changing role of nurses. A collaborative joint practice model was also established with the college.

MHBC received a grant of $500,000 for 1990 and an additional $500,000 for 1991. In 1991 development of the nursing package and consultations with two vendors continued. The plan to implement two additional units before the end of 1991 included a request from the interested nursing units to be the next site for computerization.

SELECTION AND IMPLEMENTATION

Objective When Selecting a Vendor

The most critical factor identified by the institution was the selection of a vendor whose system was compatible with HBO & Company's hospital information system. A multidisciplinary group reviewed several bedside systems before selecting the Clini-Care Point-of-Care System from CliniCom, Inc. in Boulder, Colorado. HBO and Clini-Com had already worked together at an alpha site. MHBC became the beta site for the documentation research, and the alpha site for the two-way interface. The system also should be user friendly and dynamic; we wanted a system that would not only be functional but would offer other capabilities such as critical care documentation. The system featured a hand-held device that could do bar coding of medications, and also had the potential for use by other disciplines and services. HBO & Company, which was already familiar to the information system staff, agreed to be our primary vendor and to accomplish mutual goals and conduct collaborative research. The financial viability of both vendors and the hospital was of paramount importance. The market share for each vendor, as well as their growth potential, was reviewed by the vice president for information services before verifying that this was a viable direction for the hospital. The money from the grant would only cover part of the amount needed for design, research, and education.

DESCRIPTION OF VENDORS

HBO & Company is one of the top four vendors supplying computerized systems to hospitals. Founded in 1974, revenue for 1990 was $201.5 million, placing the company in the top 100 of all computer companies in all sectors in North America. HBO has corporate headquarters in Atlanta, Georgia.

CliniCom Incorporated® is a relatively small and recent (formed in 1985) entry into the health-care systems field. Nonetheless, it has carved out a niche in the bedside terminal field and as of mid 1991 had approximately 12 installations. Headquartered in Boulder, Colorado the company is privately held and employs approximately 50 staff. The company markets one basic product although there are different hardware configurations and software modules available. In the future, the product will develop from a "nursing system" into one that is geared to all health-care disciplines.

Description of System

Currently, MHBC has the following HBO systems installed: CLINSTAR®-Patient Care, Laboratory, Radiology, Pharmacy, IFAS financials (general accounting, patient accounting, and medical records abstracting), and TRENDSTAR® decision support. From the nursing station the following functions are available: order entry, revise patient data, physician access, scheduling, census, messaging, pharmacy (including access to patient's profile) and laboratory/radiology result inquiry.

Hardware Description. Each nursing station has two Data General (DG) terminals that allow access to the HBO system, with a third terminal (Universal Terminal) recently added; the universal terminal is a 286 PC IBM compatible, with color monitor emulating a DG terminal and eventually will also be able to access the CliniCom system. Each nursing station also has a dot-matrix printer to print lab results, pharmacy profiles, census, and so forth. The terminals are tied to the computer processing unit (CPU) (Data General MV 40000) in the computer room via a broadband Local Area Network (LAN).

Each patient room of the two pilot units has a CliniView terminal mounted at eye level at the rear of the room. The liquid crystal display is 9 inches by 6 inches and touch-sensitive for data entry. When data is retrieved, the user has the option of graphics or tabular form. A battery-powered hand-held unit is mounted next to the CliniView. The hand-held unit is ergonomically designed to facilitate easy use by the nurse at the patient's bedside; when removed from the wall it communicates with the Cliniview via radio frequency. The unit contains a liquid crystal display, bar-code reader, numeric keypad and function keys. The CliniView and hand-held unit are manufactured by CliniCom. Much of the system processing oc-curs on the CliniView as opposed to processing on the CliniCom CPU (file server); each CliniView contains a 8088 microprocessor. Each of the two pilot units also has a desktop terminal (286 PC with emulation software) to access the CliniCom system. The desk-top terminal is used for functions that are more easily performed with a standard keyboard or for requesting printed output. A laser printer (Texas Instruments) is also located on each nursing unit for printing CliniCom chart forms and bar codes for patients and nursing staff. Each device on the nursing

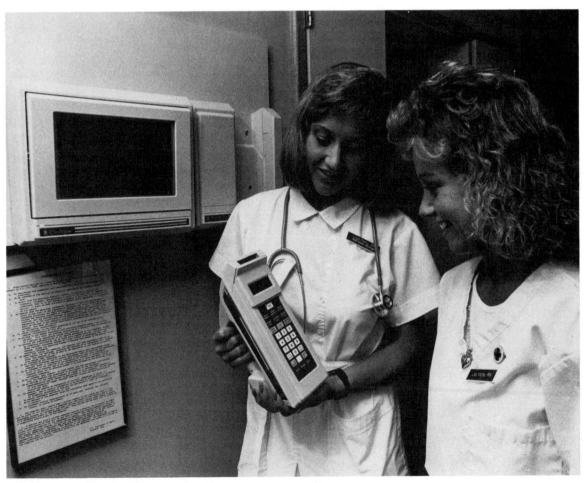

Figure 8.1 Educating nurses to use the CliniCom system.

unit is attached to a file server (manufactured by Sequent, Inc.) located in the computer room. The pharmacy contains a packaging machine which packages unit dose medications and places bar-codes on each package.

Software Description. A key concept of the system was to take information already contained in the HBO system and send it to CliniCom. This real-time, on-line, one-way interface was part of the initial installation and consists of the following: (1) ADT—when a patient is admitted, discharged, or transferred (ADT) on the HBO system, the data immediately interfaces with CliniCom; (2) Security Codes—when an employee changes his or her code on HBO it also changes on CliniCom, new employees are added to HBO and the interface adds them to CliniCom; (3) laboratory/radiology results—when tests are resulted on HBO they are sent to CliniCom and stored for four days for physician/nursing inquiry; (4) Master files—various master files are updated on CliniCom via the interface.

Pharmacy orders are also interfaced from HBO to CliniCom. Every medication order for the patient is entered by a pharmacist and generates an administration schedule on the CliniCom system; the nurse knows the proper administration time via a printed worklist. The system warns if the five "rights" are not met: right patient (by requiring the correct patient's bar-code to be read), right medication, right route and right amount (by requiring the bar-code on the medication to be read, this compares the drug to the pharmacist's order), and right time (by the system checking to see if the time is within a hospital-defined time frame).

Vital signs and fluid balance are entered into the hand-held unit directly at the patient's bedside. The system prompts the nurse for any predetermined descriptors (e.g., for site of temperature measurement) and warns if data entered is outside of unit-defined normal ranges. Once entered, this data is available for inquiry on the CliniView screen, hard-copy printouts, and the HBO system. MHBC was the alpha development site for interfacing this data from CliniCom to HBO and had input into the design. A key element of the success of this piece of the interface was to allow a group of physicians to see a prototype of the software in a test system prior to installation into the live system.

A recent addition to the system was the installation of nursing documentation, including admission history and assessment, ongoing assessment, care planning, and charting against the care plans. The care plans are based on the NANDA standards and, to date, incorporate the top 30 nursing diagnoses, with more to be added. This module has been well-received by the nursing staff, and a side benefit is that patients see the nurse in the room more often.

COORDINATION OF THE NIRA PROJECT

The grant was organized through the coordination of an interdisciplinary steering committee that served as the parent committee with several task forces reporting to it. The vice presidents for patient services and for information services cochaired the steering committee.

There were five task forces that the grant steering committee coordinated to accomplish the goals of the program. These task forces included: Joint Practice; Video—The Changing Role of the Nurse; Care Planning and Documentation; CliniCom Implementation; and Quality Assurance/Evaluation/Monitoring.

Joint Practice

MHBC is a clinical rotation site for a number of nursing programs. These include a baccalareate nursing program of Rutgers, The State University, two associate degree programs from area colleges, and LPN program from the vocational-technical school. Burlington County College (BCC), which offers a two-year associate degree program, is the nearest school and many of their graduates join the staff of MHBC. BCC students rotate through all clinical areas. In addition, LPNs and nursing assistants from Memorial continue their education to become RNs at BCC. The vice president for patient services is a member of the nursing advisory committee for the College and the president of BCC is on the board of directors of Memorial Health Alliance. A nursing educator from MHBC is on the curriculum committee at the college while two faculty members joined the CliniCom committees.

In addition, a faculty member of the College with the assistant vice president for maternal child health developed an intensive arts option, as an elective, that was designed to "develop" clinical judgment skills of the student. The students who were selected to participate indicated their area of interest and desired shift. Nurses with one to three years experience were selected to mentor these students. The students worked the same schedule as their mentor. Areas selected were as diverse as 12-hour shifts in the intensive care unit to 8-hour shifts in the labor and delivery unit. Students learned clinical judgment skills and gained exposure to a clinical area in which he or she previously had limited experience.

The students, as well as the mentors, found this to be an excellent program. The potential for this type of program is limited only by limited imaginations. Expansion of this option to nonacute care settings and community programs would expose students to additional opportunities in health care.

Video—The Changing Role of the Nurse

The role of the nurse has changed dramatically over the past 40 years but the public's perception of the nurses' role and responsibilities has not kept pace. MHBC sincerely believes that education of the public is essential if nurses are to be viewed as individuals who are decision makers and not as hand maidens to physicians. The video committee, chaired by an assistant vice president for nursing, included members of the community. The video "More Than Caring" was produced featuring staff nurses at MHBC. This video is shown daily on the hospital patient education channels and there are plans for MHBC to use it as a recruitment tool as well as a public relations film for the community.

Care Planning and Documentation

This committee is cochaired by an assistant vice president, clinical nurse specialist, and the project coordinator. This committee is responsible for reviewing screens for care planning and documentation provided by CliniCom. This committee has representation from the pilot units as well as nonpilot units representing all divisions and shifts. A consultant from the North American Nursing Diagnosis Association (NANDA) worked with the committee reviewing the use of nursing diagnosis.

CliniCom provides a very thorough nursing documentation package. Screens are customized to meet practices at MHBC. Screens are changed through a process called "screen builders." Five employees, three from nursing and two from information systems, traveled to CliniCom headquarters and attended an intensive four-day screen builder class. Although one person from information systems is involved with screen changes, it is very important that the remainder of the group completely understand the process.

This has allowed MHBC to develop additional screens.

The full documentation committee met every two to three weeks for approximately three months for all-day working sessions. In addition to reviewing and editing the changes, policies and procedures were developed for the use of CliniCom for documentation. This was an excellent opportunity to reassess the manual documentation system.

Development of an automated care plan based on a nursing diagnosis and charting against the care plan was implemented early in May 1991 and charting of ongoing assessment in June 1991. The nursing staff on the pilot unit where care planning was implemented has been very enthusiastic. The staff soon realized that unnecessary written documentation was significantly reduced while pertinent data were captured. Manual charting will be reduced even further when additional modules of CliniCom are implemented.

CliniCom Implementation

The CliniCom Implementation Committee was the nucleus for installing bedside computerization at MHBC. This was a multidisciplinary group that included a core group of nursing, pharmacy, and information systems personnel who would use the CliniCom system on a daily basis. The core group included four nurses from the pilot units and staff representatives from each division of nursing. Staff nurses were selected to represent all shifts and divisions, so that in the future when implementing the system hospital wide the policies and procedures would not have to be drastically altered. The committee was cochaired by the director of financial/clinical systems and the project coordinator.

Time Frame/Process. The CliniCom Implementation Committee was organized in January 1990 (see Figure 8.2). An overall view of responsibilities and expectations were presented to the group. In late February, 10 of the 18 members traveled to CliniCom headquarters for a four-day intensive education and training session on building and using the system. For the next two months the CliniCom account manager met with the full committee every two to three weeks for one- or two-day-long sessions. At these sessions the committee determined how CliniCom would be used at MHBC, the flow of information on the screen, and the parameters of vital signs for each nursing unit. Forms were designed that included permanent chart documents and work sheets. Print times were established for each unit. Policies and procedures were developed by the staff outside the committee. At the end of May 1990, the committee attended a "Train the Trainer" session in preparation for teaching.

IMPLEMENTATION AND GETTING READY TO "GO LIVE"

The trainers consisted of the experienced users who were members of the CliniCom Implementation Committee. Since this system would be used by staff nurses, the trainers needed to be experts. Many of these were nurses who had no formal teaching experience and were surprised to realize they really enjoyed teaching (Figure 8.1). Others used their expertise as support during "Go Live." The target group to be trained was not only the staff on the pilot units but the in-house per diem pool members and agency nurses who were assigned to those units. Trainers were provided with a lesson plan as well as a step-by-step instruction guide developed at MHBC. At the end of class, a check-off sheet was signed by the trainer and each trainee that indicated the material that was covered during the session. Class size

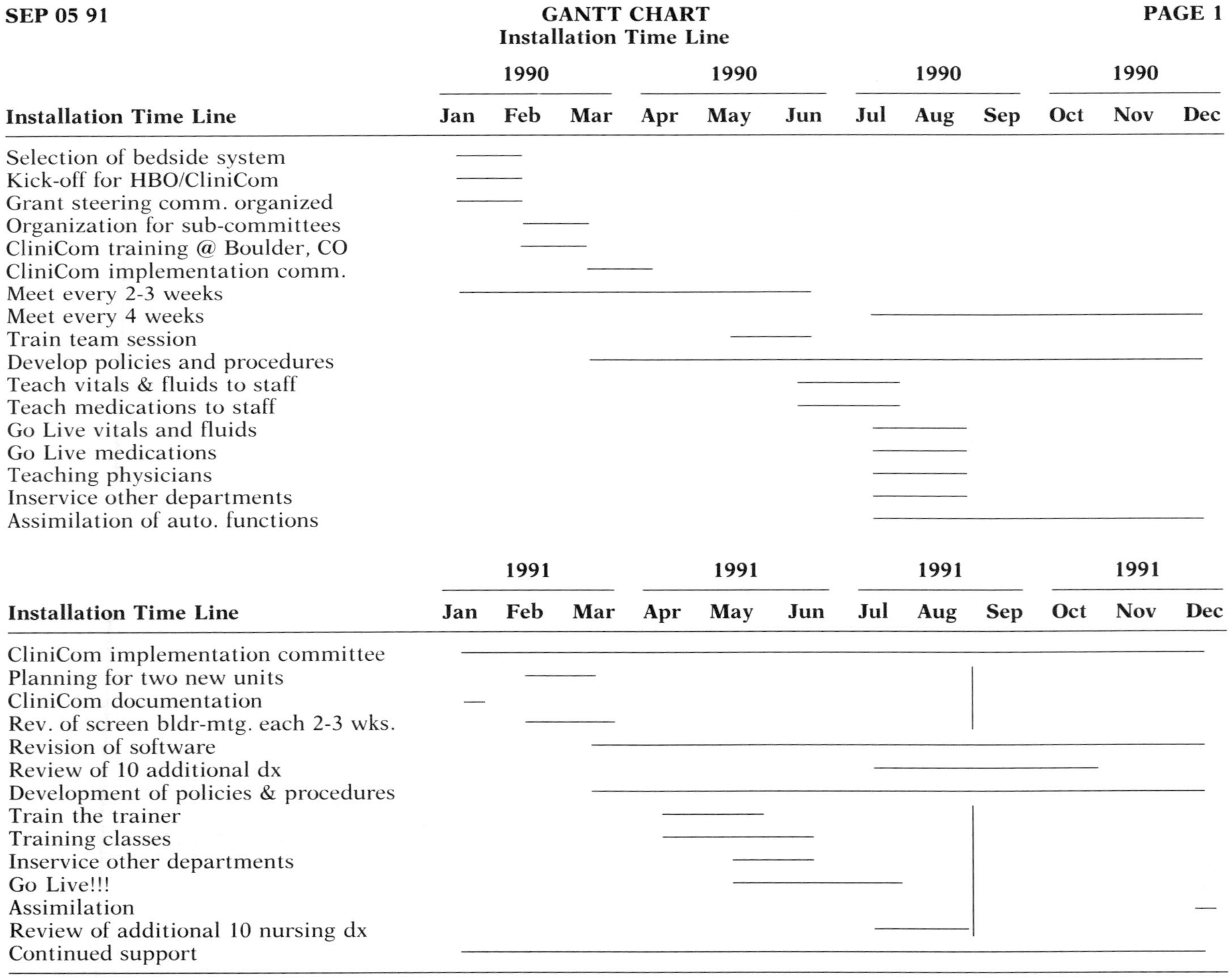

GANTT CHART
Installation Time Line

Installation Time Line	Jan	Feb	Mar	Apr	May	Jun	Jul	Aug	Sep	Oct	Nov	Dec
	1990				1990			1990			1990	

Selection of bedside system
Kick-off for HBO/CliniCom
Grant steering comm. organized
Organization for sub-committees
CliniCom training @ Boulder, CO
CliniCom implementation comm.
Meet every 2-3 weeks
Meet every 4 weeks
Train team session
Develop policies and procedures
Teach vitals & fluids to staff
Teach medications to staff
Go Live vitals and fluids
Go Live medications
Teaching physicians
Inservice other departments
Assimilation of auto. functions

Installation Time Line	Jan	Feb	Mar	Apr	May	Jun	Jul	Aug	Sep	Oct	Nov	Dec
	1991				1991			1991			1991	

CliniCom implementation committee
Planning for two new units
CliniCom documentation
Rev. of screen bldr-mtg. each 2-3 wks.
Revision of software
Review of 10 additional dx
Development of policies & procedures
Train the trainer
Training classes
Inservice other departments
Go Live!!!
Assimilation
Review of additional 10 nursing dx
Continued support

Figure 8.2 GANTT Chart.

was limited to six people. This meant one device per two students, and allowed hands-on opportunity during the training sessions. This also allowed more interaction between the trainers and the trainee and time for discussion. The small nursing computer training room which was used for teaching HBO functions to all nursing employees was reconfigured to add three CliniView devices and one desktop personal computer. The last piece of equipment is mainly used for requesting printed information. Classes were divided into two phases. One phase introduced the use of CliniCom, and taught vital signs and fluid balances, and printing functions. The second phase taught medication administration. Permeated through these three-hour classes were policies and procedures developed at MHBC.

CliniCom devices were available on the nursing units with fictitious patients. This allowed the staff to return to the pilot units and practice what they had learned in class. The nurses needed to reach a comfort level just to pick up the hand-held unit and replace it, as well as to learn how to use the bar code reader. Learning how to touch the screen to select the desired item was a new technique. Many staff members found it easier to touch the screen with the blunt end of a pen rather than their finger for greater accuracy.

During "Go Live," on-site support was provided by CliniCom. In addition, members of the CliniCom Implementation Committee who were the expert users paired up with a CliniCom representative to assist the staff with using the new technology. It was an opportunity for our in-house trainers to reinforce policies and procedures while assisting the staff. This was a time for CliniCom to teach more advanced trouble shooting techniques. In addition, change-of-shift meetings were conducted with nursing, pharmacy and information systems to resolve problems.

Trouble Shooting

When the formal support ended, a schedule was developed indicating the availability of the in-house trouble shooters. Having members of the committee from different shifts and different units really was essential. This schedule was on each of the pilot units, the computer room, information systems, as well as the nursing resource office and continued for about four months.

Trouble shooting ranged from answering questions such as, "how do you change this entry?" to fixing paper jams in the printer. If the trouble shooters were unable to handle the situation, they contacted the project coordinator or the senior systems analyst. On off-shifts or weekends, CliniCom was contacted for assistance. All calls for CliniCom and HBO problems were funneled through the information systems staff to identify recurrent problems.

Communication with pharmacy has been paramount to implementation. Since pharmacy now entered schedules that had impact for medication administration there had to be complete agreement between nursing and pharmacy. Because of the many meetings that occurred between these departments there is a greater appreciation of each other's role. A 24-hour pharmacy coverage enhanced the installation.

The hardware support staff of information systems have become expert in maintaining the hardware both in the computer room and on the nursing units. They have devised a schedule for ongoing preventive maintenance of the equipment.

Security

CliniCom can only be accessed for secured information by the use of a bar code and an identification number through the hand-

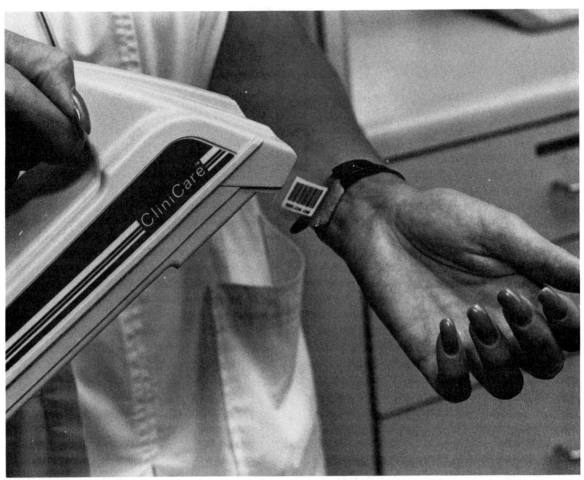

Figure 8.3 Reading a bar code with the CliniCom hand-held unit.

held unit or by an identification number and a secret code on the CliniView or desktop (Fig. 8.3). This is an electronic signature. Each employee who accesses the system completes and signs an employee data form and a user agreement form usually during training. The user agreement form indicates that the employee may not share his or her identification, bar code, or secret code with anyone. If this occurs, the person will be disciplined and possibly terminated.

Information from the data sheet is entered into the employee file on HBO which generates an identification number. This information is sent to CliniCom. A bar code can then be printed for the employee. Each person develops his or her own secret code. This secret code must be updated every 30 days and can be changed on HBO at any time.

SURVIVING INNOVATIONS

Obtaining and Retaining Administrative Support

Support starts at the planning phase, when time commitment, the information systems priority, the need for consultants, education needs, and a financial monitoring system are considered. The effect on the hospital goals, as well as particular areas within the hospital such as nursing, pharmacy, medical records, and the physicians and patients, should not be underestimated. The VP for patient services was able to coordinate the hospital goals with the computerization goals of the nursing department to produce better patient care as well as retention of qualified staff as a recruitment tool.

The goals of the bedside system were to extend professional productivity, increase quality and quantity of patient time with the nurse, decrease hall traffic time, improve documentation, decrease medication errors, decrease intershift report time, decrease legal risks, and decrease lost patient charges. The system needed to be able to accept future requirements and developments, have a positive impact on employee and patient satisfaction, have an impact on staff requirements, and to provide a competitive edge. Constant communication and reports were necessary to keep the momentum from waning when other projects competed for priority.

CLINICOM IMPACT

Nursing Staff and Physicians

CliniCom was viewed as a nursing system when it was selected to interface with HBO. Although physicians were involved from the beginning it was not until CliniCom was installed and functioning that physicians recognized the impact to their practice. They had to read an automated medication administration record (MAR) that was very different from the manual medication kardex. No longer could they glance at a kardex to determine if a medication had been administered but had to read the legend on the MAR.

Vital signs and fluid balance records that previously hung on a clip board at the bottom of each patient's bed now could be accessed on CliniCom in the room. In order to access CliniCom, physicians had to sign in the same way as they signed onto HBO with security. After many conferences with physicians, CliniCom developed a quick log-on function. Any unsecured data, vital signs, and fluid balances can be viewed by touching quick-view on the screen and selecting the desired patient vital signs or fluid balances. It shows either the last 48 hours or is date specific; either a graph or a tabular presentation is available. What is available with quick-view is definable by each hospital.

Originally the scale on the vital signs graph was too wide so small changes were difficult to detect on the screen. CliniCom developed a method that allowed the individual hospital to determine the eight intervals on the graph. Another example of vendor response was changing the order in which laboratory and pharmacy data displayed. A small pocket-sized card was developed with instructions for accessing both HBO and CliniCom to assist the physician.

The printed graph sheets presented the first set of vital signs taken in four-hour blocks. The complete information was in a tabular format. Physicians preferred a graphical display of the complete information. CliniCom worked with the physicians to design a new form that reflected the complete information.

Nursing also had a list of changes and enhancements that they wanted to see in the system. Easier and quicker access was a very high priority. The updated version met this requirement. Being able to enter the reason a medication was not given from the hand-held unit rather than at the desk top was another high priority. This became available in May 1991. A newsletter, "Communique for

CliniCom," was developed to communicate correct and consistent information for these updates.

Other Departments

Other departments within the hospital were given a review and demonstration of the printouts that would be a part of the patient's chart. Certain disciplines such as dietitians and discharge planners were given access to CliniCom to review information that was pertinent to their work. Dietitians now have access to CliniCom to enter a patient's weight during consult.

WORKING WITH TWO VENDORS

MHBC has committed itself to achieving maximum benefit from the HBO and Clini-Com systems and from both vendors. However, the companies are quite different in many aspects which occasionally impedes smooth progress. The vendors' "corporate cultures" are different due to their sizes, marketplace orientation, and even the geographic location of their headquarters. A simple tactic to resolve differences was to schedule face-to-face meetings between the two vendors and the hospital. Although this is a simple concept, geographic distances can make it difficult to achieve. The meetings provided a forum to iron out concepts such as: should care planning occur in the patient's room or at the nursing station. It was finally agreed that the entry and inquiry of Activities of Daily Living (ADLs) needed to be on both systems; although this entailed much programming effort for the vendors they agreed to perform this. The ideal scenario would be for each system to store, receive, and display the other system's data. However, the era of "open" systems is in the

future not the present, so in the meantime, clients must be satisfied with the interface of specific data elements in specific formats.

Although HBO and CliniCom run on different hardware/software platforms (HBO on Data General MV series with proprietary maximumps operating system and CliniCom on Sequent with Unix operating system) the vendors have done an admirable job in interfacing data. Problems also had to be overcome in the area of data communications; HBO terminals run on a broad-band Local Area Network (LAN), while the CliniCom terminals require an Ethernet Network. The hospital was able to use its existing LAN cabling (backbone) for the CliniCom terminals by installing converters at the file server and nursing station ends.

In summary, the steps to ensure success with multiple vendors are: face-to-face meetings; not allowing one vendor to say "the other vendor said . . ."; documenting and receiving sign-off of all significant agreements; communicating ongoing system enhancements to hospital staff; and vendors responsibility for co-coordinating third-party suppliers (such as printers). The hospital strengthened its relationships with the vendors, the user groups, and with the clients during the implementation; thereby ensuring on-going system development.

As we have begun care planning and charting against the care plan we recognize that greater collaboration with other departments can be enhanced with the charting and planning functions. This ultimately will positively affect patient care.

EXTERNAL EVALUATION

The State of New Jersey selected Health Research Program of New York University for an outside evaluation component of the NIRA Program. NYU was charged with comparing results from various projects to determine which had greater impact for recruitment and retention—the reason for the dissemination of NIRA grants.

NYU provided an interim report in February 1991. Their scheduled final report will be published in June 1992. Since many of the projects that have been selected by the various NIRA hospitals take time to develop as well as to allow for the change process, it may be some time before the full impact of these projects is realized.

INTERNAL EVALUATION

As part of the NIRA project, an internal evaluation component was essential to determine if anticipated changes were achieved. An Evaluation/Monitor and Quality Assurance Committee was established. This committee included staff nurses from the pilot unit, the clinical nurse specialist responsible for nursing quality assurance, the manager of the quality assurance department, the nursing director of finance and resource management, the management engineer, and the project coordinator. It was chaired by the assistant vice president for surgical services. She was selected for this because of her assumed neutrality; she did not have responsibility for a pilot unit. The Evaluation/Monitoring/Quality Assurance Committee was responsible for developing an evaluation component that addressed the desired goals as outlined in our proposal. Working with a nurse consultant from Andersen Consulting, measurement tools were developed. The tools included surveys for nurse, pharmacy, physicians, and patients; work sampling which involved 8,000 observations; and frequency studies for activities on the unit that would be impacted by bedside computerization.

In the second year of the NIRA program,

evaluation components addressed the impact of automated documentation on other departments. We see collaboration with other disciplines as an essential outgrowth of nursing's automation. If nursing automation helps to fulfill regulatory agency requirements, allows other departments within the hospital to work more efficiently when information is consistent, readable and available, many of our goals will have been achieved. Patients overwhelmingly rated the computers high and were satisfied with the nurse being in the room more. It is most important that automation positively impacts patient outcomes in a cost efficient manner so that there is a greater opportunity for success.

LESSONS LEARNED

1. Make certain that vendors have read the proposal and are in agreement with it.
2. Keep encouraging physicians to be involved from the beginning since it affects their medical practice.
3. Secure and sustain hospital administrative support, especially from the Chief Executive Officer and Chief Operating Officer.
4. Utilize those units that truly want the system—request letters of intent from staff to show support for the initiation of a pilot project on their unit.
5. Keep staff nurses involved. They are the backbone of the project and they know their practice.
6. Anticipate unexpected costs; training includes not just salaries but frequently involves trips to vendor headquarters.
7. Keep active in user groups. Vendors may make changes based on suggestions from a hospital's nurses and

physicians but to really provide product direction, a united voice from client hospitals is important.

8. Network with other users. Make contacts at user groups and develop relationships. If another hospital has a module or function that your hospital is considering, get that contact name from vendor.

9. Make certain that information systems is involved from the beginning of any automated system.

10. Do not underestimate the impact that this will have on daily routine practices of the nursing and physician groups.

11. The medication administration process was the most difficult to implement because it required communication between two departments. The medical administration process should not be installed in the beginning because it is important to get some early "wins."

12. Physicians and nurses are accustomed to rapid response to problems and anticipated faster turnaround on enhancements or changes in the system. The nature of designing and implementing new computerized tools is usually a slower process, emphasizing the need for communication.

13. Plan for 24-hour pharmacy service for effective system operation of Clini-Com.

14. Have adequate numbers of trainers/troubleshooters to support implementation.

FUTURE

At this writing we are planning our continued relationship with the two vendors and the feasibility of when and if we can continue to expand to other areas of the hospital. We recognize the financial and time commitment impact of more design and research.

Short-term goals would be to place existing capabilities on other medical–surgical units, and to review the critical care modules. The most important criteria will be to make sure that all future applications have interface capabilities.

Future goals include: linking the system to the physicians' offices; predetermining charting quality indicators for each department to make retrieval less time intensive; making it possible to retrieve past information from repeat admissions on the units; weighing certain charting elements that automatically create an acuity value for patient classification; printing or reviewing policies and procedures at the nursing station or patient room; using the existing terminals as a vehicle for continuing education at the nurses' station; exploring the possibility of voice recognition capabilities; and preparing for the eventual introduction of a completely automated electronic medical record.

Section Three
Nursing Information Systems
for Care Planning

The seven chapters in this section focus on nursing information systems which impact upon care planning by nurses and nursing students. Nursing information systems assist the nurse in planning care more effectively, but present dilemmas as well. The authors of the first chapter, Bliss-Holtz, et al., explain how the software entitled "Professional Care System" was developed using a process and practice model based on Self-Care Deficit Nursing Theory. The software is designed to be used by bedside nurses to make decisions about self care limitations of patients and create a written care plan.

Care planning in nursing homes is discussed in the next two chapters. Downey and Hood provide a model for the development of computer assisted care planning. Computer screens for multi-disciplinary care planning and protocols are provided. Miller and Giamporcaro described how information among nursing home care givers was organized and integrated into a relational database and used for reimbursement to providers. These authors worked together in the development, testing, and implementation of care plans for nursing homes resulting in their use in ten nursing homes in the state of New York.

The creation of a microcomputer database for tracking home care workers across multiple vendors by a home health agency is discussed by Chalmers and Brady. The methods of development and implementation are addressed.

Smaldone and Greenberg explain the decision-making process for either developing or purchasing a computerized care planning system. Both the system features and nursing practice issues associated with automated care plans for an acute care setting are discussed. The design of a relational database for generation of care plans and its use with nursing students is addressed by four authors in Chapter 14.

The effects of using nursing information systems, both good and bad, are presented by Yoder in the final chapter of this section.

9

Development of a Computerized Information System Based on Self-Care Deficit Nursing Theory

Jane Bliss-Holtz
Susan G. Taylor
Katherine McLaughlin
Patricia Sayers
Lynne Nickle

INTRODUCTION

This chapter discusses the development of a computerized nursing information system (CNIS) based on self-care deficit nursing theory (SCDNT). The initial system was developed for use with a postpartum population. Although the separate phases of this software's development have been described elsewhere (Bliss-Holtz, McLaughlin, & Taylor, 1990; Bliss-Holtz, Taylor, & McLaughlin, in press; McLaughlin, Taylor, Bliss-Holtz, Sayers, & Nickle, 1990), this will be the first documentation of the process from inception to initial clinical testing.

The system was produced under the auspices of Nursing Systems International Incorporated of Bordentown, N.J. and partially supported by a small business Phase I grant awarded by the National Center for Nursing Research, a Small Business Innovative Research (SBIR) Bridge Grant and an Innovative Partnership Grant from the New Jersey Institution of Science and Technology.

The software, Professional Care System™, runs on an IBM or IBM-compatible 80386-SX or 80486 system. The software is menu-driven throughout, with access to all levels of screens in no more than three key-strokes. Users can enter most documentation through menu choices in one key-stroke, although they also can enter data in free-form text.

The phases of development included: (1) articulation of data relationships, which incorporated process model formulation and derivation and validation of the practice model; (2) identification of system content, which included the steps of choosing a prototype population and structuring the content into theory-related categories; (3) establishing clinically relevant data relationships; (4) developing a user-friendly interface; and (5) initial clinical testing.

ARTICULATION OF DATA RELATIONSHIPS

That there is a relationship between data and information and knowledge is the premise that supports computerized information systems. Data are objectively described, discrete entities; when they are interpreted or structured they become information (Blum, 1986). In most cases, the user enters data into the computer system. Structure or organization is given to the data either through choices made by the user, as prompted by the software, or from a base that is built into software which defines the relationship of entered data.

Computerized nursing information systems (CNIS) allow users to input data in a manner that will allow it to be reorganized into information useful for nursing practice. For a CNIS to be a data-based system, types of relevant data and possible relationships among data must be explicitly defined within a logical framework. For nursing, as with any discipline, the meaning of data is dependent on the theoretical or conceptual model which frames data gathering and analysis. However, one of the problems inherent with nursing models is that they, by definition, are too broad to use as a base for data relationships. For a CNIS to be theory-based, the relationship between data and the theory must be articulated.

Bliss-Holtz et al. (1990) described a process by which data was related to SCDNT. The process will be summarized in this section of the discussion. Self-Care Deficit Nursing Theory, a synthesis of three theories, guides nurses in gathering appropriate facts and articulating relationships between them in order to plan effective nursing care (Taylor, 1988). In her theoretical formulation, D. E. Orem (personal communication, 1988) moved beyond the traditional definition of nursing as a linear problem-solving process and reconceptualized it as a matrix process. Nevertheless, before the conceptualized SCDNT matrix could be actualized as a CNIS structure, three steps were necessary: (1) a process model that explicitly identified the processes of nursing practice was formulated from SCDNT; (2) nursing experts derived a practice model; and (3) the practice model was validated as one that reflected nursing practice.

Process Model Formulation

Formal derivation of the process model began at theory development sessions sponsored by Nursing Systems International in 1988. The original theory development team included the authors and D. E. Orem. During these meetings, the group examined the dimensions of nursing practice and developed a three-stage process model, called the SCDNT Process Model (Bliss-Holtz et al., 1990).

Practice Model Derivation

In developing the practice model, the team interviewed expert nurses and analyzed cases to determine what information they used in their practice and how they used the information in relation to the processes encompassed by the SCDNT matrix and the SCDNT Process Model (McLaughlin et al., 1990). Clinical decision-making processes described by the practitioners were compared with the clinical decision-making processes postulated as inherent in the theory.

Practice Model Validation

By the end of 1988, the SCDNT Process Model was defined sufficiently to permit validation of its effectiveness in reflecting nursing practice in an acute care setting. The team designed a validation procedure and performed an initial trial, using a panel of six nurses expert in postpartum care. The trial tested, with positive results both the SCDNT Process Model and the validation procedure. Consequently, validation of the

Process Model for use with acute care patients with various medical diagnoses was a success.

IDENTIFICATION OF SYSTEM CONTENT

Choosing a Prototype Population

The previously described work provided the basis for the structuring of the CNIS platform, but it did not provide the specific content of the system. In order to continue the system's development, the group needed to select a patient prototype population. Orem's (1991) classification of seven nursing situations by health focus was used to delineate their characteristics. It was decided that a Group I nursing situation was an appropriate starting place for the development of content for the CNIS. Patients in Group I situations generally are in good health and represent relatively "uncomplicated" nursing situations, but still capture aspects of general information areas that would subsequently be used when developing the system to address the remaining six nursing situations.

After choosing a Group I situation, the team had to decide on the patient population that would represent it. Patients in Group I are in good to excellent general health and are experiencing life cycle changes (Orem, 1991). The CNIS was initially targeted for use with patients receiving nursing care on an "in-patient" basis. Therefore, the prototype population needed to be one that was experiencing a life cycle event that affected anatomic, physiologic, and psychosocial parameters; needed nursing care; and typically was seen in an "in-patient" setting. Healthy postpartum patients met the above criteria and thus were chosen as the prototype patient population.

Structuring Content into Theory-related Categories

Establishing the content of the system as it related to the specific population was the next phase in the development process. This process was described by Bliss-Holtz et al. (in press) and is summarized below.

Theoretical elements of SCDNT and the designated relationships between the elements were used as a base from which to identify concrete conditions and factors of nursing practice situations. Using certain theoretical elements and their designated relationships, patient information was categorized as it related to or provided data to aid in formulating the purpose for individualized health care. The theoretical elements which provided the framework for the development of the content were the Basic Conditioning Factors (BCF), and the three sets of Self-Care Requisites were Universal Self-Care Requisites (USCR), Developmental Self-Care Requisites (DSCR), and Health Deviation Self-Care Requisites (HDSCR).

The specific factors operating within the prototype population were established, and representative data elements and values were identified by an expert panel of seven nurses. The panel represented three health care institutions: an urban regional center for perinatal care, a suburban hospital, and a hospital serving an urban area. The panel was asked to consider each general category of BCF and identify specific factors, their related data elements, and possible range of values. Panel members worked in small groups over a two-week period after which the panel reconvened and the results were shared. At that time the panel reached a general consensus on the factors, the associated data elements, and value ranges representative of their patient population. In a similar manner, the panel also identified appropriate factors, related data elements, and ranges of values for Self-Care requisites.

ESTABLISHING CLINICALLY RELEVANT DATA RELATIONSHIPS

The above-described process related clinical data to theoretical categories. In order to produce information useful to nursing practice from the entered data, decisions were made regarding the relationship between the assessed patient-specific requisites and the patient's self-care operations. Because the software does not represent an expert system, these decisions are made by the nurse-user, with appropriate system prompts that allow these decisions to be made more easily. For example, the nurse is asked to make a decision about the patient's ability to meet each requisite. If the patient's self-care operations are not adequate, the nurse identifies the nature of the limitations. These limitations can be categorized as limitations in knowledge (K), judgement and decision-making (D), and/or the ability to perform appropriate action (A) (see Figure 9.1). A summary of these identified limitations can be generated by the system; the summary can be used for identifying the required patient action and nurse action. With further system development, the amount of nursing time needed for each patient could be derived as well.

DEVELOPMENT OF A USER-FRIENDLY ENVIRONMENT

In addition to development of the data relationships that represent the system base, the user needed to be considered. The software is menu-driven throughout, with access to all levels of screens requiring no more than three key-strokes. Most documentation can be entered through menu choices in one key-stroke. To save nursing documentation

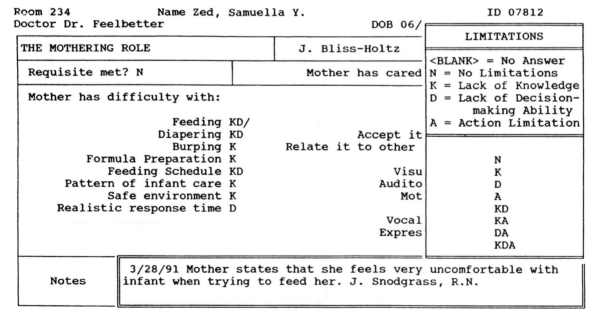

Figure 9.1 Screen documenting self-care operations regarding the mothering role. Shown with "help" menu.

time, the system is designed so that when data is entered on any screen, it is automatically transferred to any other appropriate screen in the system. Although data entry currently is exclusively through keyboard, development of touch-screen data entry is being planned.

Figure 9.2 shows the main menu of the system. Before data can be entered, the user must identify the patient to which the data refer. This is done with the "SELECT PATIENT" option. Once a patient is selected, the patient's name and identification number appear on every screen. This feature reminds the user which patient's file is currently being addressed.

The main menu lists broad data categories identified in the theory. For example, the main menu item "Universal Self-Care Requisites" gives the user access to the options "fluid intake," "nutrient intake," "fluid output," and "maintenance of a sufficient intake of oxygen." Menu options can be chosen by typing the first letter representing the category or by moving the cursor to the desired category and pressing "ENTER." The chosen category is highlighted and the submenus contained within each highlighted category are shown at the bottom of the screen.

The first section of the main menu screen (ADMISSIONS and SELECT PATIENT) allows admission information to be entered or displayed or patient files to be chosen. The second section of the main menu (MONITORING and OTHER BASIC CONDITIONING FACTORS) allows information to be entered for which there is little user interpretation beyond that associated with patient assessment and monitoring (see Figure 9.3). For example, figure 9.3 shows the screen used for recording fluid intake. There is little interpretation needed by the user to record the type of fluid, amount, date, and time administered. The "help" screen gives the user the choices of types of fluid available under a particular category (in this case, in-

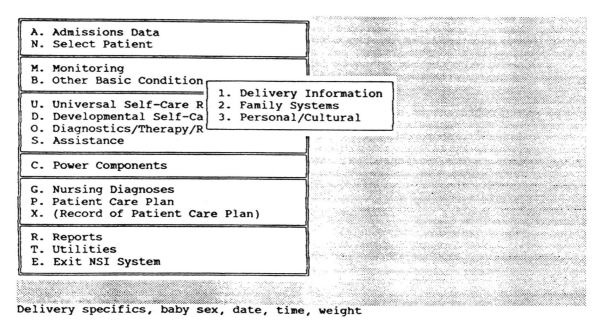

```
A. Admissions Data
N. Select Patient

M. Monitoring
B. Other Basic Condition ┌─────────────────────────
                         │ 1. Delivery Information
U. Universal Self-Care R │ 2. Family Systems
D. Developmental Self-Ca │ 3. Personal/Cultural
O. Diagnostics/Therapy/R └─────────────────────────
S. Assistance

C. Power Components

G. Nursing Diagnoses
P. Patient Care Plan
X. (Record of Patient Care Plan)

R. Reports
T. Utilities
E. Exit NSI System
```

Delivery specifics, baby sex, date, time, weight

Figure 9.2 Main menu of the system.

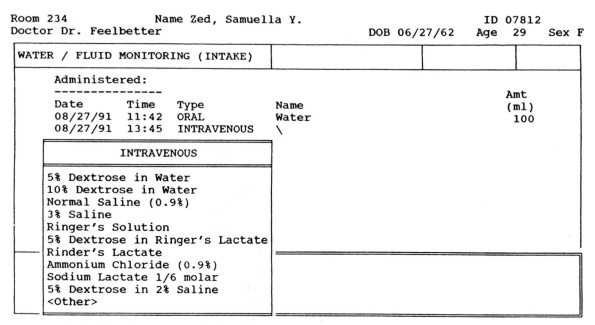

```
Room 234              Name Zed, Samuella Y.                    ID 07812
Doctor Dr. Feelbetter                        DOB 06/27/62   Age  29   Sex F
```

Figure 9.3   Fluid intake screen with "help" menu.

travenous fluid) and also allows the user to enter that choice with a key stroke. The third and fourth sections of the main menu contain screens which prompt the user to make a decision about the self-care limitations of the patient (see Figure 9.1). The user's decisions are supported by information previously entered in the second section of the main menu. The decisions entered, in turn, can be summarized in a self-care operations report. This report, as well as others, can be generated by selecting it from a submenu in the sixth section of the main menu (REPORTS). The fifth section (NURSING DIAGNOSES, PATIENT CARE PLAN, and RECORD OF PATIENT CARE PLAN) of the main menu allows the user to obtain a summary of nursing diagnoses or a patient care plan. These can be displayed on the screen or printed for hard copy. The UTILITIES section allows new users to be entered into the system, as well as the time and date to be easily corrected.

INITIAL CLINICAL TESTING

The monitoring section of the system currently is being tested at two clinical sites in a total of 26 patient rooms, which involves approximately 30 staff nurses on the postpartum units. Classes for nursing staff have included an introduction to computer use, as most staff were uncomfortable with using computers. The class then covered an overview of the system, with specific focus on the second section of the main menu (MONITORING). All registered nurses assigned to patients in the rooms containing the system were then asked to: (1) perform documentation using the system, (2) use the old documentation forms, and (3) fill out an entry log form designed to monitor any problems the nurses encountered. Although the system of double documentation was laborious for the nurses, it was vital to detect any problems with capturing and storing data. After several weeks of trial, no problems with data integrity have been encountered.

CONCLUSION

This paper described the development of a computerized nursing information system (CNIS) based on Self-Care Deficit Nursing Theory (SCDNT). The system's relational base is theory-driven, which supports data gathering and prompts nursing decisions. Because data relationships are based on a nursing framework, the data can be structured in a way that creates information which is readily accessed and useful to nursing practice. Further work on the system includes the development of a patient classification system and formulation of nursing diagnoses congruent with the nursing theory (Taylor, 1991).

REFERENCES

Bliss-Holtz, J., McLaughlin, K., & Taylor, S. G. (1990). Validating nursing theory for use within a computerized nursing information system. *Advances in Nursing Science, 13*, 46–52.

Bliss-Holtz, J., Taylor, S. G., & McLaughlin, K. (in press). Nursing theory as a base for a computerized nursing information system. *Nursing Science Quarterly.*

Blum, B. (1986). *Clinical Information Systems.* New York: Springer-Verlag.

McLaughlin, K., Taylor, S. G., Bliss-Holtz, J., Sayers, P., & Nickle, L. (1990). Shaping the future: The marriage of nursing theory and informatics. *Computers in Nursing, 8*, 174–179.

Orem, D. E. (1991). *Nursing: Concepts of practice* (4th ed). St. Louis: Mosby-Year Book.

Taylor, S. G. (1988). Nursing theory and nursing practice: Orem's theory in practice. *Nursing Science Quarterly, 1*(3), 111–119.

Taylor, S. G. (1991). The structure of nursing diagnosis from Orem's theory. *Nursing Science Quarterly, 4*(1), 23–32.

10

Development of Care Planning Software for Nursing Homes

Edward H. Downey
Gail Hood

INTRODUCTION

New York State requires the periodic completion of a utilization review document (UR) for all nursing home residents. The UR and the New York Quality Assurance Standards (NYQAS) guide the multidisciplinary care planning process. A team of clinicians (nurses, therapists, dieticians, and social workers) review the UR, using the NYQAS to determine the areas that a care plan must address. The recently introduced Federal Minimum Data Set (MDS) and Resident Assessment Protocols (RAPS) will be used in much the same way to produce multidisciplinary care plans for nursing home residents throughout the United States. New York State has its own version of MDS called MDS+. This is currently being implemented as a computer application for electronic submission of MDS+ data to the state. Eventually the MDS+ will also be integrated into computerized care planning.

When done manually, the care planning process is time consuming and costly. Therefore, the development and implementation

of computer-assisted care planning software has the potential for increasing the productivity of nursing home clinicians and improving the quality of care. Improper development and implementation, however, will probably have the opposite effect. This chapter describes how administrators, nurses, and clinical staff members at two New York State Nursing Homes worked with academicians and programmers to develop care planning software currently being used in ten nursing homes. These efforts were coordinated by the software developer, P&NP Computer Services, Inc. This chapter presents a conceptual framework for similar endeavors.

CRITERIA FOR COMPUTER APPLICATIONS DEVELOPERS

The six criteria discussed below helped determine whether or not the computer-assisted care plan project could be accomplished.

Manual systems must be effective, prior to computerization. The computerization of any system requires that it have a well-defined set of decision rules that can be conceptualized as a decision tree with certainty or known probabilities. When the team first examined the care planning process it appeared as though many of the decisions made did not follow well-defined rules. From the systems analyst's point of view, the care planning process seemed too vague to allow construction of clear system specifications. Despite this, the manual system did produce effective care plans.

On the positive side the people who are on multidisciplinary care planning teams (e.g., nurses, therapists, dieticians, and social workers) all come from disciplines that stress, where possible, the importance of clear and unambiguous standards in decision making. Second, the NYQAS are a logical set of triggers that unequivocally indicate when a care area should be addressed by the multidisciplinary care team. Third, state auditors from the Department of Health review care plans on a regular basis to determine their appropriateness. Thus, the team receives regular feedback and has the opportunity to constantly improve their care planning techniques.

Text management must be feasible. While the programmers had developed many nursing home systems, multidisciplinary care planning appeared to be an area that required a totally new approach to text management. The vast majority of other applications were fixed field oriented—the number of fields per record and their lengths were predetermined. The care plan is a document that can have any number of data fields of varying lengths. In essence the care plan lacked the structure required for a convenient, menu-driven computer application. While the academicians and programmers had long standing relationships with a broad range of nursing home professionals, they were not immediately encouraged by the extent to which nursing home professionals understood the text management problem.

Computer applications must result in direct and obvious benefits to the user. These benefits are of two types: time savings and information that results in improved outcomes. Because the care plan is frequently revised during its initiation and updating and a care planning team is usually composed of four or five members, there is a great deal of editing and retyping. The task is time consuming and tends to detract from team concentration on patient needs.

The goal was to design an efficient program that would produce complete and revised care plans immediately. One alternative would be to use commercially available word processing software to decrease the time spent preparing the document. Although the software saved time, it still took too long to produce final care plans at the team meeting.

The team developed a system that allowed for the choice of predetermined text which could be quickly modified with a word or phrase. This design met the team's goal since it was quick enough that final care plans could be completed as team decisions were made. The result was finished care plans at the end of each meeting, as well as a marked decrease in the time required to complete each document.

The users must have computer capability. The higher the levels of computer capability, the better. Both of the nursing homes involved in the project to develop the computer-assisted care plans already had experience with our computerized patient care system (PCS). PCS is a complex system that processes admissions, discharges, readmissions, census, patient histories, UR, Resource Utilization Groups (RUGs is the patient review system employed by the state for reimbursement), patient spending accounts, billing and accounts receivable, and a host of other functions (Miller, Guhde, & Downey, 1986).

Users must have enthusiasm for the development of computer applications. One of the best ways to ensure staff enthusiasm is to be sure that they have experienced previous success using computer applications. As previously mentioned both of the nursing homes we worked with used PCS. Their responses to this experience were positive and resulted in the enthusiasm that was necessary to sustain the development process. In addition, at both homes the administrators supported development of automated multidisciplinary care planning.

Time must be available for the development of computer applications. Software development is a time consuming process. The time required can be broken down into five parts: systems analysis, programming, bench testing, beta testing, and writing a user manual. Systems analysis requires that user needs be translated into system specifications that a programmer can use to write the software. The systems analyst must learn precisely how user decisions are made. The user must also learn how to specify decision rules to the degree of precision needed for computer applications. Since the teams were composed of four or five clinicians from various disciplines, this required more time than usual.

As already mentioned, this application required managing text to allow for any number of fields of varying length. Unfortunately programmers usually work with records containing a fixed number of fields of predetermined length. As a result, a great deal of time was spent learning how to accommodate new text management demands. One-half of the approximately 500 hours in programming time was spent solving text management issues.

The team bench tested the software by running simulations in our computer lab. The beta test was administered at two nursing homes, where the system was used to produce actual care plans. The test resulted in many programming changes and some changes in the systems analysis. There are so many possibilities in systems that require the use of any number of fields of varying length that testing is difficult and time consuming.

Since the six criteria for computer applications developers were met or the problems could be overcome, the team determined that the environment was suitable for the development of computer assisted care plans. Some difficulties were anticipated, since even in the best of circumstances the development of complex software applications is difficult. Nonetheless the team encountered unanticipated problems that are important enough to examine.

SYSTEM DESIGN ISSUES

One of the biggest challenges to developing computer applications is translating the way people make decisions into a format that allows for software development to begin. A high level of objectivity is required in computer applications, since computers are not capable of intuitive decision making. Because care planning requires some intuition, the software has to be designed to assist this process, not replace it. The members of care planning teams are disciplined by virtue of their training and experience. Despite this the developers encountered difficulties in understanding the decision-making process employed by the team. In the final analysis there was difficulty understanding even the fundamental framework within which the decisions were made.

The structure provided by the NYQAS triggers was very helpful. For example, NYQAS are triggered if the UR shows high scores for the activities of daily living (i.e., eating, mobility, transfer, and toilet). Despite this level of structure, when care planners were asked how they organized their meetings and in what order patient concerns were considered they were surprisingly vague. In addition, the process of working through a care area was also vague. At this point we became very concerned about our ability to reach the level of objectivity required to write care planning software.

In considering the surprising vagueness of team responses to queries about decision making, the development of a new understanding of how care planning teams operate was necessary. Many of the issues faced by a team consisting of nurses, therapists, dieticians, and social workers are very complex since the approaches of one discipline necessarily impact those of the others. This makes it difficult to develop system design specifications with the exactness programmers and systems analysts prefer. To meet the levels of objectivity required would probably have the effect of suffocating the team's decision-making abilities. This may have resulted in a decrease in the quality of care. The use of subtlety and intuition in developing care plans had to be allowed for in an effective computer assisted system.

For the above reasons developers determined that a considerable amount of flexibility had to be built into the system, thereby reducing the inherent system structure. Unfortunately the increased flexibility also increased the complexity of the system and therefore generated more computer code. It also made the system somewhat more difficult to learn. However it allowed the care planning team to work effectively.

First, a set of protocols for all twenty eight NYQAS care areas were carefully specified by the care planning team at one of the homes. Then, flexibility was increased by developing a whole subsystem that allows a team to edit and modify all existing protocols. The system also includes a subsystem that can create new care areas and new sets of protocols.

A considerable amount of time was spent considering how to make the system easy to use, since the system had become more complex than we anticipated. It was felt that the best way to do this was to maximize the use of pull down menus and minimize the number of keys needed to create a care plan. As a result the whole care plan can be produced by using only two keys (F1 and F10). Once the system takes you into a care area the cursor is automatically positioned on the next logical task. The user performs the task using system prompts and moves through the care plan from one step to the next with a minimum of key strokes.

A BRIEF REVIEW OF THE CARE PLANNING APPLICATION

A brief look at the computer-assisted care planning application will assist in understanding some of the problems faced in its development. Figure 10.1 shows the entry screen used in the computer-assisted care plan.

The screen in Figure 10.1 has already been completed with predetermined protocols for Problem, Objective, Approach, Responsible Party, and Response. Progress notes can also be done on this screen but they are not shown in Figure 10.1. This screen is for the care area Elimination–UTI which was triggered for the patient, based on his UR score for elimination. The predetermined protocols were developed by care plan team members for their respective disciplines. Figure 10.2 shows an example of a menu that appears on the screen when the user chooses the Problem protocols for the care area of Elimination–UTI.

There are 28 possible care areas that can be addressed based on NYQAS triggers. Each area is broken into five sections (Problem, Objective, Approach, Responsible

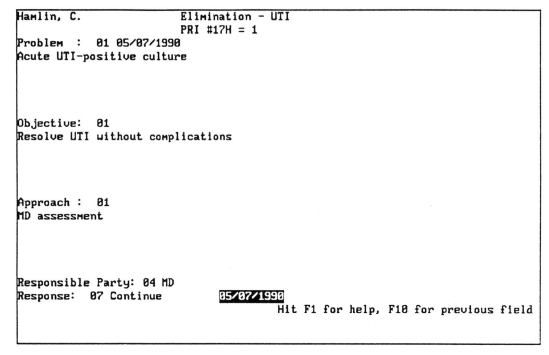

Figure 10.1 Care plan entry screen.

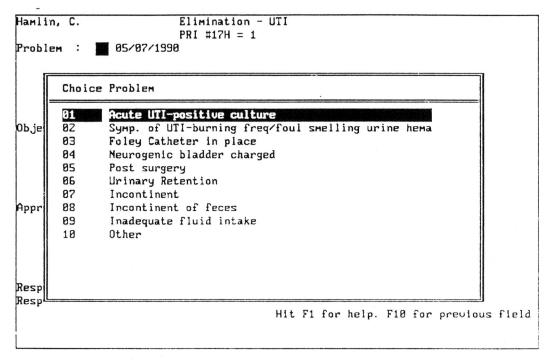

Figure 10.2 Protocols menu.

Party, and Response), which means that a minimum of 140 sets of protocols are maintained in the system.

The system allows the protocols to be edited in the care plan so team members can make unique comments. This was considered to be a critical feature since there was concern that care plans respond to the unique needs of patients. Figure 10.3 shows that after the first (01) protocol was chosen for the problem under the care area Elimination–UTI a modification was made (Note the added text "THIS IS A TEST").

The system is designed so that each care area can accommodate one or more Problems. For each Problem there can be one or more Objectives. For each Objective there can be one or more Approaches and so on. Thus the system develops a tree like structure for each care area.

IMPLEMENTATION ISSUES

Throughout the system design stage developers became increasingly aware of conflicts between people and machines. This struggle became even more evident during implementation as the project began to reach an equilibrium between two control factors in the care planning process: the system and the care planning team.

While there was an initial awareness of the uniqueness of nursing homes, it became even more evident as we began to implement the system. In one home, staff was greatly concerned about patients wandering into the remote woody area surrounding the facility. Several patients at this home seemed to prefer the woods to other parts of the facility. Patient safety was of such great concern that a complete care area was developed by the

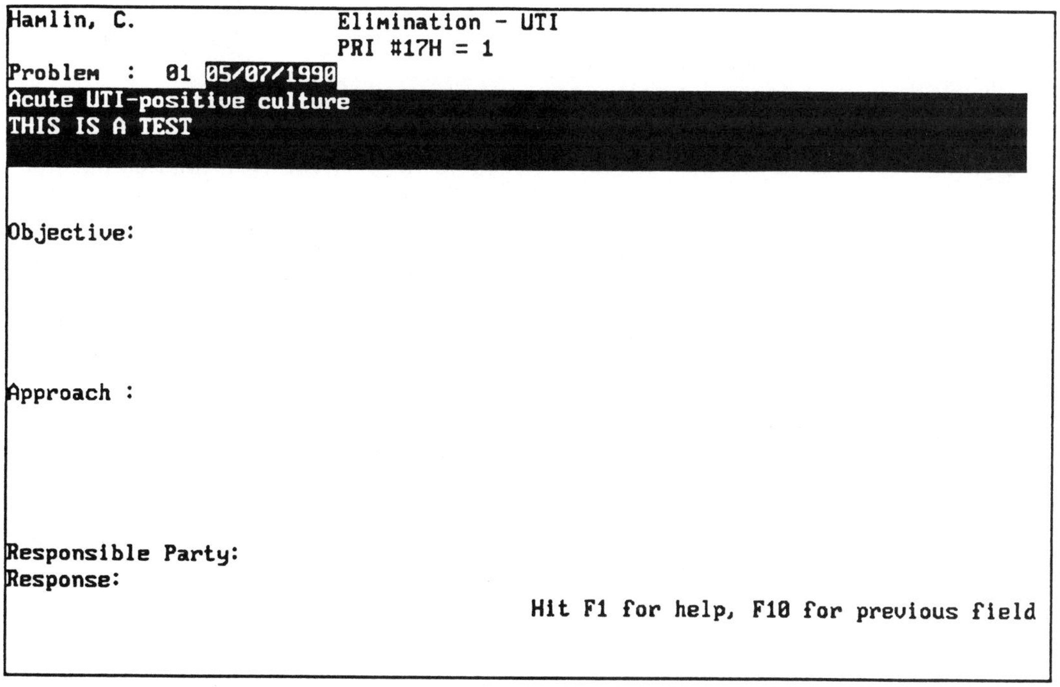

```
Hamlin, C.              Elimination - UTI
                        PRI #17H = 1
Problem  :  01 05/07/1990
Acute UTI-positive culture
THIS IS A TEST



Objective:




Approach :




Responsible Party:
Response:
                        Hit F1 for help, F10 for previous field

```

Figure 10.3 Editing protocols.

care planning team. The system had to be flexible enough not only to meet the unique needs of patients, but also to respond to the unique environments surrounding the homes themselves.

Some teams purchased an overhead screen projector to enable everyone to easily review and control what was being done. This allowed for a single input person and relieved the administrator of training everyone in the system's use. The use of the overhead screen projector also kept the entire team focused on specific tasks. This increased the efficiency of and the team's control over the group process. The projected screen acted as a dynamic agenda that immediately reflected team decisions.

In some of the nursing homes that use the system there is a conflict between quality tracking and ease of screen input. The system is structured in a linear fashion so that a tree of Objectives, Approaches, Responsible Parties, and Responses must flow from a single Problem. This maintains an internal logic that forces clear, logical quality tracking. On the other hand this does curtail the ability to do free form editing, which some users find objectionable. Developers are working to achieve a compromise in this area.

When we began developing the system we wanted to be able to produce a high quality care plan in 15 to 20 minutes. Of course we expected a learning curve, but were not certain when or precisely how this goal might be met. The project team was fascinated at how care planners used the system to increase their own productivity.

At first the system seemed to control the care planning meeting, but fortunately this soon changed so that the team took control of the system. They freely modified protocols and used reports to plan their individual contributions. Soon after implementation of the first system, team members requested modifications and new reports. For example,

one team wanted the option to produce individual care plans by team member discipline. As soon as teams in other homes heard about it they also requested this reporting option. Clearly, the teams were taking more control.

The issue of whether the system controlled the team or the team controlled the system was critical to the quality of the care plans. If the system controlled the team, "canned" care plans and a decrease in the quality of care would result. Therefore, it was gratifying to see the teams take more control. The quality of the care plans produced by the system was recently verified in one home by State Health Department inspectors, who not only gave the home a glowing report on its last three care plan reviews, but strongly recommended that other homes in the region adopt computer assisted care plans.

RECOMMENDATION: THE SEVENTH CRITERION

The six criteria for development of computerized multidisciplinary care planning led to a successfully implemented and applied program. Nevertheless, our experiences indicate the need for a seventh criterion: The success of the computer application will be determined by the extent to which an equilibrium is established over the control of the process between the users and the system.

A major difficulty encountered was the determination of what the appropriate equilibrium should be. Programmers and systems analysts will tend to favor more system control since it will, from their point of view, increase the quality of the data and the ability to analyze it. Users will want to increase their control since, to them, the quality of outcomes is at least partly dependent on their ability to make decisions based on subtle, less predictable thought processes. Despite the difficulty and frustrations associated with establishing this equilibrium, ignoring it can only be at the system developers' peril.

With the recent nationwide introduction of the Federal Minimum Data Set (MDS), which triggers Resident Assessment Protocols (RAPS), the development of computer-assisted care planning in long-term care will be accelerated. The successful development of these systems will depend on the close cooperation of clinicians, systems analysts, and programmers. The need to establish an equilibrium between user and system control over care planning decisions will be-

come even more acute. The seven criteria for computer applications developers can provide the necessary framework within which this can be achieved.

REFERENCES

Miller, R. P., Guhde, R., & Downey, E. H. (1986). Computerization of the resource utilization groups (RUGS) [Abstract]. *Proceedings of the 39th Annual Scientific Meeting of the Gerontology Society of America. The Gerontologist, 26*, 122A.

11

Computers in Nursing Homes: Impact of the Resource Utilization Groups (RUG-II)

R. Paul Miller
Christine D. Giamporcaro

INTRODUCTION

In 1986 New York State introduced the Resource Utilization Groups (RUG-II), a case-mix payment system for nursing homes. This payment system is based on the assumptions that patient characteristics and impairment levels can be measured for the intensity of nursing care required and reimbursement could be equitably adjusted by the amount of such care rendered. In 1988 New York mandated that the RUG-II data be electronically transmitted, effectively forcing the computerization of long-term care in the state.

This chapter describes a five-year experience with the use of computers in the nursing home setting. The initial goal in 1986 was to meet the projected electronic submission of the RUG-II case-mix data. As this goal was achieved, it became apparent that there was a rich information flow among care giving disciplines in long-term care that was open to analysis and could be defined and structured by principles used in data man-

agement. If successfully integrated and computerized, the information flow could be utilized for management, quality assurance, and research.

TEST FACILITIES

St. John's Home is a nonprofit, multilevel geriatric facility with 230 skilled nursing facility (SNF) beds, 241 health-related facility (HRF) beds, and 64 independent apartment units. Special programs offered to the community at the SNF level include respite care, rehabilitation, comfort care, and mental health. St. John's Home also offers home health care, a medical model adult day care center, and an emergency response system for homebound elderly. These special programs lead to an unusually large turnover rate for a long-term care facility. The Home renders services to approximately 800 to 1000 individuals per year. In 1987 the RUG-II programs at St. John's Home were incorporated into a Local Area Network (LAN) which linked the micro computers in the medical, pharmacy, business, nursing, and social service departments. The programs described below are commercially available (P & NP Computer Associates, 16434 Telegraph Rd., Holley, NY 14470).

Oneida City Hospital Extended Care Facility is a multilevel geriatric facility with 77 SNF beds and 31 HRF beds. It is part of a municipal hospital system with 101 acute beds and serves a rural population. Special programs offered to the community through this complex include outpatient services, rehabilitation, a community-oriented intergenerational day care center, and an emergency response system for homebound elderly. The computer-assisted comprehensive care plan which will be briefly described below was developed at this facility.

THE RESOURCE UTILIZATION GROUPS

The RUG-II is based on an ambitious study performed by New York State from 1983 to 1985, in collaboration with Rensselaer Polytechnical Institute (Schneider, Fries, & Foley, 1988). The clinical characteristics, Activities of Daily Living (ADL) level, and behavioral characteristics of approximately 3,400 patients at 52 selected long-term care facilities were studied utilizing an encounter form that captured 227 data elements. The impairment level of these nursing home patients was directly related to nursing and nursing aide staff time. The original 227 data elements were reduced to only those which held the greatest explanatory power for consumption of nursing resources. To these elements, other data sets were added that can serve for quality assurance purposes. These data elements are collected with an encoun-

ter form, the Patient Review Instrument (PRI) (Schneider et al., 1988).

The PRI is divided into descriptor areas that include: Demographics (16 fields), Medical Events (9 fields), Medical Treatments (13 fields), Activities of Daily Living (4 fields), Behavior Problems (4 abnormal behaviors), Specialized Services (Physical/Occupational therapy), Medications (2 fields), total number of physician visits, and the primary problem (ICD-9 diagnostic code) which consumes the most nursing time. The clinically relevant fields are listed in Table 11.1. The fields are graded numerically, and then weighed by their response.

The PRI data are collected quarterly by certified nurse assessors. All residents within the facility are screened with the PRI, and three months later data are collected only on new admissions and discharges. The cycle is then repeated. The collected data give six-month snapshots as to the actual case mix of all residents of a nursing home. The admission and discharge screen provides information on the discharge patterns of nursing homes and on their most recent admissions.

Depending on the response to key questions, an algorithm assigns the nursing home resident to one of 5 hierarchial groups and subsequently classifies the care needs into one of the sixteen different classifications (Schneider et al., 1988). Individual Medicaid payment rates are assigned to each of the 16 classifications. The average case mix is calculated for all residents at a facility, and the Medicaid rate is determined from this average case mix. This rate is prospectively paid for three months, and then adjusted according to the subsequent RUG-II screen.

Although RUG-II is a case-mix reimbursement system, not all of the data elements collected by the PRI are integrated into the algorithm that assigns residents into a payment classification. Specific clinical elements, for example, presence of contrac-

Table 11.1 Patient Review Instrument Clinical Data

Decubitus Level	(num)	Tracheostomy Care	y/n	Eating	(1-5)	
		Suctioning	y/n	Mobility	(1-5)	
		Oxygen	y/n	Transfer	(1-5)	
		Respiratory Care	y/n	Toileting	(1-5)	
Internal Bleeding	y/n	Nasal Gastric Feed	y/n			
Stasis Ulcer	y/n	Parenteral Feed	y/n	Verbal Disruption	(1-5)	
Terminally Ill	y/n	Wound Care	y/n	Physical Aggression	(1-5)	
Contractures	y/n	Chemotherapy	y/n	Disruptive/Infantile	(1-5)	
Urinary Tract Infect.	y/n	Transfusion	y/n	Hallucinations	(1-3)	
HIV Infection	y/n	Dialysis	y/n			
Accident	y/n	Catheter	y/n	Physician Visits	(num)	
Ventilator Depend.	y/n	Physical Restraints	y/n	Medication (total)	(num)	
				Meds (Psychoactive)	(num)	
P.T. Level	(1-4)	O.T. level	(1-4)	Primary Problem	(ICD-9 code)	
P.T. Days	(1-5)	O.T. Days	(1-5)			
P.T. Time	(num)	O.T. Time	(num)			

Adapted from New York State's Patient Review Instrument

tures, diabetes mellitus, total number of medications, and other data elements, are ignored in case mix. These data elements and those actually collected for case mix allow the state to computer identify quality of care issues at the individual nursing home level—the New York Quality Assurance System (NYQAS).

NEW YORK QUALITY ASSURANCE SYSTEM (NYQAS)

From the RUG-II database submitted by individual nursing homes, the state health department is able to computer identify conditions or events which will allow targeting of quality issues. The health department can set percentage corridors for these conditions which can identify facilities which may be rendering poor quality of care. The targeted conditions are termed NYQAS "triggers" and are listed in Table 11.2.

The NYQAS triggers may relate to a single data element, for example the presence of a decubitus ulcer on a RUG-II screen. Alternatively, they may relate to change in function over a six-month time span, for example, continued presence of a urinary tract infection. Computer targeting will allow surveyors to evaluate a specific resident's chart and comprehensive care plan to determine whether the staff had introduced appropriate corrective measures. The archiving of RUG-II submissions allows design of computer programs which identify NYQAS triggers and introduce a powerful nursing management tool.

It is apparent that the current NYQAS triggers are rudimentary and that individual facilities can utilize this, and other data, to develop their own quality assurance programs. It is expected that the NYQAS triggers will expand and the state will target other quality issues from the RUG-II data base. Although the value of computer-assisted quality assurance is being explored at hospitals (Wilbert, 1985; Wilson, 1987), it is indicative that a recent monograph on quality assurance at the nursing home level ignores the topic (Lesage & Barhyte, 1989).

Table 11.2 New York Quality Assurance Triggers

ELIMINATION	*NUTRITION*	*RESIDENT SAFETY*
(P) Residents with catheters	(P) Eating level = 4	(O) Accidents
(L) Continued use of catheters	(L) Deterioration in Eating	
(L) Recurrent UTI	(P) Number with dehydration	*RESPIRATORY CARE*
(L) Deterioration in toileting	(P) Number with NG tubes	(P) Respiratory care
	(P) Number with gastrostomy	(P) Number receiving oxygen
INFECTION MANAGEMENT	(P) Number parenteral feeding	(P) Tracheostomy care
(O) Evaluation of HIV		(P) Number receiving suctioning
	PSYCHOSOCIAL	(O) Ventilator
MEDICAL, DENTAL, LAB	(L) Deterioration in ADLs	
(P) Discharges to higher level	(L) New behavior problems	*SKIN INTEGRITY*
(P) In-house deaths	(L) Continued behavior	(P) Decubitus level 2 through 5
(P) Discharges to lower level	problems	(L) Deterioration in decubitus
		(P) Stasis ulcers
MEDICATIONS	*REHABILITATION*	
(O) Medications (total)	(L) Continued heavy restorative	*SPEECH, LANGUAGE*
(O) Medications (psychoactive)	(L) New contractures	(O) Not computerized
	(L) Deterioration in ADLs	
MOBILITY, RESTRAINTS		
(P) Transfer level 4		
(L) Deterioration in Mobility		
(L) Inc. in phys. restraints		
(L) Continued use of phys. rest.		

Adapted from the Long Term Care Survey Manual, New York State Department of Health
(P) = Prevalence triggers
(L) = Longitudinal triggers
(O) = On site review

COMPUTERIZATION OF RUG-II DATA

The computerization of the RUG-II database and its electronic transmission to the State Health Department was successfully accomplished during the early phases of this work (Miller, Guhde, & Downey, 1986; Miller & Guhde, 1987). A commercial relational database manager (dBMAN, VersaSoft) was utilized to perform this task. The impetus behind computerizing this task was twofold. First, the health department wanted to capture the RUG-II data in a form that could be utilized for future study and trend analysis. Second, as subsequently demonstrated (Nichols, Groupman, Miller, & Guhde, 1987), it was felt that electronic transmission of the data would relieve part of the work burden associated with the RUG-II cycles.

The relational database model was chosen because it was projected that the program would need to be expanded to meet needs that were not directly related to the RUG-II submission. This database concept was first introduced in 1967 by I. J. Codd of IBM and is deceptively simple in concept. Any grouping of data elements can be set up in a table with rows (individual records) and columns (data elements or fields). The table may be developed either as a flat file (non sequential) or as a transaction file (sequential). As long as a common data element exists between each table, or data set, two or more tables can be linked, merged, and explored for relationships. Although commercial relational database programs in the personal computer (PC) environment do not fulfill the stringent criteria set by Codd's theoretical approach (Pascal, 1989), they remain powerful and flexible tools (Goley, 1989).

The database management program stays in the background and is exploited through a command or program language. A variety of functions including date, arithmetic, logical, and string operators (alpha-numeric characters) are available to explore the captured data elements. A powerful feature of the database manager is its indexing capabilities. Any database file can be reordered by indexing on one or more key fields. This allows almost instantaneous access to any record. The design of simplified sequential data input screens allows clerical personnel to input the data. Thus, the program appears to be a package specifically designed for a task. The database manager's command and query language remains in the background for developmental work, special reports, and idiosyncratic queries of the collected data.

The architecture of our initial program has been described (Miller & Guhde, 1987). The anchor of the program is the admission file which contains the demographic data associated with each resident, as well as a series of volatile fields such as current room, first admission date to a building, and most recent readmission date. This is a real time file, reflecting the most current resident status. Linked to this file are a series of databases that capture the history of resident (transactional), the current PRI score (flat file, real time), the archived PRI data (transactional), diagnosis (transactional), pertinent family information (flat file), and others.

DATA MANAGEMENT

From the initial experience, it became apparent that a rich but disparate and difficult to integrate information flow exists within nursing homes. The information flow has characteristics of distributed databases, with discrete domains, core data sets, and definable tasks where the data sets are repetitively utilized.

It was thought that the RUG-II data, with only minor modification, could serve as "core" data. When tasks within a nursing home were examined, there was a hierarchy, with three layers of core data, which had to be satisfied before any application could be developed. The first layer consisted of the name, unique identifying number, and location of a resident. The second included the RUG-II demographics, which were expanded by adding key information from the medical records face sheet. The third was a historical record, which would capture location, financial status, and specific event or relevant transaction (see Table 11.3).

Multiple, task-oriented functions and applications were identified which used this core data, ranging from the actual collection and submission of the PRI for the RUG-II screen, to the generation of an electronic medical records face sheet. Examination of the core data set and individual tasks allowed the introduction of two key concepts: identification of domains and promotion of investment.

A domain is a department, or work group, which has administrative responsibility for a data set. For example, the identification of the Medicare number may start in the social service department, but the ultimate responsibility for the correct identification of the number rests in the business office. The identification of key family members is the responsibility of the social work department. The responsibility for identifying diagnoses is the function of the medical department. Thus, any data element, or groups of elements (data sets) can be identified with a corresponding responsible domain. Such partitioning of a complex database such as the RUG-II system should increase its accuracy.

Table 11.3   Historical Database

Field	Functions
Patient I.D. Number	Social Security or med record
Date (Date field)	Date of transaction
Location (Text)	Room number, building (Operating Certificate)
Transaction (Text)	Initial Admission
	Readmission from hospital
	Readmission from Community
	Room Change
	Discharge with bed hold
	Discharge without bed hold
	Insurance Change
	Diagnosis Change
	Program Change
To/From (Text)	Home
	Hospital (by name)
	Other facility
	Previous room, building
Bed Hold	Private Pay bed hold
	Medicaid bed hold
	Administrative leave
	Facility bed hold
	No bed hold, priority return
	Discharge, no expected return
	Discharge, Death
Insurance Status	Private Pay
	Medicaid
	Medicare
	Other
ICD-9 code	4 fields
ICD-9 (Text)	4 text fields

A single record in the History database will contain all listed fields, with any of the variable functions. For example, a Room Change may or may not be associated with an Insurance Change, Diagnoses Change, and/or Program Change. The Room Change and Insurance Change would be batch updated to the RUG-II databases.

The accuracy of the database can be further enhanced by identifying and promoting investment. Investment is defined as a domain or work group perceiving the accuracy of a data set to be of personal importance. For example, both the nursing department and the medical department share a need for accurate data centering on accidents and incidents. Thus, as a domain is identified, if another domain has investment in the accuracy of the data, formal and informal error checking mechanisms that cross domains can be instituted.

Once domains and investments are identified, data input can be initiated by any work group. The introduction of computer LANs, which require minimal financial investment, force the examination of domains, investment, and, more importantly, the management structure for the database. The LAN allows data elements to be distributed to individual work groups, and thus data elements can be retrieved by domains, independent of other work group involvement. For example, the nursing domain can retrieve the RUG-II data, the social service domain can retrieve the responsible party and family data base, and the medical domain can update significant diagnoses when they occur.

CLINICAL DATA BASES IN NURSING HOMES

A series of functions, listed in Table 11.4, were identified as being linked to potential quality issues in nursing homes. These functions are either mandated by the federal or state regulations which govern nursing homes or impose internal clinical and management requirements. They vary from highly structured functions which include standardized data elements, such as the RUG-II system, to unstructured functions with idiosyncratic data elements, such as the comprehensive care plan. All the functions use segments of the three layers of core data elements, simplifying computerization with a relational data base.

The data elements of utilization review (UR) are indistinguishable from those of the PRI used to submit RUG-II. Thus, these two functions can be managed independently of each other, or can be computer integrated. As the cycles of UR are shorter than those of the RUG-II, this database contains more current information. Depending on the stage of the cycles of these two databases, one can be used to "refresh" the other through batch update procedures. Such an approach avoids redundancy of data input and decreases error rates in the databases.

The records of these functions are either chart specific, for example the comprehensive care plan of a resident, or location specific, for example the filing of accidents and incident reports for review by state inspectors during the annual survey process. Despite being heavily text oriented, some of the functions can be computerized. For example, using a data dictionary (look-up table) that contained 98 key words, accident and incident reports were computerized to allow retrieval by desired resident, nursing unit, or characteristic of an event (Miller, Won, Kollar, Nichols, & Clark, 1988). Similarly, the monthly pharmacy review was computerized and linked to the RUG-II data (Miller, Coblio, Bellnier, & Veneron, 1989).

Within the medical department, a series of partial state-mandated or nonmandated

Table 11.4 Mandated Data Gathering Functions

Function	Data Base Characteristics
PRI Data set	structured, defined data elements
Utilization Review	structured, defined data elements
Minimum Data Set	structured, defined data elements
Pharmacy Review	structured, defined data elements
Staff physician visits	Medicare, limited structure
Physical Therapy	Medicare, limited structure
Comprehensive Care Plan	unstructured, text
Accidents/Incidents	unstructured, text
Clinic visits	partially structured, text
Ancillary Services	partially structured
Infection Control	partially structured
Quality Assurance	variable, partially structured

data-gathering functions can be identified that have quality of care implications, including the capture of physician visits, clinic visits (dentistry, podiatry, ophthalmology, and so forth), and the data generated from ancillary services (laboratory, electrocardiography, radiology, and so forth).

In approaching the computerization of these nonstandardized databases, the key questions are those of overhead (maintenance of the database), functionality (does computerization introduce time saving), and whether there are identifiable gains in patient care in relating these databases to existing ones. Although patient care issues may not be a major factor, management issues may force computerization of these areas. In turn, ad hoc establishment of relationships with other databases with computer queries may lead to identification of patient care issues.

Perhaps the greatest challenge is to link the multiplicity of the actual and potential computerized data elements to the resident's comprehensive care plan. This document must be updated at least quarterly, and after every significant event. For example, transfer of a resident from one level of care to another, a significant medical event, or changes in ADL function, all should lead to review and updating of the plan.

COMPREHENSIVE CARE PLAN

The comprehensive care plan (CCP) is an interdisciplinary document, invariably generated by a team reviewing and focusing on the strengths and impairments of a nursing home resident. It is text oriented, patient specific, and parcels out responsibility and tasks to individual disciplines. The members of the team include dietary, medical (physician, physical therapy, occupational ther-

apy), nursing, recreational therapy, social work, and on occasion pastoral care and mental health staff. Unlike all the other functions and databases listed in Table 9.4, where a single individual extracts data on an encounter form for subsequent computer input, the information for the CCP is generated in a real time mode and in an interreactive fashion. Thus the computerization of the CCP poses both technical and human factors problems.

The integrity of the team is maintained by utilizing overhead projection of the computer screen and choosing a recorder. This allows unimpeded verbal team interaction. Central to the generation of the CCP is the identification of a *Problem* which the team can address. The core data for the computer-maintained problem list is the PRI data set. To this core data, users can add problems (such as sensory impairments or discharge planning) that are not listed in the PRI. This problem list is kept in a look-up table, which is displayed during care planning. The program allows the recorder to check off the problem areas the CCP team wishes to address. Before initiating the CCP, the resident's computer-identified NYQAS triggers are transferred to the resident's problem look-up table from the UR database, forcing the team to either examine the trigger, or override the program by eliminating the problem area from consideration.

Once a *Problem* is identified, user defined look-up tables allow setting of *Objectives*, *Approaches*, and the *Responsible Team* members. The *Approach* is defined (e.g., implement, continue, inactive), the action is dated, and a short space for free text is available. Each resident's CCP is stored in a transaction file, using a tree structure to retrieve the data for analysis and modification. The development of the computer-assisted comprehensive care plan is described by Downey and Hood in Chapter 10.

MINIMUM DATA SET

In 1987, Congress passed the Omnibus Reconciliation Act (OBRA '87) which contained significant new regulations governing nursing homes. The centerpiece of this legislation was the Minimum Data Set (MDS), a compilation of data elements which would introduce uniformity in care planning. The Health Care Financing Administration (HCFA) was charged with developing the MDS and implementing the Congressional mandate.

Based on the Congressional mandate, HCFA contracted to develop the MDS, which was to serve as a uniform resident assessment tool. The experience in developing, validating, and field testing the instrument has been published (Morris, Hawes, Fries, Phillips, Mor, Katz, Murphy, Drugovich, & Friedlob, 1990). Although individual states were given the option of developing variants of the MDS, all fields of the MDS had to be included. New York State opted to add a series of fields to the basic instrument, and this is termed the MDS +. This instrument was implemented by the New York State Health Department in January of 1991.

The MDS has eleven logical groupings covering administrative data, psychosocial functioning, ADL capabilities, nutritional identifiers, specialized services, and others. As in the RUG-II program, the fields are defined and graded either numerically (0 to 4 for ADL function) or in a "yes" or "no" fashion. The MDS is to be completed on admission or readmission of a nursing home resident, following a major health event, and annually. An abbreviated instrument is to be completed quarterly. A workbook has been published which details field definitions (Morris, Hawes, & Murphy, 1990).

The most innovative aspect of the MDS is that specific fields, or groups of fields, will trigger a Resident Assessment Protocol (RAP). Within the information generated by completion of the MDS, there are a total of 18 RAPs, some of which interdigitate with each other. Each RAP carries a statement of the problem, the triggers from the MDS, a set of guidelines, and those areas of the MDS which contain key questions that interdigitate or confound the condition. The guidelines, potential investigations, and possible interventions are detailed in the MDS workbook (Morris, Hawes, & Murphy, 1990).

On the completion of an MDS, the Resident Assessment Protocol Trigger Legend, which is a summary sheet listing the RAPs, is completed. On this sheet, the team preparing the comprehensive care plan lists whether a RAP will be included or excluded from the plan. The surveyors from the State Health Department will focus on the RAPs and utilize them as a key for outcome measures.

The concept of care issues (RAPs) being identified from a standardized encounter form (MDS) parallels the identification of NYQAs from the submitted RUG-II data. Similar to the described RUG-II programs, the data elements of the MDS have been computerized. Algorithms have been designed to computer identify the RAPs, which are then presented for either their inclusion or exclusion in the comprehensive care plan (Guhde, Downey, Carlo, & Miller, 1991).

CONCLUSIONS

Databases in the acute care hospital setting are driven by finances or the needs of individual disciplines. Unlike nursing homes, where the team approach to patient care is emphasized, the acute care setting is fragmented by discipline and specialization, leading to multiple independent databases. Such databases are difficult to integrate as they cross computer platforms and do not achieve common field definition (Mendenhall, 1987).

Although the long-term care setting has features which would prove attractive to explore health care informatics, including low turnover rate, clinical fields which can be narrowly defined, and the ability to longitudinally study cohorts of patients under controlled circumstances, it has escaped the attention of investigators interested in computer use in health care. This is probably related to the fact that most nursing homes are small in size, and their operations can be managed by manual systems.

The introduction of the RUG-II reimbursement system in New York State forced computerization of nursing homes by mandating that the case mix data be electronically submitted. As pointed out by Cotterill (1984), case mix payment systems are inherently more attractive than a flat per diem rate because they do not discriminate against the individual who may consume significant nursing resources by their care needs. The RUG-II data set, or its variants, is being explored as a payment system by both Medicare (Fries, Schneider, & Foley, 1989) and states other than New York. It is apparent that this mechanism of reimbursement will spread (Butler & Schlenker, 1989).

Inherent in all case mix payment systems is the ability to computer identify quality of care issues. As the data can be transmitted electronically, the burden of data input by the regulatory body is obviated. Mandated onsite chart audits ensure accurate submission of the data sets, and computer algorithms check the field integrity of the submitted data prior to storage in the central banks. Thus, a relatively accurate database is available for targeting of quality of care issues.

The incorporation of the RUG-II data set into the comprehensive care plan is an evolving process. OBRA '87 mandated the creation of a Minimum Data Set for care planning in nursing homes. The breadth of this data set, and the practice protocols that it will create will mandate its computerization (Tishman, 1991).

A remarkable parallel exists between the team concept in long-term care and the work group concept fostered by networked computers (Tazelaar, 1988). The centralization of core data at the described nursing homes and their subsequent distribution to members of the team allow individual disciplines to develop their own applications, permit sharing of discipline specific data, and avoid redundancy of data input. The identification of tasks which can be computerized at long-term care facilities, other than those mandated by state or federal agencies, is still in its infancy. The challenge is to integrate these disparate databases for research, management, and quality assurance purposes.

REFERENCES

Butler, P. A., & Schlenker, R. E. (1989). Case-mix for nursing homes: Objectives and achievements. *Milbank Quarterly, 67*, 103–36.

Cotterill, P. G. (1984). Provider incentives under alternative reimbursement systems. In R. J. Vogel & H. C. Palmer (Eds.). *Long term care: Perspectives from research and demonstrations*. Baltimore: Health Care Financing Administration.

Fries, B. E., Schneider, D., & Foley, W. J. (1989). A classification system for medicare patients in skilled nursing facilities: The Resource Utilization Groups (RUG-T18). *Medical Care, 27*, 843–858.

Guhde, R., Downey, E. H., Carlo, S., & Miller, R. P. (1991). Comprehensive care plan. Unpublished manuscript.

Goley, G. F. (1989, April). The dBASE: Who's the fastest gun? *Data Based Advisor*, 52–89.

Lesage, J., & Barhyte, D. H. (1989). *Nursing quality assurance in long-term care*. Gaithersburg, MD: Aspen Systems.

Mendenhall, S. (1987). The ICCS code: A new development for an old problem. In W. W. Stead (Ed.), *Proceedings of the 11th Annual Symposium on Computer Applications in Medical Care*. Washington, DC: IEEE Computer Society Press, pp. 703–709.

Miller, R. P., Coblio, N., Bellnier, T. J., & Veneron, J. P. (1989). Integration of case mix and drug utilization data in the long term care setting. In Lawrence C. Kisland III (Ed.), *Proceedings of the 13th Annual Symposium on Computer Applications in Medical Care*. Washington, DC: IEEE Computer Society Press.

Miller, R. P., & Guhde, R. (1987). Computerization of the Resource Utilization Groups (RUG-II). In W. P. Stead (Ed.), *Proceedings of the 11th Annual Symposium on Computer Applications in Medical Care*. Washington, DC: IEEE Computer Society Press, pp. 710–714.

Miller, R. P., Guhde, R., & Downey, E. H. (1986). Computerization of the Resource Utilization Groups (RUGS) [Abstract]. *Proceedings of the 39th Annual Scientific Meeting of the Gerontology Society of America. The Gerontologist, 26*, 122A.

Miller, R. P., Won T. S., Kollar, M., Nichols A., & Clark, M. (1988). Computerization of incident reports in a nursing home setting [Abstract]. *Proceedings of the 41st Annual Scientific Meeting of the Gerontology Society of America. The Gerontologist, 28*, 172A.

Morris, J. N., Hawes, C., Fries, B. E., Phillips, C. D., Mor, V., Katz, S., Murphy, K., Drugovich, M. L., & Friedlob, A. S. (1990). Design of the national assessment instrument for nursing homes. *The Gerontologist, 30*, 293–307.

Morris, J. N., Hawes, C., & Murphy, K. (1990). *Minimum data set: Resident assessment instrument training manual and resource guide*. Natick, MA: Eliot.

Nichols A., Groupman J., Miller R. P., & Guhde R. (1987). Computerization of the Resource Utilization Groups-II (RUG-II): Nursing implications [Abstract]. *Proceedings of the 40th Annual Scientific Meeting of the Gerontology Society of America. The Gerontologist, 27*, 174A.

Pascal, F. (1989, September). A brave new world? *BYTE*, 247–256.

Schneider, D., Fries, B. E., & Foley, W. J. (1988). Case measurement for nursing home payment: Resource Utilization Groups—(RUG-II). *Health Care Financing Review Annual Supplement*, 39–52.

Tazelaar, J. M. (1988, December). In depth: Groupware. *BYTE*, 242–281.

Tishman, E. (1991). Entering the age of computers. *Provider, 17*, 16–25.

Wilbert, C. C. (1985). Computers: Quality assurance application. In *Quality assurance: A complete guide to effective programs* (207–238). Gaithersburg, MD: Aspen Systems.

Wilson, C. K. (1987). Quality assurance: Should you computerize? *Journal Nursing Quality Assurance, 1* (4), 11–8.

12

Using a Microcomputer Program to Manage Contract Services in a Home Health Agency

Margaret Chalmers
*Frank Brady**

BACKGROUND OF PROBLEM

The authors worked for a voluntary home health agency that provides over one million visits a year, servicing most of the New York City metropolitan area. The volume of needed services has long exceeded the agency's personnel capacity. Therefore, the agency contracts with numerous licensed agencies to provide paraprofessional services to its patients. A cooperative, constructive approach between the manager of the quality assurance department and a consultant programmer resulted in a computerized system to track a specific indicator of quality for services under arrangement. At the time this project was undertaken, the agency was contracting with 25 vendors to provide over 110,000 hours of paraprofessional services weekly. Securing and maintaining updated documentation about the 5,000 or more workers providing these services was the responsibility of the Quality Assurance Department.

In New York State, the department of health is responsible for surveying and regulating the provision of health care services. One area of regulation and monitoring concerns personnel qualifications and health clearances for all workers providing patient care. Any certified agency is required to verify and document that these requirements have been met before accepting a worker for placement from a vendor agency. The required personnel information includes:

- date of employment by vendor
- preemployment check of references
- preemployment physical and annual health assessment
- evidence of immunity to Rubella
- TB (tuberculosis) testing by Mantoux with documented negative result or evidence of chest X-ray and treatment
- worker classification

---

* The authors worked for a large voluntary home health agency in the northeast United States.

113

- worker training and certification (date and type)
- continuing education—mandated at 12 hours per year (dates and hours)
- annual evaluations—professional and administrative

In this agency, the quality assurance department monitors this information by having vendor agencies provide a profile of information on every worker to be placed. This profile outlines the above elements and must be on file with the agency prior to placement of the worker. The department reviews all profiles for completeness and compliance with requirements and periodically audits the source documents on site at the vendor agency. The agency must make this information available on demand to department of health surveyors. In addition, the certified agency is required to make its system of monitoring available to the state at survey time.

The quality assurance department had developed a manual system for maintaining this information on the more than 5,000 worker profiles. As workers and qualifying information about them would change, new forms were submitted to the quality assurance department. The process of both reviewing and filing this information became very labor intensive due to a regular volume of between 250 and 300 forms received weekly. Since it was not feasible to summarize the data manually, the system did not provide a ready reference for agency use or for surveyors auditing the agency.

DESCRIPTION OF PROJECT

The quality assurance department made the decision to automate the flow and tracking of personnel profiles. The objectives of automation were to: (1) minimize paper filing and handling, (2) organize profile data in a discrete form in order to make information readily accessible, (3) provide an up-to-date list of information on file, and (4) provide other agency personnel with a list of qualified workers.

Background

The options available to quality assurance were to buy an existing system, develop a system in-house, have the current manager of the department develop a system, or hire a consultant to develop the system. A review of available software failed to uncover any programs that would meet the needs of the department and the agency.

Existing Software

While a limited computerized system for tracking some paraprofessional placements was available, this system could not accommodate the detail and volume required by quality assurance. As is true in many large agencies, the information systems are elaborate and handle the flow of data, particularly as it relates to billing and reimbursement. It was decided that this was not an option for the quality assurance department because the paper burden and regulatory needs were too pressing to wait.

Develop an In-house System with Agency Resources

The agency has a large information systems department, but it was decided not to use that resource because: (1) the MIS department was involved with the maintenance and redesigning of the agency's overall mainframe and information systems, (2) MIS lacked uncommitted resources, and (3) using the information systems staff would mean a large time requirement for the manager of the quality assurance department to instruct the information systems staff on all the facets of the monitoring process for services under arrangement.

Quality Assurance Manager to Develop System

Another option that small agencies or small departments in larger agencies often adopt is to have the "noncomputer" manager or staff develop their own computer application. Even for a computer-literate manager, this would involve a great deal of precious management time. In this case the manager would have had to spend many hours learning the programming language as well as developing the system. Therefore, this was not viewed as a viable option; the loss of management time could not be afforded.

Hire a Consultant

The final option, and the one chosen, was to hire a consultant to develop the program. While planning to hire someone, they explored the option of farming out the entire project to a programmer and waiting for the completed product. This option had a significant drawback. The manager would not be involved in the design phase and therefore would lose control of the process.

Generally, the professional, or responsible party provides the overall design of a project. The professional has the ultimate knowledge of how the system will help and the responsibility to accomplish the identified goals. Although the basic needs of what the system *should* do were clear, the potential of the system for streamlining related tasks was not yet apparent. That would have to wait for more specific information on what the system *could* provide.

The decision was made to use a consultant

programmer with extensive experience in home health care to work collaboratively with the manager of the quality assurance department throughout the process of development and implementation. This would allow the manager of quality assurance to retain conceptual control throughout. It also allowed for ongoing refinement of the program design as the project moved forward.

Hardware Decisions

The decision was made to develop the program for use on existing hardware in the quality assurance department. This would enable the system to function economically but it highlighted the antiquity of the existing IBM PC. The personal computer had been in place for several years and had two low-density floppy disk drives and an old, slow, dot matrix printer. In order to control costs, a simple upgrade of the personal computer was made by adding a hard disk drive adequate to the anticipated memory storage needs of the system. No immediate action was taken to replace the printer. It was felt that once the system began to operate, it would be easier to justify the cost of upgrading the printer.

Software Decisions

In order to develop a program that could be maintained by management personnel it was decided to write the program in dBase III+ by Ashton-Tate. This program allows the user to create individualized reports and provides an assistive mode to help with tasks such as data query.

It also allows for global changes in the data structure and programming. This was an important factor since it provided for flexibility and made future changes to the database possible without major rewriting of the software.

The development of the system began with several joint meetings between the staff of the quality assurance department and the consultant programmer. The goal of these early meetings was for the programmer to fully understand the operation of the current system. This process was facilitated by the fact that the programmer had many years of experience in various home care agency settings tracking and reviewing the state-mandated information. The meetings also served to begin to focus the quality assurance staff on the specifics of their current system and to think about ways that the computer system would best meet their needs.

Software Design

The most important thing the program could do was to generate a list of workers on whom the quality assurance department had received and accepted a complete profile of information.

The computer system would be used to track whether a given worker had been cleared for placement; in other words, the system tracked whether information on a file was correct. The quality assurance staff would continue to review the profile to determine whether the information about the worker was complete and met the basic requirements. In addition, they would decide when that information would become out of date and set that date as a "tickler" to trigger the system. After review and acceptance of a worker's profile by quality assurance, the worker would be "logged" into the system.

A systematic analysis of any system to be computerized must first focus on what is to be the end product, or the "outputs." In this case, the outputs were the reports, worksheets, and file control data sheets that the staff would need to keep the information accessible and meaningful. The programmer worked with the staff to determine what the specific outputs needed in order to design a program that included the specific inputs.

Each desired output required the "input" of fields of information. Table 12.1 demonstrates how the need for each data element was established.

Table 12.1 The Relationship between Input and Output

desired OUTPUTS	needed INPUT (Fields)
Alphabetical list of all workers	1. Worker last name 2. Worker first name
List of all workers by agency	3. Agency name 4. Office code
List of "OK" or "NOT OK" workers	5. Date when information "NOT OK" 6. Active or not 7. Date not active 8. "Do Not Use" status 9. Date of DNU status
A unique number identifies worker	10. Social Security 11. Worker type
Where is paper record?	12. Document Control Number 13. Input date

Initial development of the program involved a joint decision by the programmer and staff as to what the content of each of these outputs would be. These discussions led to the selection of the fields of data for each record in the system. A decision on what each field should contain determined the type and size of each field.

Usage—"Fine Tuning"

During program development ongoing meetings were held to review the developing programs and identify areas of questions or problems. During these discussions staff indicated they would enter data on paraprofessionals in batches, one agency at a time. It was because of this that it was decided to store the information from each of the then 22 different vendors in its own unique file. This would also facilitate and speed access to the records. Later developments provided further support for this decision. Several agencies changed names or restructured, and this then required only minor changes to the program. The flexibility to accomplish these changes quickly was a direct result of careful planning and continual communication between users and the programmer.

There were other programming decisions which were also made jointly by the programmer and the department manager. One such decision was to include a report that would list workers whose information would be outdated within two months of "today." This provided an easy control and worklist for the quality assurance department as well as a convenient reference for the vendor agencies involved. Another need was to provide for a simple method of backing up the information to floppy diskettes each day and determine when "old" records were to be deleted. It was apparent that a paper trail would need to be established so that each

Code	Selection
V	Select paraprof vendor agency
A	Select professional vendor agency
E	Enter data—select a vendor first
L	Look up Social Security # on worker
P	Put on Reference Registry or terminate worker
R	Reports on Para-professional workers
X	Reports on Professional workers
U	Utilities
D	Return to dBase
Q	Quit program and dBase

Enter your choice (type in the code):—

Figure 12.1 Home Care–Quality Assurance Main Menu for Vendor Program.

profile and reference in it could be tracked throughout the office.

A menu-based program was written that allowed for rapid data entry, as indicated in Figure 12.1. Every effort was made to prefill information whenever possible to reduce duplication of keyboard inputs. In addition, the program was designed to automatically check each entry against a list of workers whose past performance had led the agency to determine they would not be rehired. This was a major advantage of automation as this step had previously been manual and was made immensely faster and more effective by the program.

Modifying the Design

Further, it became obvious that during a routine day quality assurance staff would often have to look up workers' records to confirm they were on file and current. The addition of a simple "look-up" feature to the program quickly increased its popularity with staff and offered real time savings. This feature provided for quick access to important information to other quality assurance staff who otherwise would have to request a manual check of the extensive files, or do so themselves.

IMPLEMENTATION AND TRAINING

Once the program was completed it was installed on the hard drive, and the business staff of the quality assurance department was trained by the programmer. The initial input involved large numbers of profiles that had been received during program development. This had been considered in the plan for implementing the system. What had not been planned for was the extent and impact of staff resistance to the new system.

Resistance

Despite considerable thought, planning, and attempts to anticipate all problems, the programmer and department manager did not fully anticipate the resistance of the business staff to automation. Despite verbal statements that they would welcome it, the business staff strongly resisted the system's implementation. One of the major reasons for this was their anticipated loss of control.

The business staff virtually controlled all access to these essential files under the manual system. The very cumbersome and time consuming qualities that were the hallmark of the manual system were just those that caused a heavy reliance on these staff to maintain and retrieve the information as needed. The very purpose of the computer system, to speed and ease access to this body of information, was about to eliminate the control in which these staff were highly invested. To the staff involved, this was a time saver but also a threat to job security.

All staff resist changes in their work, particularly automation. It has been well documented that morale tends to drop immediately after implementation of a computerized system (Romanczyk, 1985). However, this normal drop in morale was complicated by serious resistance on the part of a central worker. The rearrangement of office responsibilities because of this automation and other changes taking place, led to a high turnover of business staff in the department. Each change of workers further delayed the full implementation of the system. Whereas the original plan called for phase-in and initial entry of all current data within one month, it in fact took four months.

The plan had been to generate a list of all workers for each vendor agency within one month and send these lists to the vendors for confirmation and updating. Because of the delay in establishing the initial database this was not done until eight months from the start of implementation. This part of the process required that someone communicate directly with each of the vendors and help them understand and respond to the new system. It was during this time that the department manager also left (for unrelated reasons) and was not replaced for several months. This led to further delays in follow-up with the vendors.

OUTCOMES

The original automation plan has been implemented. Although the evaluation of any change must be an ongoing process, some evaluations of objectives are listed below:

Objective One

The first objective, to minimize paper handling, had been met. Instead of having to alphabetize and file the 250–300 profiles it processed each week, the staff review them, log them into the computer, and then file them in the same order in which they have been entered. Not having to retrieve and associate old forms and then refile alphabetically has significantly cut down on paper handling time.

Objective Two

The information is organized and readily accessible to many more agency employees. Staff can access the program in seconds to determine whether required information about a worker is on file and current. In addition, several reports, produced on demand by the computer system, serve to facilitate communication with contract vendors. Agency staff can now keep the vendors informed of the need for updated information. This eliminated the need for duplicate forms and information which had been the hallmark of the old paper system.

Objective Three

The list of qualified paraprofessionals does now exist. Making it available to other agency personnel to use in making worker placements is currently a part of a major project undertaken by the agency's MIS department. That department is now working to access the information organized as a result of the original project into a mainframe system.

Objective Four

Not only will this allow for online, automatic checking of orders entered for paraprofessional service, but it will eventually extend to the vendors themselves, allowing them direct entry of their data in the personnel database. These features, the next logical steps in automating the information at hand, are possible because the problem has already been clearly defined and the path to its resolution by automation has been paved.

CONCLUSIONS AND RECOMMENDATIONS

The writers have presented a description of the cooperative effort that took place to develop a computer program to assist in tracking information in a large, certified home health agency. The process of manager and consultant programmer working together took time but resulted in the joint development of a program to assist with the handling of voluminous information. The incremental process used gave the staff and consultant numerous opportunities to make adjustments and customize the program. This has resulted in a program that meets many of the needs of the quality assurance department.

Computerization of a process only automates the flow of work. It does not actually do the work for the agency. It is essential to invest in managerial and staff time during program development in order to maximize the effectiveness of any computer system. This joint effort demonstrates one excellent method for accomplishing this end.

It is recommended that other agencies and organizations use the collaborative model to solve their computing needs. Particular attention needs to be paid to developing the working relationships between health care workers and managers and the growing field of consultant programmers.

REFERENCES

Romanczyk, R. G. (1985). A case study of micro-computer utilization and staff efficiency: A five year analysis. In L. W. Frederiksen, & A. W. Riley (Eds.), *Computers, people & productivity* (pp. 141–154). New York: Haworth.

13

Nursing Software: Develop Your Own

Arlene Smaldone
Carol Greenberg

INTRODUCTION

In the past ten years there has been great advancement in the use of computer technology by the health care industry. In the early 1980s only large tertiary care institutions utilized computer systems for patient care activities such as admission/discharge/transfer, order entry, results reporting, and management of financial data. Today a much larger percentage of hospitals use these systems as part of everyday operations. Even with this computer revolution well under way, nursing is still often one of the last departments to reap the benefits of automation.

University Hospital at Stony Brook was in a unique position when it opened in 1980. The hospital had purchased an IBM mainframe system and was prepared for the automation of many hospital functions. Educational programs were developed to prepare staff unfamiliar with this technology to use the system. Nurses learned how to enter orders and retrieve lab data while they continued to document their practice using handwritten notes, care plans, and flow sheets. As hospital services expanded, staff began to recognize that computers could offer them assistance with their routine functions. Nursing care plans were selected as the first component of documentation to be automated at University Hospital. It was hoped that automation would improve documentation compliance by making it easier for the nurse to develop an individualized care plan for her patients.

The purpose of this chapter is to describe the steps in both making the decision to develop an automated care planning system rather than purchase a commercial system and its subsequent development and implementation at University Hospital at Stony Brook.

THE UNIVERSITY HOSPITAL EXPERIENCE

In March 1985 the deputy director of nursing appointed a small committee and charged the members with the responsibility of recommending either purchase or in-house development of a care planning software package. Armed with an idea of what was needed, and tempered by reality, the committee conducted a literature search. Publications about automated care planning systems were extremely limited and none described the development process or use of self-developed systems. Funding for long distance site visits to evaluate existing systems was not in the budget. Instead, telephone surveys were used to gather information about existing systems, including their documentation framework, were they menu driven, what was their light pen availability, ratio of terminals per nurse and per patient, terminal location on nursing unit, how much competition was there for use of terminal and what was their percent of downtime. In addition, local site visits were made to similar teaching institutions which were using automated systems for nursing documentation functions.

The committee established criteria for evaluation of care planning software features: (1) compatibility with the existing hospital mainframe system, (2) contemporary documentation nomenclature through utilization of nursing diagnosis, (3) evidence of nursing process logic governing system flow, and (4) integration of discharge planning and patient education activities. After completing the review of existing software, none met each of the initial requirements. Nursing administration accepted the committee's final recommendation to develop an in-house automated care planning system.

INVESTIGATION

Examining and investigating the universe of nursing software is only as beneficial as one's ability to critically identify, assess, and evaluate the systems under which an institution presently functions. This includes not only the institution's hardware and software systems, but also its philosophy of nursing, present documentation format, and state regulations that govern its documentation.

Define Minimum System Requirements

Institutional needs are determined through analysis of the present documentation system and examination of manual chart forms. The following questions define minimum system requirements. When must care plans be written? How frequently must they be reviewed and updated? How much of this information is required as a permanent part of the patient care record? Must the names of all nurses interacting with the plan as well as the date of the interaction be stored in computer memory? How long following patient discharge should the plan remain online? What is the patient turnover and return rate? How acutely ill are those patients? How many patient problems are identified through care planning and what is the length of each care plan? Evaluate hospital-approved documentation nomenclature and care planning format. Compilation of this information determines whether to automate the present system or improve upon it through computer capabilities.

Research Regulatory Agency Requirements

Health care regulatory agency requirements also affect ultimate decisions. Review state and local regulations. Validity of the electronic signature in a court of law may be viewed differently from state to state, and there have been few if any legal precedents set.

Patient confidentiality mandates that user access to information stored in hospital computer systems be well defined. Registered nurses are the health care professionals who document plans of care in the format of a nursing care plan. They should have exclusive access to the care planning system. This requires that one level of the computer access code differentiate the registered nurse from other system users.

Software Shopping

When need is great and enthusiasm for change high, it is very easy to fall into the "impulse buy" trap. Software packaging and presentation can be deceptive. "What you see may or may not be what you get." The more information one has before beginning to investigate, the better consumer and decision maker he or she will be.

It is important to collect vendor-specific information and to keep these facts well-organized. Trying to make decisions based on informal anecdotes and recollections is not helpful. Develop an outline for each member of the search committee to use while previewing each vendor's system. Is the software compatible with your system? Is the system menu driven? Is there light pen capability? Is there free text entry? How much? Is it optional or required? Is the information easily retrievable? Is a programmer needed to change statements? How much does the software cost? What is included in that cost? What is the cost for system updates and maintenance? Ask for a demonstration. Try the system yourself. Is screen flow logical? Is information well-organized on each screen? This cache of information will be your basis for comparison (see Table 13.1). Sound decision making will benefit your institution both financially and from a quality assurance and risk management perspective.

Table 13.1   Software Shopping Checklist

I	**PRODUCT NAME:** VENDOR:

II	**SYSTEM FEATURES:**
	 —Selection of options
	   —menu driven
	   —light pen
	   —touch screens
	 —Free text entry
	   —how much
	   —where
	   —optional/required
	 —Ease of use
	 —Screen directions clear
	 —Screen flow logical
	 —Information well organized on each screen
	 —Customized by area of nursing practice
	 —Ease of content updating
	 —Compatibility with present system

III	**NURSING PRACTICE ISSUES:** —Discharge planning —Patient education —Measurable patient outcomes —Nursing process logic —Potential use as QA/reseach tool

IV	**COST:**
	 —What's included in purchase price
	   —staff inservice–who/for how long
	   —institution customization
	 —Updating/maintenance of software
	 —Additional hardware to support use of system

V	**DID YOU USE SYSTEM OR WAS IT A DEMO**
VI	**OTHER HOSPITALS WHICH USE THIS SYSTEM:** —Contact persons

DEVELOPMENT

Development of a nursing application such as patient care planning requires concurrent effort in two areas: system design and nursing content. It is also necessary to closely examine actual practice using the handwritten system. This captures a baseline upon which effectiveness of the new automated system can be evaluated. The systems liaison nurse is more likely to make factual rather than intuitive decisions regarding design specifications when exploration of content occurs early in the development phase. It is the integration of content with system design which yields the final software product.

System Design

Close collaboration of nurses with data processing colleagues is required in order to formulate system design specifications for the proposed system. In designing a computer system, consideration needs to be given to the following: (1) algorithm development, (2) determination of field lengths for components stated in the algorithm, (3) estimation of the extent of memory allocation, (4) determination of how the nurse will use the system, (5) screen design, (6) plan for system maintenance and updating, and (7) development of a coding scheme for choices within the system.

Algorithm Development. A computer algorithm is used to direct screen flow in the automated system. The effort spent in algorithm development is critical to the ultimate success of the new system because it will govern system logic for the user. The desire to make the flow of the care planning consistent with the premise that nursing intervention is directed toward resolution or amelioration of the cause of the patient's problem determined the need for a relationship file in the Stony Brook automated care planning system. Use of this relationship file enables the systems nurse to configure choices for nursing intervention strategies dependent upon selection of a "re-

lated to" option for completion of the nursing diagnosis statement.

Field Length. Each component of the algorithm must be assigned a field length or maximum number of characters for that component. A care planning system requires decisions about the following field lengths: nursing diagnosis name, "related to" statement, nursing intervention, intervention frequency, patient outcome, time frame for achievement of patient outcome, and "qualifiers" or free text descriptors for both nursing interventions and patient outcome choices. It is helpful to map out field lengths on graph paper to visualize their impact on content development, user comfort, and documentation adequacy prior to making final field-length decisions.

Memory Allocation. The programmer and systems liaison nurse must estimate the need for computer memory allocation for the proposed system. It is in this area where nurse system developers may discover differences in their thought process as compared with those of the programmer. System programmers raise questions to determine the average length of a care plan and average number of nursing diagnoses per plan to determine impact of the new function upon the working of the system as a whole. They expect concrete answers because there is a direct relationship between extent of memory allocation and system response time. Nurses recognize the need for precision, but may have no ready answers to the programmer's questions. The fact that University Hospital at Stony Brook is a tertiary care facility and provides services to patients with a high level of acuity provided the basis for our answers. After examining the types of patient care issues throughout the hospital, it was estimated that the average number of nursing diagnoses would be approximately five per patient and each diagnosis would have an average of 15 nursing interventions.

The length of time a care plan remains online for immediate retrieval is also a consideration in the allocation of computer memory. A decision was made to store care plans online for the six months following a patient's discharge from University Hospital. This would allow adequate time to foster system utilization for retrospective nursing research and quality assurance studies. At the end of this period, the care plan is downloaded to tape and can be retrieved upon request from the information services department.

Nurse Utilization. System design needs to incorporate features which promote both efficient use of the nurse's time in creating a care plan and selection of appropriate choices for that plan. Keyboarding free text entry is kept to a minimum in the Stony Brook system. The system is designed with light pen selectable menus in order to achieve this. Each menu item has the option to be "qualified" and nursing intervention frequencies added. The number of screen flips for nursing intervention choices within any one nursing diagnosis would not be greater than three. This limits the number of nursing intervention choices per "related to" to a maximum of 45.

Nursing diagnosis categories are applicable to all patient populations and areas of nursing practice. Certain patient populations may have unique reasons why they might be at risk for or develop a problem. Specialty databases are built into the system for "related tos," nursing interventions, and patient outcomes to deal with the unique concerns of different patient populations. There are a total of seven subspecialty databases reflecting the uniqueness of nursing practice within the tertiary care setting. Each database is shared by multiple patient care units.

Screen Design. Screen design guides the user through the system maze, informs him or her of present location within the system, and directs him or her to subsequent sequences. Basic principles of screen design are incorporated throughout the Stony Brook care planning system:

1. Place brief directions on each screen. This alerts the nurse to the task at hand.
2. Format each screen in the same manner. The use of headers and footers give inner consistency to the system. In the Stony Brook care planning system "footers" are light pen selectable choices. Directions such as "return," "enter," "view more interventions," and "continue" are placed in the same location on each screen.
3. Avoid content overcrowding. Screens that are too "busy" are overwhelming to the user.

When a nurse logs onto the computer, the system recognizes who the nurse is from the unique system ID and password. This assigns accountability for the plan. The unit location of the work station being activated designates the subspecialty database which is displayed for care plan choices. In unusual circumstances, for example, when an adult patient is admitted to a pediatric unit, the nurse has the option to override this default database by choosing "Select New Specialty Area" from the care planning master menu (see Figure 13.1). This complex relationship between subspecialty database and relationship files is transparent to the user but serves well in providing sound choices for review and selection.

Plan for System Maintenance and Updating. The care planning system developed at Stony Brook utilizes both hard coding and dynamic display programming formats. Hard-coded screens are fixed or permanent screens or

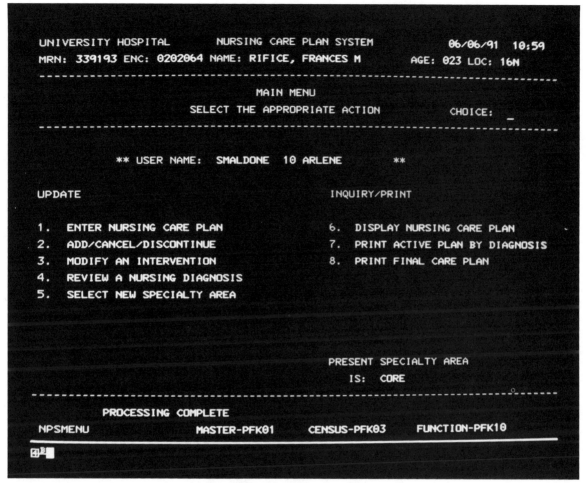

Figure 13.1   Main menu of the Care Planning System. Upon entry into the system, the user name is identified and the default database determined.

screen components. They may only be changed by a member of the programming staff. This format is used for master menus, directions, and headers and footers. This type of programming technique is not optimal for nursing content choices within the system which may need updating on a regular basis. Dynamic display is used for this purpose. The nursing system coordinator has the ability to make content updates directly into production as needed by using the care

planning relationship file database (see Figure 13.2).

Upon implementation of the system at University Hospital, nursing policy and procedure was instituted to provide for review and updating of each subspecialty database every two years. If an aspect of nursing practice changes within this period or the hospital begins to serve a new group of patients, content changes can be entered at any point in time prior to the designated two-year up-

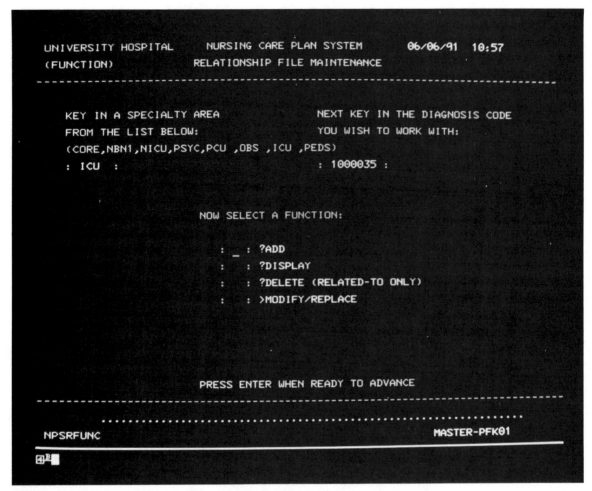

Figure 13.2 Updating the Care Planning System.

date. A unique security identification and password is assigned to the systems liaison nurse to access system maintenance functions. Accessing the maintenance system enables the systems nurse to issue code numbers to new database elements through their entry into the master file and assign these database elements to the appropriate relationship files in various subspecialty databases. (See Figure 13.3.)

Coding Scheme. Coding is an important consideration for long-range utilization of data within the system. One can learn a great deal from entries made into a nursing documentation system if they are retrievable in flexible ways. When developing a coding scheme one needs to be visionary. How will the institution wish to use this kind of information in quality assurance monitoring or in nursing research?

Each data element is uniquely coded within the Stony Brook system. The code identifies the following about each element: (1) its classification as a diagnosis, "related to," intervention, or patient outcome, (2) whether the element is universal through nursing practice or tagged to a specialty

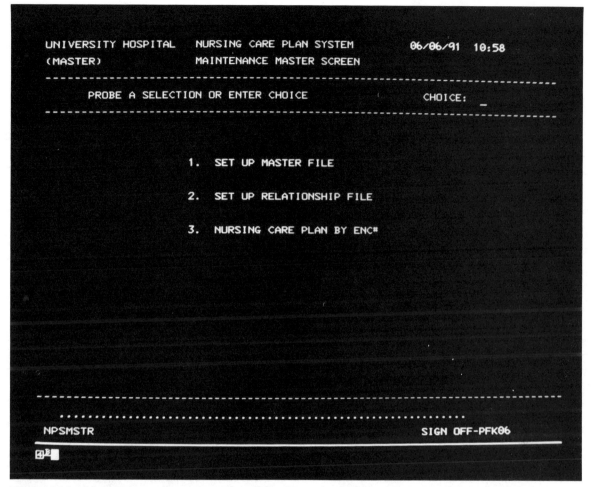

UNIVERSITY HOSPITAL   NURSING CARE PLAN SYSTEM   06/06/91 10:58
(MASTER)   MAINTENANCE MASTER SCREEN
- -
    PROBE A SELECTION OR ENTER CHOICE   CHOICE: _
- -

        1.   SET UP MASTER FILE

        2.   SET UP RELATIONSHIP FILE

        3.   NURSING CARE PLAN BY ENC#

NPSMSTR   SIGN OFF-PFK06

Figure 13.3   Master menu for assignment of database elements and incorporation of elements into the Care Planning Databases.

database, and (3) its sequential number within the classification. The intervention "Monitor intake/output" is considered universal to nursing practice and is a documentation choice on all nursing care units. It is assigned a prefix code which identifies it as an intervention statement and a service code which designates it as a component of the universal nursing database. The computer then assigns an ordinal number which identifies the element within its classification. The integration of these three coding components becomes the unique code number for

that database element. Each component has its own importance and needs to be determined based on institutional goals, philosophy of nursing and long-term plan for utilization of the nursing database which the system will create.

Content Development

In preparation for using the computer to document nursing care plans utilizing a nursing diagnosis framework, a "Nursing Diagnosis Reference Guide" was added to the University Hospital Information System (UHIS) Help Screen Index. The guide serves as a ready reference tool for staff and standardizes the meaning of each diagnostic category within the institution. Each guide consists of a category definition, a list of contributing factors which place the patient at risk for problem development and a list of defining characteristics or signs and symptoms of the problem itself (see Figure 13.4). Although staff were still using a manual care

plan system they could begin to associate care planning activities with the computer. Use of the reference guide helped them to become more familiar with the terminology which would be used in the automated care planning system. The information in this guide also served as a foundation for development of "related to" choices for each diagnostic category in the developing system.

A prototype of system content for nursing interventions and patient outcomes was developed following review of the care plan-

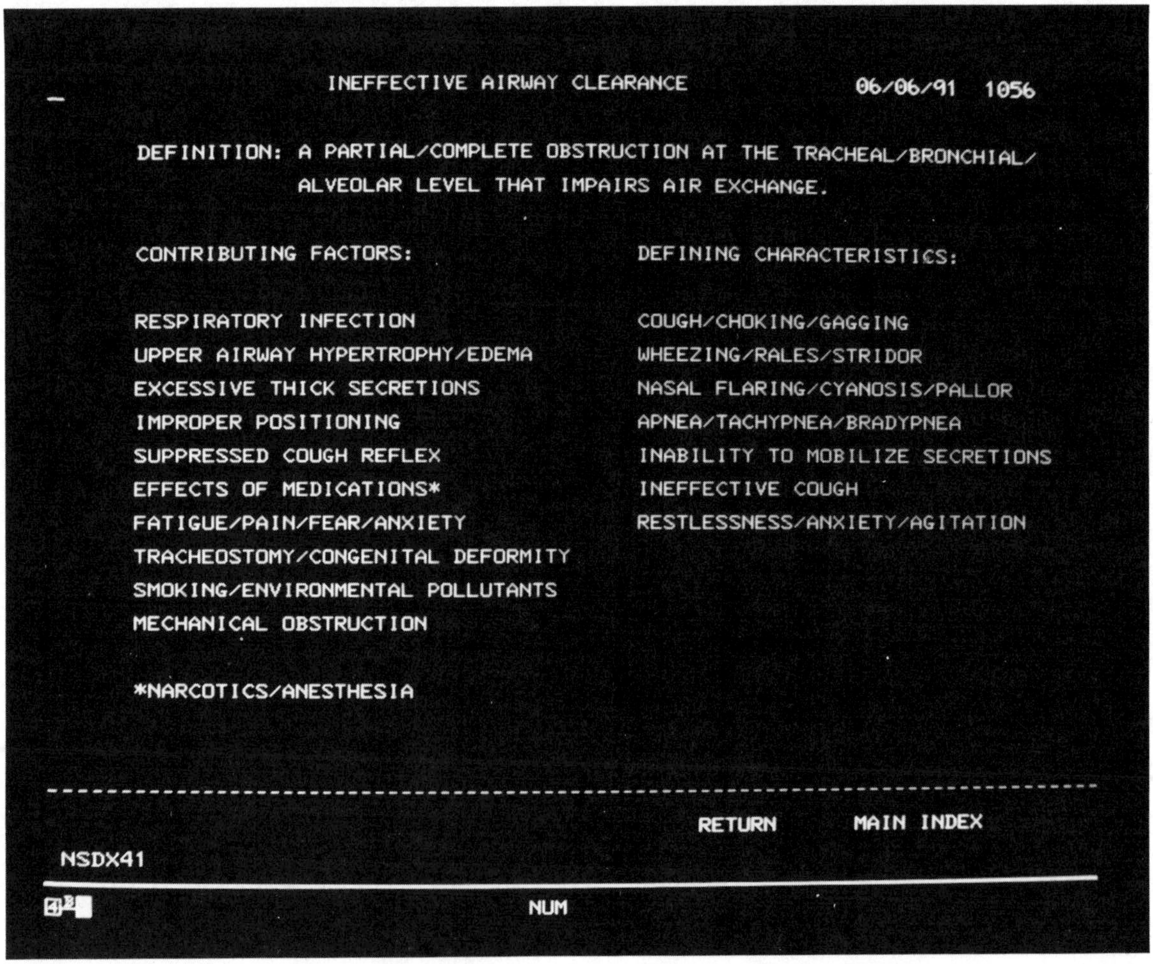

INEFFECTIVE AIRWAY CLEARANCE   06/06/91 1056

DEFINITION: A PARTIAL/COMPLETE OBSTRUCTION AT THE TRACHEAL/BRONCHIAL/
            ALVEOLAR LEVEL THAT IMPAIRS AIR EXCHANGE.

CONTRIBUTING FACTORS: DEFINING CHARACTERISTICS:

RESPIRATORY INFECTION   COUGH/CHOKING/GAGGING
UPPER AIRWAY HYPERTROPHY/EDEMA   WHEEZING/RALES/STRIDOR
EXCESSIVE THICK SECRETIONS   NASAL FLARING/CYANOSIS/PALLOR
IMPROPER POSITIONING   APNEA/TACHYPNEA/BRADYPNEA
SUPPRESSED COUGH REFLEX   INABILITY TO MOBILIZE SECRETIONS
EFFECTS OF MEDICATIONS*   INEFFECTIVE COUGH
FATIGUE/PAIN/FEAR/ANXIETY   RESTLESSNESS/ANXIETY/AGITATION
TRACHEOSTOMY/CONGENITAL DEFORMITY
SMOKING/ENVIRONMENTAL POLLUTANTS
MECHANICAL OBSTRUCTION

*NARCOTICS/ANESTHESIA

                                      RETURN   MAIN INDEX

NSDX41

                              NUM

Figure 13.4 Nursing diagnosis reference guide.

ning literature. A draft of proposed menu choices for each nursing diagnosis category was printed on graph paper to conform to system field-length specifications. This tested the adequacy of field-length allocations to operationalize the content. This content prototype was distributed to clinical service committees to review and make recommendations for revision. The coordinators of these various groups met with the nurse system developers on a regular basis to review incorporation of their recommendations into either a subspecialty or universal database and development progress as a whole. Often wording of similar ideas for nursing intervention statements needed to be negotiated by this group in order to avoid redundancy within the care plan master file. This would be invaluable later on, when using the system for nursing research.

IMPLEMENTATION

The implementation phase equals the development phase in expenditure of time and energy. It sets the stage and lays the groundwork for a smooth, successful transition from a newly developed concept to a working, productive tool.

Pilot Unit

You have diligently checked your software in the test situation and worked out any system "bugs" which have been identified. Despite this fact, you need a pilot unit in which to monitor the program in a live situation. The pilot unit is a site for testing programming and screen flow for quirks and provides an opportunity for nurses not involved in system development to evaluate its usability in the clinical setting. Select your pilot unit carefully. A positive management influence

and willingness of staff to participate are key factors to consider in making this selection.

Implementation Plan

The newborn nursery was chosen as the pilot unit to test the new care planning system at University Hospital at Stony Brook. The nursery content choices are a small subset of the total content database because of the limited realm of patient problems experienced by well newborns. By selecting this unit, programming could be checked and an educational program developed before the total content database was completed. There were fewer staff members in the nursery compared to other units. Computer terminals were easily accessible and had minimal competition for use. Their location on the unit permitted staff to observe the infants while working at the work station.

Documentation of written care plans in the newborn nursery had been limited. Essentially, well-baby care was documented on preprinted forms, signed by the nurse and placed in the chart by the unit clerk. Identification of patient problems using nursing diagnosis needed to be addressed as a component of the educational process for this group of nurses. A list of nursing diagnoses and their equivalent infant care labels was developed to keep near each terminal to assist staff in their transition to the use of nursing diagnosis. Care of the circumcised infant would be identified as an Alteration in Comfort and/or Impairment of Skin Integrity. Bonding concerns would be addressed as an Alteration in Parenting. Feeding problems and interventions would be labeled an Alteration in Nutrition.

An automated system can be technically wonderful but if it is not used for the purpose intended it is neither successful nor effective. Making the function useful and needed by the staff nurse will help to increase staff receptivity. The care plan must be presented as a usable tool. There must be discussions about how the care plan can be incorporated into practice as a guide to the shift report, as a reference when writing progress notes, and as an indispensable tool to carry out patient care activities. The care plan becomes the all important vehicle to facilitate improved communication, consistent care and accurate documentation. If you learn to rely on the plans, you have given them value and purpose. If you cannot practice effectively without them, compliance and quality will naturally improve.

EVALUATION

The automated documentation function has been implemented. Is it successful? Has the documentation of nursing practice changed? Was the past few years' endeavor worth the effort? Preautomation data has been kept in abeyance. It is now time to collect postautomation data to make some comparisons.

Preautomation Study

Five months prior to initiation of the automated care planning function a study was conducted at University Hospital at Stony Brook to examine staff compliance with the documentation policy for nurse care planning. One medical unit, one surgical unit and one pediatric unit were selected as study sites to obtain a window of nursing care planning compliance within the hospital. Twenty current hospital records were reviewed monthly for a period of four months (April through July, 1987) on each of the study units. Patients hospitalized for less than 72 hours were excluded from this study. Each record was reviewed using an 18 criteria data collection instrument. A total of 232 records were reviewed in the preautomation phase. Nursing care plans were present in 150 (64.6%) of the records reviewed. Examination of these 150 plans in detail revealed that 13 (8.7%) plans had been reviewed within the past 72 hours (hospital policy at that time). The plans addressed a total of 415 nursing diagnoses for a preautomation average of 2.76 per patient. Individual unit results are illustrated in Table 13.2.

Postautomation Study

Following implementation, each unit was followed on a monthly basis to determine the impact of automation on care planning activities. A total of 840 records were reviewed from the three units selected for the pre-

Table 13.2 Nursing Care Plans Preautomation

Unit	Sample	Care Plans Present		Care Plans Reviewed		Diagnoses/Patient Plan	
		Number	Percent	Number	Percent	Number	Percent
Medicine	80	43	(53.8)	5	(11.6)	125	(2.9)
Surgery	80	62	(77.5)	4	(6.4)	216	(3.48)
Specialty	72	45	(62.5)	4	(8.8)	74	(1.64)
Total	232	150	(64.6)	13	(8.7)	415	(2.76)

automation study. Hospital policy regarding frequency of review of nursing care plans had changed from seventy two to twenty four hours; therefore, those hospitalized less than 24 hours were excluded in the postautomation phase of the study.

Study Unit Results. Nursing care plans were present in 787 (93.7%) of the 840 patient records reviewed, an increase of 29.1%. Because the system uses nursing diagnosis as a framework, 100% of the patient problems were identified using a complete diagnostic statement. 592 (75.2%) of the 787 patient plans had been reviewed within the past twenty four hours, an increase of 66.5% despite the increased frequency of required review. Of added interest is the fact that not only did an increased number of patients have a nursing care plan present but those plans also addressed more patient problems. The 150 preautomation plans addressed a mean number of 2.76 problems per care plan whereas the 787 postautomation plans from the same three study units addressed a mean number of 3.7 problems per plan thus making the automated care plan a more comprehensive document as well. Direct comparison of each study unit postimplementation of the automated system may be seen in Table 13.3. The study did not include discontinued problems in the nursing care plan

which had been resolved by the nurse during the course of the patient's hospitalization.

Hospitalwide Results. Records of 4376 patients from 26 inpatient units were studied over a period of 18 months in the postimplementation phase. Records of 3908 patients (89.3%) had a nursing care plan present. Nurses reviewed 2383 (77.49%) plans within 24 hours. The average number of nursing diagnoses per patient plan was 3.38. In October, 1989 a spot audit was conducted on the entire hospital census, excluding patients admitted within the previous 24 hours, to determine whether the improvement in documentation of the nursing care plan had been sustained. Upon examination of 414 patient records, 356 (85.9%) patients had a nursing care plan present, 269 (75%) plans had been reviewed during the previous 24 hours and the average number of nursing diagnoses per plan was 3.12. We conclude from this data that nursing behavior regarding documentation of the nursing care plan has changed in a positive manner and has been incorporated into the practice of nurses at University Hospital.

The opportunity to develop a computerized documentation system challenges the nurse to critically analyze what exists, modify components that don't work well, and communicate specifications to system ana-

Table 13.3   Nursing Care Plans Postautomation

Unit	Sample	Care Plans Present		Care Plans Reviewed		Diagnoses/Patient Plan	
		Number	Percent	Number	Percent	Number	Percent
Medicine	290	279	(96.2)	226	(81)	925	(3.3)
Surgery	408	388	(95)	272	(70.2)	1733	(4.47)
Specialty	142	120	(84.5)	94	(78.3)	250	(2.08)
Total	840	787	(93.7)	592	(75.2)	2908	(3.7)

lysts who are unfamiliar with the nursing process. In good working relationships, the nurse becomes more sensitive to the value of algorithms in defining nursing practice and the programmer becomes sensitive to the fact that systems need to be flexible to accommodate patient care issues that are not totally predictable. This dialogue is critical to developing systems that will be welcomed by nurse users. In the future, more and more will be involved in some way with utilization, purchase, or development of compo-

nents of information systems. The challenge is ours.

BIBLIOGRAPHY

Smaldone, A., Greenberg, C., & Walsh Perez, P. (1988). A new language: Translate please! *American Journal of Nursing, 88,* 363.

14

Implementing an Automated Care Planning System in a Nursing Curriculum

Patricia Curry
Diane Elliott
Erlinda Wheeler
Robert Guhde

Tomorrow's nurses must acquire skills to handle the technology that is driving the future of health care. An important component of this expanded technology has been the introduction of computers into the health-care arena. Computers show significant potential for use in nursing education as well as in service settings. Numerous studies have compared the effectiveness of computer assisted instruction (CAI) to more traditional teaching methods. CAI has been found to be equally effective or more effective in knowledge attainment and retention than the more traditional forms of teaching (Day & Payne, 1984; Neil, 1985; Yoder & Hellman, 1985; Sizemore, & Pontious, 1987; Gaston, 1988). However, the continued integration of computers into nursing education remains a challenge. The faculty of our nursing and public administration departments decided to accept this challenge.

Our goal was to develop a computerized nursing care planning system that would allow nurses to design individualized care plans for acutely ill clients based on nursing diagnoses. Our project was divided into three phases. Phase I was the design of a comprehensive relational database care plan program and to integrate this program into nursing education. Phase II will consist of a formal research study comparing students' care plans when using computers and when not using computers for accuracy and completeness. The sample will include students from both the baccalaureate and associate degree level of nursing education. Phase III will expand the database, producing a system for use in the acute care nursing service setting.

PHASE I

This is a report on our progress in Phase I of the research in which we attempted to achieve the primary goal of helping nursing

Reprinted with permission of *Computers in Nursing* (July/August, 1991).

students learn the care planning process and produce higher quality nursing care plans. The secondary goal was to assist them in understanding the benefits which can be derived from using computer software which has both relational database content and an expert systems consultative component. Our specific objectives were to:

1. Design a computerized care plan generator which is both time-efficient and cost-efficient.

2. Write PC-based software for the care plan system.

TRADITIONAL APPROACH

A common practice in nursing education is to present students with a series of lectures on the components and implementation of the nursing process. An integral part of this content is an overview of nursing care plans—their basis in data gathered through the nursing history and physical assessment, their identification of nursing diagnoses and expected client outcomes, and their prescription of recommended nursing interventions. During such lectures, students may be shown examples of completed nursing care plans, and perhaps offered the opportunity to practice designing a care plan of their own.

Students are then expected to design nursing care plans for all assigned clients. This is a multifaceted task, requiring that students examine the entire medical record of usually complex and acutely ill clients. Nursing texts, often hundreds of pages long, are then used in selecting relevant client outcomes and interventions. The instructor's comments on the success of these efforts may take a week's turnaround time for the students to receive. In essence, students are presented with the theory of a learning task and then asked to apply this theory with minimal or no structure.

CAI care planning formats provide a beneficial intermediary level of structure. Presented with hypothetical case studies of controlled complexity, students design a care plan using a predetermined, limited universe of expected client outcomes and interventions from which to choose. Expert feedback on selections can be provided immediately by the system. The students have thus completed the process in a controlled, structured fashion numerous times before progressing to the unstructured care planning required in the actual clinical setting.

PHASE I DESIGN PROCESS

The team concept was primary to the design stage of Phase I of the research project. Our research team consisted of two nursing educators, a professor of information management systems, a public administration staff programmer and a public administration graduate student with a nursing background. Immediate access to content area experts in both nursing and information management systems proved to be a strength in translating the clinical decision-making process to a CAI format.

Three local hospitals and one baccalaureate nursing school were enlisted as participants in this design process. Information obtained from the hospitals and from the college included nursing history forms, admission forms, morbidity/mortality statistics and specific formats used in teaching the care planning process. These were used as a basis for developing nursing history and assessment screens and deciding which diagnosis related groups (DRGs) to address in the study's care plans. Client charts at participating hospitals were reviewed for assistance in designing hypothetical client situations. Client information was altered to maintain confidentiality.

Twelve DRGs were selected for case study design, reflecting commonly occurring illnesses in the medical–surgical area. Actual client cases reflective of these DRGs were reviewed and edited to include only data that could be handled by a junior level nursing student, since the care planning process is most usually learned at the beginning of an upper division baccalaureate curriculum.

Each case study included hypothetical client demographic data, a brief admission note, and an abbreviated nursing history and physical assessment. A videotape of simulated interaction between a nurse and client was produced to underscore the salient points in the nursing history. For each case study, all possible nursing diagnoses were delineated by the investigators. A priority set of the three top nursing diagnoses was then determined; both expected outcomes (goals) and nursing interventions were identified for each diagnosis.

OVERVIEW OF SYSTEM

The software itself was heavily influenced by text management software used in other vertical applications. It was written in structured database language (dBMAN Verasoft Corporation) so that it can eventually be ported from DOS and Novell OS's to Unix. Particular attention was paid to keystroke conventions, making sure that they were typical of mainstream PC programs. We used pop-up windows and help screens so that mouse drivers could eventually be used as an alternative control device. The overall architecture of the program was influenced by the relational database model which is becoming more common in hospital mainframe software. The basic model is shown in Figure 14.1.

Students see three major databases as they do their care plans. They can scan the patient's admission record, have access to important historical assessment data, and view the patient's nursing assessment. They are then presented with the screen generator main menu shown in Figure 14.2.

Students begin the care planning process by selecting the menu option that displays functional health patterns as identified by Gordon (1982). Students are asked to identify the functional patterns that are compromised, according to their clinical judgment. When the user selects a functional health pattern category, the system displays the nursing diagnoses nested under this category (Gordon, as adapted by Carpenito, 1989). Students select the nursing diagnoses (see Figure 14.3) relevant to the individual case study. The system prompts for incorrect diagnosis selection, providing immediate feedback based on the expert-identified priority set.

The system then presents a list of all expected outcomes and interventions potentially relevant to this functional health

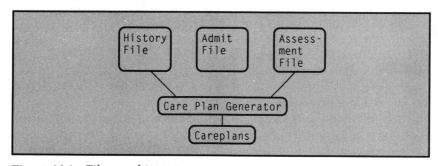

Figure 14.1 Files used in system.

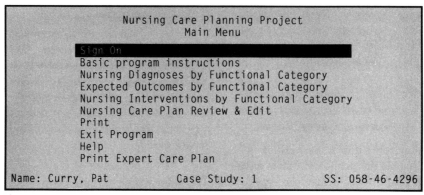

Figure 2. Generator main menu.
Figure 14.2 Generator main menu.

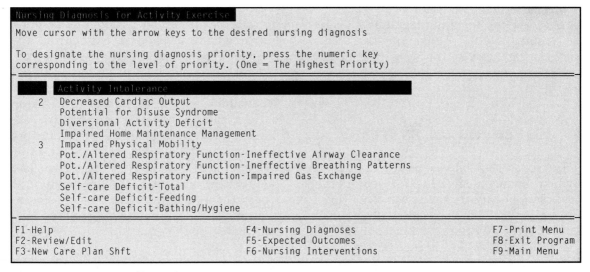

Figure 14.3 Nursing diagnosis screen.

pattern, from which the user may select. Any entry can be individualized through an edit option. Hard copies of completed care plans are available through a print option. At this point students can compare their care plans with hard copies of an expert-designed care plan.

Hard copies of student-produced care plans are submitted for detailed instructor feedback. In addition, the system tracks all incorrect diagnoses selected by the student during the planning process. Instructors can then discuss with the learners why rejected diagnoses were not relevant for inclusion in the priority set.

INITIAL PILOT RESULTS

This system was pilot tested with junior nursing students at the baccalaureate level. The students had completed the care planning module in the regular nursing curriculum, so were familiar with the process. Only one student had substantial computer experience; the rest were novices. After a 30-minute orientation to the keyboard and software, the students were given 90 minutes to complete four care plans. Results indicate that students spent the majority of this time reading and digesting the case studies. The speed with which students completed the care plans increased dramatically with experience. The computer system stored the start and end time for each discrete task, allowing the researchers to track how long each care plan took to complete. On the average, students completed the first care plan in 45 minutes, the second and third in 30 minutes and the fourth in 15 minutes. A qualitative evaluation after the session indicated that the students were tremendously pleased with the system. Using a Likert-type scale, students' responses to the system were exceptionally positive, as evidenced by the following percentages:

My nursing diagnoses selections were among the possible nursing diagnoses list provided with each case study.

Strongly agree   Strongly disagree
    1   2   3   4   5
90%

I found the functional health pattern categories effective in reviewing the lists of nursing diagnoses.

    1   2   3   4   5
90%

How would you rate the care plan generation software overall?

    1   2   3   4   5
90%

These responses to Phase I of our endeavor have served to redouble the research team's continued efforts. In our next two phases we shall attempt to apply our ideas to both a more rigorous research venue and the world of nursing practice. We are confident that this software development project will help prepare students for contemporary roles in the nursing profession.

BIBLIOGRAPHY

Carpenito, L. (1989). *Nursing diagnosis: application to clinical practice*, (2nd ed.). Philadelphia: Lippincott.

Day, R., & Payne, L. (1984). Comparison of lecture vs. computer managed instruction. *Computers in Nursing, 2*, 236–240.

Gaston, S. (1988). Comparison of computer-assisted instruction and lecture on knowledge, retention, and attitudes. *Proceedings of Nursing and Computers. Third International Symposium on Nursing Use of Computers & Information Science*, 735–744. St. Louis: Mosby.

Gordon, M. (1982). Historical perspective: The National Group for Classification of Nursing Diagnosis. In M. J. Kim & D. A. Moritz (Eds.). *Classification of Nursing Diagnosis*. New York: McGraw-Hill.

Neil, R. (1985). Effects of computer-assisted instruction on nursing student learning and attitude. *Journal of Nursing Education, 24*, 72–75.

Sizemore, M. H., & Pontious, S. (1987). CAI promotes nursing student mastery of health history-taking. *Journal of Computer-Based Instruction, 14*, 62–67.

Yoder, M., & Hellman, F. (1985). The use of computer-assisted instruction to teach nursing diagnosis. *Computers in Nursing, 3*, 262–265.

15

Computerized Nursing Information Systems: Benefits, Pitfalls, and Solutions

Marianne E. Yoder

Naisbett (1982) has identified a "high tech/high touch" future, proposing that for every technological advance (high tech) that is introduced, a counterbalancing human response (high touch) must occur. Nursing has traditionally been an art of high touch. With the introduction of computerized patient information systems, nursing must counterbalance the dehumanizing effects of computerization with the humanizing effects of nursing. Hospitals have lagged considerably behind other businesses in integrating computers (Aiken & Mullinix, 1987). But as more and more hospitals incorporate computerized patient information systems, nursing will become highly dependent upon computer technology (Bongartz, 1988), much as our society is now highly dependent upon electricity. Computerization has the potential to greatly benefit patients and nurses alike. On the other hand, computerization has potentially detrimental effects. Nurses need to recognize some of these pitfalls and

then prevent them through appropriate planning.

This chapter will delineate some of the benefits for nursing, along with possible dangers related to the development of computerized nursing information systems. Also, solutions to these dangers will be proposed. Each of these factors will be examined in terms of the effect on patient care, nursing research, nursing management, and quality assurance.

PATIENT CARE

The advantages of computerized information systems for patient care are many. Health care from many different providers can become coordinated; pertinent information about past history and allergies is readily available; and scanning patient files to select those susceptible to an illness is easily possible with such systems (Creighton, 1978; Happ, 1983; Hiller & Beyda, 1981; Norris & Szabo, 1981; Snyder & Galante, 1984).

Computerized information systems also have the capability of extending nursing patient care through enhancing nursing efficiency and increasing productivity (Ed-

The author wishes to thank Rose M. Gerber, PhD, RN, for her constructive criticism in an earlier preparation of this manuscript.

munds, 1984; Jenkins, 1988). Increased accessibility to patient data, automated ordering methods, along with computerized entry of progress notes, care planning, vital signs, medication administration, and online medication, dietary, or clinical reference libraries are but a few of the possibilities of such systems (Edmunds, 1984; Johnson, 1987).

Research has shown that computerized information systems decrease the amount of time nurses spend on the performance of clerical and communication activities, such as time spent communicating with other departments, telephoning, and searching for test results and laboratory reports (Hendrickson & Kovner, 1990; Staggers, 1988). Mowry and Korpman (1987) have estimated that 1½ hours per nursing service employee per shift could be saved by using appropriate information technology. Although such systems have not decreased the amount of time nurses spend documenting care, research has supported the findings that computerized systems improve the quality and accuracy of patient record documentation by improving the completeness, legibility, and quality and number of nursing observations (Hendrickson & Kovner, 1990; Staggers, 1988).

The computerization of patient information, however, magnifies an age-old dilemma: the professional need for information versus the patient's right to privacy and confidentiality. The potential diminution of patients' rights brought by such systems has long been recognized. In the 1970s, the Department of Commerce's National Bureau of Standards appointed Alan F. Westin, professor of law and government at Columbia University, to study the effects of computerization on confidentiality of patient records. In the 381-page report, Westin concluded that the computerized health data systems were being created without (1) advance consideration for patients' rights, (2)

sufficient consideration to what kinds of data were really necessary, and (3) sufficient control of confidentiality (National Bureau of Standards, 1976).

Hiller & Beyda, (1981) echo Westin's concerns about what they describe as a universal unease asbout which patient information is "being tabulated and used, the extent of its accuracy, the necessity to control its dissemination, and the extent to which patients may have access to, and the opportunity to verify and correct, their personal medical records." No patient information system, whether manual or automated is 100 percent invulnerable to access by unauthorized personnel. The amassing of large amounts of data in a centralized location poses a greater threat to patient privacy than written information that is scattered geographically and is often disjointed. Without safeguards in place, anyone having access to the computer can have unlimited access to the data collected about patients. Levine (1980) cautions that the task of protecting patients' confidentiality remains an integral part of the relationship nurses share with patients.

Another hidden danger for nursing is the provision of patient care with limited access to the computerized patient information. If nurses are to adequately care for their patients, nurses must have the same access as physicians to the patients' data. Yet equal access to patient information is not seen as a universal right for nursing. Some would propose a hierarchy of information access with physicians having access to nurses' notes, but without nurses having access to physicians' notes (Dawson, 1983). One computerized system known to this author, used at a large teaching hospital in the southwest, allowed physicians and medical students access to laboratory reports, but denied access to nursing personnel.

The solution, then, is for nurses to have an active role in deciding what data should be collected, ensuring that the data is accurate, and determining who should have access to what data for what purposes. Strategies to prevent the identified pitfalls include surveillance, patient advocacy, and decision-making participation.

Nurses can help limit unauthorized use by seeking and supporting surveillance procedures such as user logs. Access to patient information should be attainable only through passwords or other levels of security (Romano, 1987). Nurses should not let others use their passwords and should not leave an active terminal running unattended. A solution could be terminals that have an automatic sign-off if left unattended for a set minimal time (Romano, 1987).

By far the most important way nurses can protect patients is through patient advocacy. Nurses as patient advocates must ensure that the patients' rights to privacy and confidentiality are not compromised during the creation and use of automated computerized information systems. Patient advocacy also includes offering explanations to patients about the collection and uses of data (Romano, 1987) and promoting patients' prerogative for access and verification of accuracy of the data collected.

Nurses should serve on the committees which decide what types of data are to be included in the information systems. Criteria for inclusion of particular data include not only relevancy and legality, but also consideration of the potential of patient harm in the event that information became accessible to an inappropriate source. Data should therefore be classified according to sensitivity (Romano, 1987). Not only will these criteria help protect patients, but they will also increase the relevancy of the data nurses will be entering into the system (Johnson, 1987).

Finally, nurses must take an active role in establishing who should have access to what patient information, and ensure that nurses attain and retain access to the patient data

necessary for care. One solution is to have nurses serving on the information system committees in order to claim equal access to patient information.

RESEARCH

The development of large banks of computerized patient information offers the promise of new directions for nursing research. Although current information systems have not been designed to allow for easy retrieval of research data, the data will become available in a more organized form as these systems are further developed. The automated patient information system can be a valuable tool for research, possessing the capacity to save time and money (Kovner, 1989), especially in some types of research such as time series, retrospective, and secondary or meta-analysis. Such large data banks even provide the possibility of new types of research yet to be conceived.

Pitfalls exist in accessing the computerized information for research whether anonymity can or cannot be maintained. If anonymity cannot be maintained, then the problems of conducting research with computerized information is the same as with any research study, automated or not. However, when the data are so masked as to provide anonymity, guidelines are less clear. The assurance of anonymity does not necessarily guarantee the ethical use of the data. Demographic data can be analyzed (either accurately or inaccurately) to support conclusions about particular groups of patients which can lead to their stigmatization. The data are neither inherently good nor evil—only the uses determine the social significance.

The issue, therefore, is how to protect patients without stifling the advancement of nursing knowledge. Davis (1984) acknowledges that researchers accessing computerized information can invade patients' privacy. However, she also points out that a case can be made for the need of researchers to have access to the data for the advancement of knowledge. If nursing is to be research based, then the nurse–researcher must have access to available data. Strategies to prevent these problems involve the protection of human rights.

Whether using anonymous or known subjects, the procedures already in place to protect human subjects should be retained. Human subjects committees should screen all requests for access to the data for research purposes and weigh any possible risk against the possible benefits. Subjects must continue to give informed consent in those studies where anonymity cannot be maintained. In studies with anonymity preserved, the human subjects committee members must still consider the possible ramifications that any of the proposed variables may have, and the researcher must provide evidence of protection of patients' rights. Overall, research committees must discuss and establish ethical standards for conducting research using computerized data. Simultaneously, the issues of authority for access and assurance of scientific merit must be addressed, including what groups should have access to what information. The possibility of researchers' unethical utilization of data is no reason to prevent any utilization of the data for research purposes.

MANAGEMENT

The development of computerized patient information systems also provides the promise of many benefits to nurse managers. Automated systems can improve nurse–managers' efficiency and effectiveness by the way important information such as staffing patterns, nursing staff characteristics, nursing care efficiency, and client care costs are stored, organized, and retrieved (Kline, 1986). These systems decrease the time lapse between collecting data and making it available to the nurse–manager (Romano, 1990), thereby improving organizational problem solving, institutional planning, budgetary patterns, and needs projections (Kline, 1986). In addition, the information systems will make it easier to calculate a fee for nursing service (Johnson, 1987), and accurately assess the acuity level of patients' and thereby the staff's needs. Various staffing and scheduling programs that allow matching of patient acuity with staffing needs are already in place (Batchelor, 1985). Courtemanche (1986) reported that the installation of an automated nurse staffing schedule reduced the time managers spent on staffing from two days per month to two hours per month.

The programs in use, however, are prescriptive and not predictive. The staffing is therefore based upon the acuity levels measured daily, rather than upon the predicted acuity the patient will have. With the development of more extensive information systems, management will have a capability for even more precise staffing and scheduling. Such capabilities present a hidden source of harm for nursing service. Will the promised efficiency of such systems compromise the effectiveness of nursing care? Reliance on such scientifically precise data available through computerized scheduling has the potential to increasingly fragment patient care if, for example, staff nurses would continuously be "floated" to meet the designated "best" staffing/patient ratio to help contain costs.

The dilemma, then, is how to prevent fragmentation of nursing care through exclusive examination of the "bottom-line" when staffing. Such fragmentation of nursing care can lead to the depersonalization of the nurse and the patient, and can lead to a decrease in the effectiveness of nursing care given. Strategies to prevent this outcome entail better predictive scheduling.

The development of computerized patient information systems allows nurse–managers to uncover the relationship between patients' medical and nursing diagnoses and patient acuity, leading to better forecasting of staffing needs. For example, a patient with a particular medical diagnosis and particular nursing diagnoses predictably would need a certain amount of nursing care the first two days, a certain amount the next three days, and so forth. With the development of better forecasting, staff scheduling will become predictive, rather than reactive. Reliable forecasting can lead to more even workloads for units and provide a more rational basis for a patient admission to the skilled care of a particular cadre of unit-based primary care nurses. Fragmentation of nursing care will be prevented, while containing staffing costs.

QUALITY ASSURANCE

Existing computerized information systems can be used for quality assurance. An automated patient information system has the ability to provide for evaluation and substantiation of the accountability of nurses and their practice. Such ability can be either enriching or detrimental for nursing, depending upon the purposes of the evaluation. The information system can contribute to the scientific base of nursing by providing a richness in description of what goes on between a nurse and a patient and by providing solid documentation of nursing outcomes. Also, manual data collection techniques for quality assurance is time consuming and expensive, but using information

already contained in the automated systems can decrease collection time and expense (Kovner, 1989).

The major pitfall facing nurses is the misuse of the data in ways that can lead to the dehumanization of nursing and the possibility of an uncaring, mechanized state. Nurses have been taught to use the nursing process to solve problems and provide autonomous, theory-based or traditionally grounded care. Nursing has progressed beyond the rote learning of nursing techniques. Instead the teaching of scientific concepts and reasons behind the techniques associated with them enables a nurse to be flexible and adaptable in a variety of situations. However, computerization of patient information provides easily accessible data for which the productivity of individual nurses could readily be monitored and evaluated. Standards of care can be quantified and each nurse's performance "objectively" evaluated only "by the numbers."

Unfortunately, poorly thought out "objective" methods of evaluation can have potentially adverse effects on nursing because they threaten to stifle flexibility and adaptability. Nursing care would likely become increasingly standardized, rather than individualized. If employee productivity is closely monitored by management, will quota setting be far behind? Too frequently physicians and nurse practitioners in Health Maintenance Organizations already are expected to see a set number of patients in a set amount of time. Will bedside nursing become a set number of baths, dressing changes, and vital signs per unit of time? If so, then misuse of computer data will cause further depersonalization of the patient and dehumanization of nursing care. Nursing care will become task-"quota"-centered and not patient-centered.

The dilemma for nursing, therefore, is to find methods of evaluating and improving patient care without impacting negatively on patient-centered nursing. As Zielstorff (1983, p. 573) has stated, "the more humanistic [nurses] remain, and the deeper [their] skills in empathetic understanding and support, the less likely [nurses] are to be supplanted by computers." Strategies for preventing dehumanization of nursing consist of emphasizing patient outcomes, rather than nursing tasks.

Evaluation of nursing care should be based upon observable, measurable patient outcomes, and not upon quota-setting for nursing tasks. Patient outcomes must be established by a committee composed of patient–care nurses, nurse–managers, physicians, administrators, and consumers. Data management technology is not limited to numbers, so the outcomes established can include qualitative measures coupled with quantitative measures to further document the richness of nursing care.

SUMMARY

Computerized patient information systems are two-edged swords. They hold considerable potential advantage to nursing, but they also have potential disadvantages that can be detrimental to nursing. Computerization holds many benefits for patient care, research, management and quality assurance. Some of these benefits include a decrease in the amount of time spent on paperwork, along with assistance in planning nursing care. Further, computerization promises to offer vast patient databases from which researchers can design multivariate investigations involving large numbers of patients. Automated information systems also have the potential for improving forecasting and report generation and assisting in decision-making while decreasing time

spent on tasks. Finally, patient databases can facilitate evaluation and substantiate accountability of nursing practice.

Computerized information systems, however, bring potential pitfalls such as invasion of patient privacy, unethical conduct of research, fragmentation and dehumanization of nursing care, and quota-setting based upon nursing techniques, which must be recognized and planned for. Although there are specific strategies for dealing with the individual dangers, nurses can help surmount any pitfall arising from computerization by taking an active role, rather than allowing others to set the agenda for nursing. Measures, such as educating themselves to some of the potentially detrimental effects and then preventing them through appropriate planning, will help prevent the dangers computerization can bring. Only by becoming actively involved in the planning and implementation of computer systems affecting their patients can nurses ensure that computeriization will benefit nursing care.

REFERENCES

Aiken, L., & Mullinix, C. (1987). The nurse shortage: Myth or reality? *New England Journal of Medicine, 317* (10), 641–45.

Batchelor, G. J. (1985). Computerized nursing systems: A look at the marketplace. *Computers in Healthcare, 6,* 55–56, 58.

Bongartz, C. (1988). Computer-oriented patient care. *Computers in Nursing, 6,* 204–210.

Courtemanche, J. B. (1986). "Gearing-up" for an automated nurse scheduling system in a decentralized setting. *Computers in Nursing, 4,* 59–67.

Creighton, H. (1978). The diminishing right of privacy: Computerized medical records. *Supervisor Nurse, 9* (Feb), 58–61.

Dawson, J. (1983). Can computers replace doctors? *Private Practice* (June), 68–71.

Davis, A. J. (1984). Ethical issues in nursing research. *Western Journal of Nursing Research, 6*, 351–353.

Edmunds, L. (1984). Computers for inpatient nursing care: What can be accomplished. *Computers in Nursing, 2*, 102–108.

Happ, B. (1983). Should computers be used in the nursing care of patients? *Nursing Management, 14* (7), 31–35.

Hendrickson, G., & Kovner, C. T. (1990). Effects of computers on nursing resource use: Do computers save nurses time? *Computers in Nursing, 8*, 16–21.

Hiller, M. D., & Beyda, V. (1981). Computers, medical records, and the right to privacy. *Journal of Health Politics, Policy and Law, 6*, 463–487.

Jenkins, C. (1988). Automation improves nursing productivity. *Computers in Healthcare, 9*, 40–41.

Johnson, D. (1987). Decisions and dilemmas in the development of a nursing information system. *Computers in Nursing, 5*, 94–98.

Kline, N. W. (1986). Principles of computerized database management: Considerations for the nurse administrator. *Computers in Nursing, 4*, 73–81.

Kovner, C. (1989). Using computerized databases for nursing research and quality assurance. *Computers in Nursing, 7*, 228–231.

Levine, M. E. (1980). The ethics of computer technology in health care. *Nursing Forum, 19*, 193–198.

Mowry, M., & Korpman, R. (1987). Evaluating automated information systems. *Nursing Economics, 5*, 7–12.

Naisbett, J. (1982). *Megatrends.* NY: Warner Communications.

National Bureau of Standards. (1976). *Computers, health records and citizen rights* (SD CAT C. No.: C13.44:157). Washington, DC: U.S. Government Printing Office.

Norris, J., & Szabo, D. (1981). Removing some impediments to development of America's third- and fourth-generation health care delivery systems: Legal aspects of computer medicine. *American Journal of Law & Medicine, 7*, iii–viii.

Romano, C. A. (1987). Privacy, confidentiality and security of computerized systems: The nursing responsibility. *Computers in Nursing, 5*, 99–104.

Romano, C. A. (1990). Innovation: The promise and the perils for nursing and information technology. *Computers in Nursing, 8*, 99–104.

Snyder, K. M., & Galante, M. M. (1984). Medically intelligent computer systems—a nurse's view. *Journal of Clinical Computing, 12* (6), 185–192.

Staggers, N. (1988). Using computers in nursing: Documented benefits and needed studies. *Computers in Nursing, 6*, 164–170.

Zielstorff, R. D. (1983). Microtechnology and the future of nursing, in R. E. Dayhoff (Ed.). *Proceedings of the Seventh Annual Symposium on Computer Applications in Medical Care* (pp. 572–577). Silver Spring, MD: IEEE Computer Society Press.

Section Four
Computer Applications in Nursing Administration

This section focuses on decisions nurses make about the selection, installation, and evaluation of a nursing information system. Guidelines for selecting and implementing a staffing and scheduling system are provided by Wells and Haynor. As nursing administrators, these authors share experiences which include development of request for proposal, selection committee, and relations with vendors and nursing staff.

No computer application is complete without evaluation. A generic evaluation model based on objectives is provided by Brett and McCormac. This chapter provides the reader with parameters for demonstrating benefits of computerization in an acute care setting.

16

Selecting a Computerized Staffing and Scheduling System

Patricia M. Haynor
Robin W. Wells

INTRODUCTION

Rarely a month goes by that current nursing literature does not contain articles pertaining to computer applications in nursing. Much of the literature seems to discuss mainframe hospital information system applications and their impact on patient care and hospitals' financial well-being. Articles concerning computerized staffing and scheduling systems are sparse even though they can have a significant impact on the fiscal well-being of nursing departments.

Budd and Propotnik (1989) believe that "identifying nursing costs, resources utilization, and nursing contributions to hospital revenue have [sic] become essential to effectively preparing and monitoring hospital budgets" (p. 17). Johnson and Bergmann (1988b) further point out that "staffing is an extremely important responsibility of nursing administration and managers, which greatly affects costs, standards of care, nursing staff job satisfaction, morale, and development" (p. 59). Additionally, Johnson and Bergmann (1988a) note that "staffing the

hospital nursing service is the most difficult challenge. . . . what other industry can claim such a dynamic workload!" (p. 28).

With today's financial accountability, chief nurse executives must do all in their power to demonstrate their credibility and expertise in managing multimillion dollar budgets. According to Christensen and Rupp (1986), it is the "responsibility of nursing administrators to ensure that these dollars are well spent in the pursuit of departmental and organizational objectives" (p. 173).

One tool that chief nurse executives can use to generate timely financial reports and demonstrate appropriate nursing personnel usage is a microcomputer-based staffing and scheduling system. Christensen and Rupp (1986) felt that this is "perhaps the most frequently discussed computer application for nursing management" (p. 173). A staffing and scheduling system: creates unit personnel schedules; monitors staffing and identifies personnel needs; generates projected and actual staffing reports, including patient care hours provided; and produces user-defined financial reports. Nevertheless, Haynor and Wells (1988) have noted that "although computerized systems for staffing and scheduling have been around for almost a decade, many nurse administrators have not faced purchasing one" (p. 1).

WHY WOULD ANYONE WANT ONE?

Staffing and scheduling are the backbone of the nursing department's plan for an effective care delivery system. They also form the basis for an intelligent approach to budget control to the point where it is possible to manage compliance. A computerized system provides chief nurse executives and their staff a manageable resource for planning to meet patient requirements in a cost effective manner.

In the planning phase of the staffing and scheduling process it is possible to use the computerized system to model different staffing scenarios against various budget parameters. This type of modeling of staffing with budget compliance would be very difficult, if not impossible, with a paper and pencil approach. Once the chief nurse executive knows the staffing parameters that ensure budget compliance, he or she can authorize the staffing office to implement the plan. The chief nurse executive and clinical nursing directors can then monitor budget compliance on a shift by shift basis and explain budget variances in a timely manner. These variances are usually related to a change in patient requirements or staff mix.

A computerized staffing and scheduling system allows the chief nurse executive to review both the projected quantity and quality of care at a glance. An integral part of any software designed to plan staffing must permit the users to incorporate budget parameters and pertinent information about the care providers. It is necessary to include sal-

ary levels, including all aberrations in the base rate, skill inventories, shift preferences, certifications, work preferences, foreign language abilities, and charge capability. This type of information permits staffing office personnel to match qualified care providers (including agency personnel) with patient requirements.

IS IT WORTH THE TIME AND MONEY?

Effective budget monitoring must include qualitative and quantitative approaches. The major difficulty with reports and tools usually available to the chief nurse executive to carry out this function is that they are retrospective. The data is usually a minimum of four to six weeks beyond the events or expenditures. But a microcomputerized system enables the user to have reports on the status of care provision as projected, delivered, and required. Variances can be controlled and rectified by adjusting the next shift or day's staffing.

A second advantage is the creation of a microcomputerized database. Manual recordkeeping does not permit easy retrieval or manipulation of data elements. Although creating a computerized database takes time, any combination of data elements can be easily achieved. This makes it possible for staffing office personnel to generate reports, using an inexpensive microcomputer, that otherwise would have been too time consuming to produce manually and too costly to produce on a mainframe system. The staffing office personnel can use the reports to ensure compliance within budgeted and acuity-driven parameters.

A third advantage is the use of the system to generate the staff schedules. This saves the nurse manager 8 to 16 hours of repetitive work each schedule period. A fringe benefit for the staff is that they can receive a personalized schedule to carry with them. The schedule generated by the system requires minimal input from the nurse manager, and allows him or her to fine-tune it while maintaining control. Additional and last-minute schedule changes are easily made so that computer-generated 24-hour or shift rosters are accurate.

Another advantage is the projection of fiscal competency by all members of the nursing management team. In times of industry upheaval and fiscal constraints it is imperative that the leadership team in nursing have timely, meaningful, and accurate financial data. Such information will allow the hospital management team to make informed decisions which will positively affect patient care. Nursing resource requests are more likely to be approved if they are based on objective data from fiscally responsible department personnel.

The computerized database and record-keeping system, in addition, ensures ready access to information requested by regulatory agencies. These reports can include licensure expiration dates, CPR and specialty certifications, staffing rosters, acuity reports, vacancy reports, and productivity reports. Regulatory personnel are favorably impressed by an ability to quickly access the information which they request and to demonstrate the incorporation of the data in day-to-day operations.

DETERMINING YOUR NEEDS

The impetus for a computerized staffing and scheduling system usually comes from the chief nurse executive. Several concerns arise when the budget reports generated by the finance department differ from the care hour and budget reports manually calculated within the nursing department. This often leads to a discussion of whose numbers are correct. It is usually the hand-calculated numbers that are suspect! To prevent the game of finger pointing, it is best to be proactive. For a modest financial investment, the chief nurse executive can secure timely reports, demonstrate budget compliance, ongoing position control, and timely variance adjustment with numbers that have credibility.

The first step is for the chief nurse executive to meet with the director of nursing resources (or the nursing department finance manager) and the staffing and scheduling coordinator. The purpose of this small focus group is to determine the resources for data and report generation currently in use, to identify information gaps, and to determine the cost of the existing system. Begin the process by listing the types of data requests which you are currently receiving from the hospital management team. How many of these requests are you able to fulfill? Are the requests repetitive or varied? List the requests you receive from accrediting agencies, from local schools, students, nurse managers, surveys, and so forth. Where are the data to answer the requests? How accessible are the data? How much time does it take to generate the answers?

Assemble all reports that you currently receive or generate on a routine basis. For example, staffing rosters, personnel and unit schedules, productivity reports, float pool and contract agency reports, position control reports, acuity reports, and staff development activities. The admissions department usually generates census information, the finance department generates monthly budget compliance reports, and the operating room generates a utilization report which affects staffing. Ask yourself whether these reports really give you the information you need in a format that you can use in a time frame that is manageable. Also ask yourself how long it would take you to receive a customized report from another department. Do the reports you receive actually help you manage better? Do they warn you of impending fiscal impact?

Look at where these reports are stored and the time period of storage. Are they easy to retrieve and can the data be readily collated? Do you have direct access to a database to generate reports? Do you have independent verification that the data in the reports which you receive are accurate and reliable? If you disagree with the data, what happens? If you have answered several of these questions with: not timely, not available, not enough, limited access, or not helpful, you have just identified your major information needs.

GATHER MORE INFORMATION

Internal

Begin your search by assessing your organizations' internal strengths and weaknesses. Most of the resources are frequently found in a data processing department and with your own staffing and scheduling professionals.

1. Who are the microcomputer system experts and how available are they to you?
2. Talk with your in-house data processing experts. Find out what they and the rest of your nursing administration team know about the staffing and scheduling programs already on the market. Determine if anyone has had first-hand experience with any specific product or vendor.

3. Assess the in-house computer systems already available. Is there a mainframe? How accessible are the microcomputers? What are the current microcomputer resources within the nursing department? What software packages are currently in use?
4. Has this hospital ever had a computerized staffing and scheduling system in place? Was it mainframe- or microcomputer-based? If so, what happened to it? How do people feel about it? Why?

External

Once the internal resources have been identified it is time to gather information which will broaden your perspective. Use your best networking skills to learn from your colleagues.

1. Run a literature search and gather pertinent articles. Read them before talking to your colleagues or vendors.
2. Attend a conference to gather more information (e.g., Computers in Nursing or Symposium on Computer Applications in Medical Care). Spend time in exhibit halls examining and discussing products with vendors.
3. Seek out your colleagues. Ask other chief nurse executives if they are currently using a system and what their experiences have been. Find out what hardware their software requires.
4. If they have a working system in place, ask for a demonstration of its capabilities and ease of use. Ask to see some of the reports the system generates. Discuss the "pros and cons" of specific vendors.
5. Locate reputable vendors. Your search should have revealed the names and ad-

Table 16.1   10 Hallmarks of Reputable Vendors

1. Have been in business for several years.
2. Responsive to the clients' needs.
3. Produce regular product enhancements and updated versions.
4. Have satisfied customers.
5. Have a critical mass of systems installed.
6. Support user-groups.
7. Invest in product research and development.
8. Hire credible nursing professionals to develop, market, and install their products.
9. Provide immediate service either in person or via telephone or modem.
10. Understand the hospital environment.

If you answered "yes" to each of these ten hallmarks, you should consider the vendor reputable.

dresses of several vendors. Contact them either in writing or by telephone. Ask them to send you information about themselves and their products. Refer to Table 16.1 for the ten hallmarks of reputable vendors. Now it's time to make some judgements about them.

MAKE YOUR WISH LIST

Prioritize your needs. Keep a running list of your desires. Incorporate ideas which you have gathered from the literature, your nursing colleagues, vendor information, and your in-house experts. Break them into categories: reports, staffing, scheduling, record keeping, database, budget, acuity, hardware, and others. Determine your "must haves" and separate them from your "nice to haves." Remember that this is your starting point, not your endpoint.

The following features are frequently requested:

1. Retention of at least one year's worth of data.
2. A "smart" scheduler which automatically can generate a four-week schedule using artificial intelligence rather than following preestablished patterns created by the nursing department. It should have the ability to pull all prn or agency personnel available for the scheduling period and transfer time and costs to a specific unit's schedule.
3. Allocation of hours or dollars to the appropriate cost center when a staff member is floated to another unit or when a prn or agency person is assigned to a unit.
4. The maximum amount of information that can be stored for each employee, for example, name, address, specialty skills, skill level, certifications, shift preference, and so forth.
5. Standard reports that are easily generated by the system.
6. A report-writer to create user-defined, custom reports.
7. An acuity system that will accept a variety of concepts and interface with the mainframe hospital information system.
8. Password security system to prevent unauthorized access and use.
9. Easy system maintenance routines.
10. Mean time between system problems and vendor response.
11. Interface to hospital information or patient care system.
12. System expendability through other modules which complement the staffing and scheduling functions.

13. The capacity to network the software with other microcomputers.

14. Detailed tracking of sick time, vacation, and holidays.

You probably will have to adjust your expectations to the vendor's offerings and your budget. Nevertheless, it is appropriate for vendors to hear requests for items currently not available. This is part of their product development process and while some of your requests might be in a developmental phase, you must make your decision to buy based on what is actually available. It is important to know in what direction the software is developing.

FORMULATE SYSTEM OBJECTIVES

After the small focus group finishes with the wish list, it is time for them to formulate objectives for the selection committee to use. Objectives are crucial because all systems and vendors are judged against them. The system or vendor who meets the most objectives should be the one selected by the selection committee.

Here is a list of reasonable objectives for a state-of-the-art staffing and scheduling system:

1. Meets needs and desires on the wish list

2. Expandable with the addition of other modules

3. Frequently upgraded to remain state-of-the-art

4. Strong track record: debugged; stable; minimum down time; many users

5. Good vendor support

6. User friendly: easy to use

7. Generates the reports needed accurately, without additional programming

8. Large, expandable data capacity

9. "Smart" schedule

10. Vendor market endurance: financial stability and produce commitment and enhancement

11. An active user or vendor group used to share information and enhance the product design

12. Fast transactions: no long pauses or blank screens between key strokes and machine activity

Now that the objectives have been formulated, it is time to designate the selection committee.

THE SELECTION COMMITTEE

The selection committee will be provided with the literature review and focus group findings. Their charge (presented to them by the chief nurse executive) will be to operationalize the objectives set by the focus group, review vendor materials, refine the system parameters, and select the system.

Choose the members carefully! Keep the committee size to a workable number! The committee should include personnel who work with data processing or the hospital information system, the staffing coordinator, a clinical nursing director, a nurse manager, a nursing quality assurance coordinator, and a representative from budget or finance. The chief nurse executive does not necessarily need to be a committee member, but needs to retain veto power. A project director should be appointed by the chief nurse executive to be responsible for the day-to-day workings of the committee and eventually to coordinate the installation process.

Although the suggested selection committee has ten members, there are only six unique roles. Five members provide information from different sources, and two mem-

Table 16.2 The Selection Committee Members and Their Roles

Title	Role	Function
CHIEF NURSE EXECUTIVE	Ex officio with veto power	Cheerleader
PROJECT DIRECTOR	Committee and work organizer	Project mover
DIRECTOR OF DATA PROCESSING	Resource and information provider	Systems expert
CLINICAL NURSING DIRECTOR	Information provider	Seller
NURSE MANAGER	Information provider/user	Reality checker
SYSTEMS ANALYST	Information provider/user	Systems installer
STAFFING AND SCHEDULING COORDINATOR	Information provider/user	Seller/trainer
COORDINATOR OF NURSING SYSTEMS	Systems analyst	Systems trainer and maintainer
QUALITY ASSURANCE COORDINATOR	Systems analyst	Standard keeper
BUDGET/FINANCE	Information provider	Credible seller

bers analyze the manual system. The director of data processing is key to the success of the project because of the resources and information at his or her disposal. The project director organizes the work to keep the selection process moving while the chief nurse executive acts as the project "cheerleader." See Table 16.2 for further role definitions.

REQUEST FOR PROPOSAL

A request for proposal (RFP) is the document the selection committee prepares and sends out to vendors. It outlines your needs and wants and asks the vendors how their product measures up to them. The RFP will include:

1. An overview of your institution
2. The purpose of the RFP
3. The hospital information system
4. The response time frame
5. Specific vendor information

6. Required and optional features such as whether the schedule generator is static (repeats preset patterns) or "smart" or dynamic (uses artificial intelligence)
7. System design including hardware and software description
8. System maintenance and expansion capability
9. System installation requirements
10. System costs
11. Vendor suggestions
12. Reference and user list

Ask other in-house people to review the RFP for clarity and completeness. Incorporate their suggestions. Select a limited number of vendors whose products seem to meet your most critical requirements. For example, if a critical parameter for you is the smart/dynamic scheduling capability, it would be pointless to send an RFP to a vendor whose product only has a static scheduler. Remember to send out the RFP with a

adline for response by the vendor.
l permit you to schedule dates for the
n committee's meetings.

NARROW THE NUMBER
OF VENDORS

the responses to the RFPs have been
, it is time to evaluate them. In the
election process consider the follow-

posal met deadline

npleteness of the proposal

ıdor experience and number of in-
lations

ancial viability of the vendor

lity to satisfy the functional require-
ıts in the RFP

ephone or modem service support

e of installation and use

tract terms and conditions

t of acquisition, installation, and
ntenance

ınctional requirements should be
 a side-by-side comparison of ven-
s will allow the committee to objec-
w the strengths and weaknesses of
dor's product. If the committee has
;, it is appropriate to contact the
ır clarification. The committee must
hether each product is still in con-
ɔr adoption. This process narrows

SITE VISITS

the remaining vendors that they
ived the initial cut. Ask them to set
visit. Make sure that you visit an

institution that is similar to yours in size and
services, whose installation has been completed, and who is experienced in using the
system. Ideally, the system's requirements
should be similar to yours. Don't go alone!
Take along two or three members of the selection committee. But, to prevent bias, try
not to go with a vendor representative.

Before you go on your site visit, do your
homework! Prepare a list of questions, determine which reports you want to ask for, and
read the vendor material carefully. Another
benefit of a site visit is that it will expand
your vision of system use.

While you are on the site, listen and observe carefully! Very seldom will people
directly tell of dissatisfaction with their
choice. Nevertheless, this will be evident in
the way they talk about, handle, and use
their system. Ask open-ended questions like,
"What do you wish that this system could do
that it can't?" "Do you attend user group
meetings?" "What problems have you had
and how did the vendor respond?" "How
much of the system do you actually use?"

Remember to assess the level of expertise
of the user. Do not misjudge a vendor's product because the user does not have the expertise or knowledge to use the system well.
Ideally, two site visits per vendor should be
made. Often the vendor will share the costs
of the site visits as long as they feel they are
serious contenders.

SELECTION

After site visits and interviewing a few customers by telephone, the only thing left to do
is to decide! The committee should select the
vendor who best meets the institution's
needs, who is able to provide the level of
support needed, and whose reports give the
best information base possible. At this point,
the committee needs to make a formal pre-

sentation to the chief nurse executive. The formal presentation should include the results of the RFP, summaries of each site visit, a functional comparison report, and the committee's selection recommendation and reasons for their support for the system. If the selection is acceptable to the chief nurse executive, an additional presentation to the hospital administrative team is advisable. Once their support has been reconfirmed, contract negotiations should begin.

CONCLUSION

Once you have an operational computerized staffing and scheduling system which generates reports, schedules, and budget models, you will wonder how you ever managed without it! An effective care delivery system is based upon the wise allocation of resources. A computerized staffing and scheduling system permits you to control your budget in a timely and proactive manner. The purchase of a "smart" or dynamic scheduler that uses sound scheduling principles will prevent burnout of your staff and will save recruiting dollars. Adjusting staffing needs to meet patient acuity will en-

hance patient satisfaction and retention of nursing staff. The automatic record-keeping system will be a lifesaver for the staffing office personnel and will satisfy the regulatory bodies. In short, there are no losers with a computerized staffing and scheduling system.

REFERENCES

Budd, M. C., & Propotnik, T. (1989). A computerized system for staffing, billing, and productivity measurement. *Journal of Nursing Administration, 19* (7), 17–23.

Christensen, W. W., & Rupp, P. R. (1986). *The nurse manager's guide to computers.* Rockville, MD: Aspen.

Haynor, P., & Wells, R. (1989). *Taking the plunge: Selecting a computerized staffing and scheduling system. Aspen's Advisor for Nurse Executives, 4* (4), 1, 6–7.

Johnson, J., & Bergmann, C. (1988a). Managing staffing with a personal computer—Part I. *Nursing Management, 19* (7) 28–32.

Johnson, J., & Bergmann, C. (1988b). Managing staffing with a personal computer—Part II. *Nursing Management, 19* (8), 55–61.

17

Making It Real: Installing a Computerized Staffing and Scheduling System

Robin W. Wells
Patricia M. Haynor

INTRODUCTION

Installing a successful staffing and scheduling system just doesn't happen—it is a carefully planned event. As Maylen (1990) noted, "even the best system can fail if it's not implemented carefully. Doing it right takes a lot of work" (p. 35). The best time to develop an installation plan is after the purchase decision has been made and before the estimated date of arrival.

The committee members who selected the system should comprise an implementation task force with a nurse as the project director. If a selection committee was not used, now is the time to create a task force. Choose members of this committee carefully because they will cause the success or failure of the system. Members should include a data processing or hospital information systems analyst, the computer systems nurse or unit nurse manager, the nursing standards or policy and procedure coordinator. The project director should be the person who is administratively responsible for the staffing and scheduling activities of the nursing department.

The mandate of the task force is to develop a time line, analyze how the system will be used, determine what information must be gathered, and plan the installation phases. According to Denger, Cole and Walker (1988), the implementation plan should combine careful planning, institution wide teamwork and accountability, and a cooperative partnership with the vendor. The ongoing support of the chief nurse executive and senior hospital management staff will be essential to the installation process because the relationship of quality to cost and the management of resources are addressed by the task force and built into the software.

DEVELOPING A TIMELINE

Remember that it takes many years to select and purchase a staffing and scheduling system, and it will be several months before

Table 17.1 Implementation Tasks and Time Frame

Tasks	Sept.	Oct.	Nov.	Dec.	Jan.	Feb.	Mar.	Apr.
Vendor selection and contracting	█	█						
Analyzing current system	█	█						
Pre-install visit								
Negotiating the software delivery			█					
Paper planning process			█	█				
Hardware delivery			█	█				
Software preparation			█	█	█			
System testing				█				
Procedure writing				█				
Training					█			
System finalization					█			
Pilot units						█		
Live (remaining units)						█	█	
Sustained implementation						█	█	█

it is functional. First and foremost, have an end and sustained implementation date two months prior to the start of the new fiscal year. This will allow the new system to capture data from one complete year and to generate quarterly as well as annual reports. Begin by listing the tasks to complete and then assign them dates.

Table 17.1 lists implementation tasks and time frames. Certain tasks that tend to be related will overlap. Do not make the mistake of underestimating the time that certain tasks, for example, data entry and system testing, require. It is better to overestimate and bring the system live earlier than to underestimate and create tremendous anxiety within the department. The time frame developed in Table 17.1 covers an eight month period.

The vendor, task force members, and project director create the timeline. Nevertheless, once it has been created, it is the project director's responsibility to ensure that the timeline is followed. Notice that the time frame specifies months but not dates.

This limited flexibility is necessary because tasks are not totally under the control of the nursing staff.

CREATING THE CURRENT MANUAL SYSTEM DOCUMENT

The systems analyst is usually responsible for assessing how the department currently handles staffing and scheduling events. The analyst creates a document by breaking these events down by major activities, associated tasks, and reports and forms used. Major categories to take into account are listed in Table 17.2.

Each major activity has several associated tasks. It is important to capture what each task is, where the task occurs, who performs it, and how the data are recorded or to whom they are reported. Both the reports generated using the data and the forms used to collect or transfer data should be referenced and attached to the document. If this has

Table 17.2 Typical Nurse Staffing and Scheduling Activities

I. Scheduling employees
II. Scheduling PRNs
III. Scheduling agency personnel
IV. Prepare student rotation roster
V. Prepare two-week block manual
VI. Update bi-weekly time pay period
VII. Complete schedule changes
VIII. Fill schedule to replace employees "calling out" sick
IX. Update weekend "call-out" list
X. Calculate payroll hours
XI. Calculate patient care level hours
XII. Verify agency personnel bills
XIII. Prepare monthly agency hours utilization report
XIV. Contract agency personnel

never been done before, the task force will be astonished at the complexity of the tasks (see Table 17.3).

This level of detail is not critical to the selection of the staffing and scheduling system because the major activities were assessed previously. During installation, nevertheless, the detail becomes the guide and must accurately replicate the manual system.

The importance of this current manual system document cannot be overemphasized. It permits the task force to realistically view the task of staffing and scheduling before trying to incorporate the tasks into a new system. It also forms the basis of com-

parison between what is currently done and what the selected computerized system will be able to replicate.

The last section of the report should compare the staffing and scheduling desires and concerns with the system's capabilities. This becomes a road map and must be completed before the preinstallation visit and the software delivery.

THE PREINSTALLATION VISIT AND NEGOTIATING THE SOFTWARE DELIVERY

Purchasing the system does not mean immediate use of the software. The system should arrive when the nursing and data processing departments can allocate the personnel and resources required for a successful installation. The process often includes a visit to the vendor's training and development center.

In-depth discussion of the nursing department's structure, needs, and details of the matching software design specifications occur during this visit. This is an opportune time for the vendor installation team and task force members to assess each other's strengths.

During the preinstallation visit, the workload distribution between the vendor and the task force is negotiated. The vendor may be able to enter data off-site so that later on-

Table 17.3 Example of Major Activity Analysis

Item	Activity	Report Forms
A	Receive "call out" from employees to work weekend	
B	Fill in information on Daily Roster Sheet	Employee Roster Report
C	Distribute copies of Daily Absentee List to Unit Supervisors on a weekly basis	Daily Absentee List
D	Unit Supervisors responsible for weekend make-up	

site visits are more productive. Data often include: number of units and names; levels of personnel; types of personnel information to be captured; skill level and special abilities; certifications; licensure information; budget parameter; acuity system specifications; and so forth. Having the vendor enter this type of data off-site, before the system is even delivered, is more cost-effective than doing it in-house. Data entered also tend to be more accurate because the vendor is familiar with the system and is not learning during the entry process.

During the visit, vendor representatives can illustrate how other institutions have handled specific issues. This will provide the task force with successfully implemented models which demonstrate how to fully use the system's capabilities. From among those models, the task force can choose which most closely match their own needs. There are often a variety of data collection forms currently in use which can be modified.

Use this opportunity to have the vendor representatives double-check the hardware order. The hardware is usually ordered from a separate vendor. The worst thing that can happen at this point is to order the wrong hardware and find the error during the first software installation visit. This wastes everyone's time and creates needless frustration.

At the end of the on-site visit, the vendor and the project director should have a timetable for the installation and a clear understanding of each participant's role and tasks. From this visit until the first installation visit most communication will occur via telephone with follow-up confirmation letters.

THE "PAPER PLANNING" PROCESS

The difficult task of putting the existing staffing and scheduling system on paper so that it can be imbedded in the software re-

quires diligence and provokes the most controversy among task force members. The stakes are high—if errors are made in this process, the numbers will be wrong and the staff schedules will be worthless.

During this phase, the project director plays the role of referee. The chief nurse executive is most frequently consulted to finalize decision-making. The chief nurse executive and the project director are often the only two members of the management team who have the entire picture of the varied uses of the data and the inconsistencies within the department. The other team members often see things only from the perspective of their own departments and units. For the system to adequately meet the needs of both types of users these two conflicting views must be reconciled. If these issues are not resolved, the system is designed for failure.

Some specifics which must be planned include: the staff mix per unit; the staffing/shift/budgeted care hours; shift types and length; cost centers/unit designations; number of beds/units; staff demographics and profile; and staff weekend schedule. The clinical directors of nursing contribute the individual unit budget parameters in dollars and care hours and the desired staffing mix and budget. The unit nurse managers need to design the staff demographic and time preference forms.

Table 17.4 contains nursing personnel demographic information. These data are essential because they allow the staffing coordinator, manager, or house supervisor to readily identify specific staff members with specific skills to meet patient and unit needs. Additionally, they are frequently used in emergency situations, such as major accidents, industrial disasters, or severe weather conditions to mobilize the appropriate staff in a timely manner.

Determine the work rules. This is where staff retention and satisfaction are created.

Table 17.4 Nursing Personnel Demographic Information

UPOS # _____

UNIT _____

NAME _____

EMPLOYEE # _____

HOME PHONE # _____

ALTERNATE PHONE # _____

EMG CONTACT _____

ADDRESS _____

_____

_____

LICENSE # _____

LICENSE EXPIRATION DATE _____

BLS EXPIRATION DATE _____

ALS EXPIRATION DATE _____

SKILL LEVEL _____

CAREER LADDER LEVEL _____
(ENTRY 1, 2, 3, 4)

STATUS _____
(FULL TIME, PART TIME, PER DIEM,
24/40 FULL TIME, 24/40 PART TIME,
24/40 PER DIEM, 19/30)

HIRE DATE _____

BIRTHDATE _____

SS # _____

SEX _____

MARITAL STATUS   S   M   D   W

EVALUATION DATE _____

QUALIFICATIONS - PLEASE CHECK

☐ A. ACLS CERT
☐ B. BLS CERT
☐ C. CHEMO CERT
☐ D. DIALYSIS CERT
☐ E. CRIT CARE
     EXPERIENCE
☐ F. FOREIGN LANGUAGE
     ☐ POLISH
     ☐ SPANISH
     ☐ ITALIAN
☐ G. NATIONAL CERT
☐ H. MEDICATION CERT
☐ I. LPN IV CERT
☐ J. ARRHYTHMIA CERT
☐ K. BLS INSTRUCTOR

☐ L. ACLS CERT
     INSTRUCTOR
☐ M. MCH EXPERIENCE
☐ N. INSTRUCTOR
     TRAINER
☐ O. OR EXPERIENCE
☐ P. PSYCH EXPERIENCE
☐ Q. CHARGE CAPABLE
☐ R. RN IV CERT
☐ S. PEDS EXPERIENCE
☐ T. LIKES OVERTIME
☐ U. PERCEPTOR
☐ V. DIPLOMA
☐ W. ADN
☐ X. BSN

☐ Y. MSN
☐ Z. DOCTORATE
☐ 0. BONUS $50
☐ 1. BONUS $100
☐ 2. 5–15 MINS FROM
     HOSPITAL
☐ 3. 15–30 MINS FROM
     HOSPITAL
☐ 4. MANAGEMENT
     EXPER
☐ 5. TEACHING EXPER
☐ 6. LOCAL CERT
☐ 7. CHILD BIRTH
     EDUCATOR

Issues here include: how many days in a row can nurses work; how many hours between shifts; how many shift changes per week; number of required evening and night shifts per schedule; and number of required weekend shifts per schedule.

Often managers and directors wish to avoid these decisions for fear of getting trapped by them. The major fear is that during shortages they will be unable to staff their units if the staff finds out about or gets used to these work rules. The chief nurse executive must intervene and impose work rules if the others cannot.

After the paper planning process is complete, the off-site vendor data entry can continue until the hardware is delivered.

HARDWARE DELIVERY

As soon as the hardware arrives, it should be assembled into a working unit and thoroughly tested by the systems analyst. It should be kept in a locked storage area and access allowed only to the computer systems nurse and the systems analyst. All warranties should be completed and coordinated with the data processing department's maintenance plan. The software vendor representatives should be notified of its arrival.

Placement of hardware in the nursing administrative offices should take the following into consideration: the room must be climate controlled; the dedicated power line must be of the correct voltage; the hardware should not be installed in a high traffic area where it may be bumped or have liquid spilled on it; placement should allow the staffing and scheduling coordinator a peaceful work area; there should be accessible storage areas for the diskettes, special computer paper, printer ribbons, and other supplies; and, it should allow proximity to a telephone so that the coordinator can verify information and make changes easily.

The peak use time of the system will occur on the day shift when the managers, directors, and the staffing and scheduling coordinator are present. During this time, the system should only be used for staffing and scheduling. During the evening shift, the reports are generated by the system. No other applications should run on the system during these times. Because this hardware becomes dedicated to staffing and scheduling

applications only, it should not be available for word processing use.

Now that the hardware is ready for action, the on-site software installation can proceed as scheduled.

SOFTWARE PREPARATION

The software that is purchased from the vendor is called "open architecture." This is similar to a house plan that an architect designs. Fitting in the institution's layout, idiosyncrasies, staffing permutations, and budget and scheduling parameters is a major task. If the institution is not accurately portrayed, the vendor's system will never work. And, it will not be the fault of the open architecture! Next to the system selection decision, these are the most important decisions to ensure the success of the system. Take sufficient time when making them. Use the written analysis of your current nurse staffing and scheduling system and incorporate the scheduling concerns and recommendations.

The vendor representative is an invaluable resource during this phase. Elicit suggestions, examples, and rationales from this person. There are often compromises which need to be made. For example, there may be four types of personnel categories available to you, but you have six different names for them; what is the best way to fit them into the system? Ask how similar situations were resolved and why.

Calling the personnel that the selection committee met with on institutional site visits is also helpful during this stage. They have lived through this process and can help avoid time-consuming mistakes. They can also tell you of the impact of their decisions and whether they would make the same decisions again. Do not be afraid to ask for as-

Table 17.5   Staff Time Preferences

Number of Shifts Worked Per Pay Period ____   ___   ___

Workstretch _____ (number of days preferred to work in a row)

Daily Doubletime Start _____

Weekly/Biweekly Doubletime Start _____

Non Duty Shift Length (Minutes) _____

Maximum 1st Shift Workstretch _____

Maximum 2nd Shift Workstretch _____

Maximum 3rd Shift Workstretch _____

Fixed Skeleton

Week 1	S	M	T	W	T	F	S		Week 2	S	M	T	W	T	F	S
	–	–	–	–	–	–	–			–	–	–	–	–	–	–
Week 1	S	M	T	W	T	F	S		Week 2	S	M	T	W	T	F	S
	–	–	–	–	–	–	–			–	–	–	–	–	–	–

sistance—internally or externally. The credibility of the system and its subsequent output or reports are at stake.

During this phase, use for scheduling purposes the data collection sheets, created earlier by the nurse managers for staff information, and the planning sheets (see Tables 17.4 and 17.5). Often these are modifications of those currently in use or they are the result of all the information the staffing coordinator and nurse managers wished they had in one easy-to-access place, but did not. It is best to collect more information than less. This will avoid going back to your managers and staff several times and having them question your approach.

If the institution did not have a position control procedure, now is the time to create one. These parameters ensure compliance with budgeted positions, staff ratios per shift and per patient, and needs to be carefully negotiated with the clinical directors and the nurse managers. Resistance will be encountered here if this is a newly introduced concept. If so, the chief nurse executive may need to intervene. If the institution already has a position control procedure in place, work with the human resources and finance departments to be certain that the nursing department's approach is consistent with theirs.

And, last, create back-up procedures. This is the daily duplication of system transactions in case the computerized system malfunctions. Most vendors have specific approaches which they strongly recommend. There is a difference between daily back-up and archiving. Daily back-up can reconstruct the events of the previous day and can update the system to the point of the malfunction. Archiving, on the other hand, is the compilation of data from a longer time frame (such as a month) and from which monthly or quarterly reports are written.

Now that these preparations have been made, the on-site vendor installation visits can occur.

VENDOR INSTALLATION, ON-SITE VISITS

The vendor comes to the institution to install the staffing and scheduling system in several steps. Each visit has a specific agenda and tasks to accomplish. The success of each vendor visit depends upon freeing key personnel, determining the role of the staffing coordinator, and having the requested data prepared and ready for input.

During the first visit, the software is installed and the system's functions and support documentation are overviewed. There is hands-on training for data entry, data modification, back-up, and archiving procedures. During this visit it is important to accurately estimate the number of hours it will take to input the data. In a large institution (400–500 beds), this may be as many as 30 man days for all three vists with some data having been entered by the vendor. The systems analyst should determine if any of the institutional or departmental data on other software systems can be downloaded directly into the staffing and scheduling system.

At least three people should know the system and the data entry process. Ideally, this should be the staffing and scheduling coordinator, the computer systems nurse, and the systems analyst. When the workload can be rotated, the accuracy of the data entry is less likely to be compromised because there is less fatigue and boredom.

At the end of this first visit, there needs to be a clear understanding of the tasks to be completed, the number of hours required, knowledge of procedures to test this portion of the installation, and the preparation required for the second visit. Via modem, there is often a direct telephone line link between the on-site system and the training center headquarters. This permits simultaneous troubleshooting and an off-site assessment of progress. During the second site visit, the vendor representative reviews the tasks that have been performed since the first visit and meets with nurse managers to explain the new scheduling procedures, to demonstrate the process, and to clarify their roles. A schedule is actually created interactively on this visit. Reluctant nurse managers are often converted to believers during this visit.

Additionally, all on-site staff demonstrate their ability to perform functions without assistance from the vendor representative.

During the second visit the installation of the staffer and the report writer takes place. The staffer is run daily to collect acuity information, calculate target staff, collect time and assignment changes, prepare the daily roster, and write daily reports. The report writer generates end-of-period reports or other cumulative reports as required. Data required for entry is discussed.

In the course of the third visit, the scheduling process is reviewed and the schedule updated in order to prepare it to generate the schedule for the next period. Training to perform daily staffing and scheduling activities occurs as well as the printing of staffing work sheets, productivity reports, and the new schedule. At the end of this visit, the staffing and scheduling and report writing activities are totally computerized and paper and pencil systems are gone.

If other modules were purchased, they are often installed after the entire staffing and scheduling modules are up and running.

SOFTWARE SYSTEM TESTING

Software testing occurs at specific times during the installation. After each data set has been entered, it must be verified for accuracy, and the function requiring the data must be activated. Compare manual data to the data set generated by the system. If there are discrepancies, it must be determined whether is was a case of bad data (GIGO— garbage in and garbage out) or whether the function did not capture the data set accurately. Testing occurs in an incremental fashion; going from the simplest to the most complex function.

For example, first look at the structure where the data is to reside, then print out the data in a raw form, then have the system manipulate the data, and finally have the

Table 17.6   Software System Testing

STEP I	DATA ENTRY SCREEN	
NAME	**LICENSE NUMBER**	**EXPIRATION DATE**
ROBIN WELLS	266351	7/93

STEP II	DATA FILE	
NAME	**LICENSE NUMBER**	**EXPIRATION DATE**
ROBIN WELLS	266351	7/93
PATRICIA HAYNOR	269467	5/93
MARY JONES	217629	7/93
JOHN MAY	199652	5/93

STEP III	DATA MANIPULATION (LICENSES EXPIRED AS OF 6/27/93)	
NAME	**LICENSE NUMBER**	**EXPIRATION DATE**
PATRICIA HAYNOR	269467	5/93
JOHN MAY	199652	5/93

STEP IV	DATA PREDICTION (LICENSES THAT EXPIRE JULY '93)	
NAME	**LICENSE NUMBER**	**EXPIRATION DATE**
ROBIN WELLS	266351	7/93
MARY JONES	217629	7/93

system predict from the data. Table 17.6 illustrates system testing. The first step is to print out the data entry screen with one nurse's name, license number, and license expiration date. The second step is look at the complete data file by printing out all nurses by name, license number, and license expiration date. The third step is to assess data manipulation by printing out all nurse names and license numbers whose licenses are expired as of today's date. The fourth step is to test data prediction by printing out the names and license numbers of all nurses whose licenses will expire next month. Each step is compared with the manual data set which existed prior to the system installation.

If there are discrepancies or the system does not seem to be performing according to the manual, it may be necessary to activate the modem. A call to the vendor representative to discuss the problem may result in a request to permit the vendor representative to simultaneously view the process. This two-way view of the system is often the most expedient way to solve the issue. Usually it is not the system which is malfunctioning, it is the human component. Remember, the rule is *stop*, *fix*, then *proceed*. Do not proceed to enter the data until the problem is resolved.

Again, to avoid the problem of the human component, it is best to restrict access, inputting, and testing to the staffing and scheduling coordinator, the computer systems nurse, and the system analyst. Most importantly, do not permit the entry team to move ahead of the tasks which were agreed upon with the vendor representative. A staged installation is usually the most successful because it permits adequate testing of each function and prevents the need to reenter data. It also permits the team to see whether the data collected and entered was adequate for the function.

The next step is to codify the new procedures required by the system and the nurs-

ing department's enhanced approach to staffing and scheduling.

PROCEDURE WRITING

During the software development and installation, a variety of data collection forms will be created. These will be used to collect general and specific information about each staff member and their scheduling preferences. Other forms will be used by the nurse managers to create their schedules, positions, budgets, changes, special time requests, and so on. And still others will be used by the staffing and scheduling coordinator to keep track of data and reports. It is important to collect any form and save it for the policy and procedure manual. Try to draft the ideas behind the forms as they are created. This will help reconstruct the purpose and philosophy behind the policies and procedures.

System forms are often hybrids of the manual forms, log books, three-ring binders, and clipboards which abound in most manual staffing systems. It is important to assess each item in light of the software capabilities and to use this opportunity to eliminate redundant data collection or storage and to collect the data that always seemed to be missing or out of date.

Current policies and procedures must be reviewed carefully and broadened to incorporate the concepts inherent in a computerized system. In addition to the usual manual system policies and procedures, there are several specific policies and procedures which must be created for a computerized system. These are data access levels and data storage and archiving systems.

Most manual systems did not incorporate information regarding budgets, salaries, employee demographics, and other confidential information. Permitting only certain classifications of the nursing management team access to specific types of data solves this problem. Nevertheless, it is often a hotly debated topic; everyone wants to have access to everything. This is not a realistic expectation and should not be indulged. Leaked confidential information can destroy the credibility of the system and the nursing department's management team. It is better to be too restrictive with information and to broaden access later than to try to remove access once people are accustomed to having it. This is another area where the chief nurse executive may need to set the limits.

Data archiving and storage also bring up issues of confidentiality and restricted access. Data tampering is a dangerous event which also can destroy the credibility of the nursing management team. If the stored data is lost, the monthly, quarterly, and annual reports cannot be generated for use by the chief nurse executive and other members of the hospital management team. The issues again are where do you place archival and back-up diskettes and who has access to them. They need to be in a fire-proof, waterproof, locked storage container, in a cool environment, away from magnetic fields, with the archival and back-up diskettes physically separated from each other.

MANAGEMENT SYSTEM TRAINING

In terms of knowledge of the computer system, the task force members are the most experienced members of the nursing management team. To reward their hard work and to show the others that the system is manageable, task force members should be showcased during the training. Usually a one-day training session with the entire nursing management team is sufficient. The training session should be held after the first section of the software has been installed

and the unit-specific information has been entered and edited. This makes the system more tangible and the management team can see their data "live." The training session should be planned as a celebration of a long-awaited event with a sense of accomplishment attached to it.

The chief nurse executive should begin the training with an introduction and an overview of the uses of the data from the computerized staffing and scheduling system. It is important that he or she present the "macropicture": the reasons behind the purchase and installation of a new system, what the expectations of its use are, and what the rewards will be for the department. This introduction sets the tone and ensures that the rest of the presentation will be taken seriously by the nursing management team.

Next, the new system should be described, differentiating it from other systems on the market. This information is important if the new system is replacing an older one or if it has key differences from the others on the market. This will reassure the nursing management team that this was a positive choice and not just a cheaper or "lesser of two evils" choice. This will also answer the question of "we used X where I worked before, why didn't you buy that one?"

The third section should present the implementation time frame, the roles of the participants, and the associated policies and procedures. This begins to set the stage of how nursing management will use the system and what the expectations and guidelines will be. In an open forum, the implications of the policies and procedures can be addressed with the chief nurse executive present to hear them first hand and to explain the need for them.

The major portion of the training session is then devoted to defining codes, reports, and work sheets. This is the hands-on portion of the session and allows the nursing management team to familiarize themselves with the needs of the system, the reports which they will be able to generate, and the work sheets they will fill out for the system.

Working in small groups on specific types of tasks in a nonthreatening situation removes a lot of anxiety. It begins to make the unknown known and the situation manageable. Seeing specific unit data on printouts and learning how to manipulate the data increases users' comfort level. Nurse managers need to experience success in this way so that they will experience success again in the real situation. They also quickly learn that they maintain control over and full responsibility for their schedules and staffing and that they cannot blame the computer if their staff does not like their decisions.

PILOT UNITS

Using criteria to determine the selection of the pilot (test) units is important. The pilot units should represent the best and the worst of the institution both in terms of size and complexity. The nurse manager should show interest in the system and have a high tolerance for trying new things. This is not the time to work with a nurse manager who has yet to be convinced that the staffing and

scheduling system could be a good thing. The units should be notified of their selection and the nurse managers should work together to determine which unit should "go live" first, second, and so on.

Beginning with the most straightforward, small unit with adequate permanent staff is a good idea. Then, bringing up the units by their degree of complexity should occur. This permits a successful experience and increases the comfort level of those with more complex staffing issues to deal with. Learning how to solve simple problems leads to more creative problem-solving when complex issues arise.

Stagger bringing the units online. Bring up the first unit; debug it. Then bring up the second unit; debug it. This process should only take one or two days per unit. It is reasonable to have four pilot units on the system and functioning within 10 working days. As soon as possible, have the system generate customized schedules for each staff member (see Figure 17.1). The customized schedule can be printed in four-week blocks on a sticker or index card. This makes individuals' work and time-off schedules portable and readily accessible. There can be no more excuses like, "I didn't know when I was working." This is a nice way to introduce the benefits of the new system to the staff and,

EISLER, MICHAEL							RN 1.0 FTE						2-19-93
S 19 N	M 20 E	T 21 E	W 22 N	T 23 N	F 24 X	S 25 X	S 26 X	M 27 N	T 28 N	W 1 N	T 2 N	F 3 X	S 4 N
S 5 N	M 6 N	T 7 N	W 8 X	T 9 N	F 10 N	S 11 X	S 12 X	M 13 N	T 14 N	W 15 N	T 16 N	F 17 X	S 18 N

N = Nights
E = Evening
X = Off

Figure 17.1 Individual staff schedule.

when they show these to other staff members on other nonpilot units, requests to go online will start coming.

As a result of the pilot units' successes and their staffs' demonstration of system-generated individual schedules, many of the other nurse managers will clamor to "go live" next. Resist the temptation to put them all up at one time. Proceed in an orderly fashion and debug as you go.

"GOING LIVE"

"Going live" means every unit in the nursing department is using the staffing and scheduling system. Changes to schedules are being entered on a daily basis, new schedules are being generated by the system (not manually), all prn staff costs are being allocated to their appropriate units by the system, the daily staffing roster is being generated by the system, and other types of reports are available. The manual system is no longer in use even as a back-up.

Paid time-off can now be tracked including surrounding events. For example, are sick days falling on Mondays, after holidays, or other days off? New hires' data sheets are entered directly into the system so that new schedules can be generated for the nurse manager. Daily productivity reports, acuity summaries, and termination reports are used on a regular basis.

For the chief nurse executive "going live" means *no surprises from the monthly finance reports*. It means objective data with which to teach managers and directors how to live within their budgeted resources. It means a nursing department success story because fixing budget or staffing variances while the problem is still small and manageable can be accomplished. It means reliable reports from the nursing department which do not

conflict with reports from the finance department. It means freedom to manage intelligently and proactively.

SYSTEM FINALIZATION

As stated previously, it's important that the system installation, debugging, and ongoing use be timed to precede the start of the new budget year. This will provide a full year of computerized data and will not require going backwards to enter data from the current budget year. If there are major changes in the new year budget, there will still be time to enter them. If there is a major problem with the installation, there will be time to fix it before the new budget year begins.

At six months, compare the hopes for the system with the actuality of the system. If there is disappointment, it is usually the human component which is to be reckoned with. After all, the system is at their command and mercy. At first, the system often gives managers information which they do not like (e.g., their staffing is out of compliance with budgeted parameters or their scheduling attempts are not in synch with the new rules). During the first six months, managers need to be gently guided to see this as an opportunity to learn and not as a tool for their superiors to use as punishment. If this is achieved, resistance or sabotage of the computerized system will be minimized. If the computer becomes a tool for punishing, the system will never achieve the intended effect.

At the six-month point, there is a need to make refinements, bring on new functions, and perhaps expand the database. Do so only where necessary, and remember to explain to the nursing management team why and how things were done. Do not alter the quarterly reports so much that the earlier ones cannot be compared to the later ones. Remember, the goal is to have one year's worth of data which matches the budget of the department and can be used to prepare the management team to successfully navigate the new budget year process with credible numbers and clearly defined needs.

SUSTAINED IMPLEMENTATION

What is the sense of installing the system if there is no continual use of it or updating of the database? This is a common fate of staffing and scheduling systems usually induced by a nursing management team who is passively resisting the objective data which the system can produce.

Just as it was important to carefully plan the installation, it is crucial to plan the sustained use of the system and to implement ways to ensure nursing management compliance with the use of the system. The chief nurse executive must be the enforcer of these standards.

Ongoing support of the system requires continued allocation of resources in terms of personnel and consumable supplies. The type of personnel hired as staffing and scheduling coordinator may need to be reassessed. At six months and at 12 months, the staff should be assessed for level and type of personnel, not necessarily for number of persons needed. You may find that hiring one data entry person will now make more sense than using a nurse for the input function.

Additional modules, if available, may need to be planned into the next budget year. If the system has credibility, expanding its function should not meet with much resistance. As system updates become available, the vendor will contact the project coordinator for installation instructions. Up-

dates are usually included in the cost of the software maintenance contract. Updates are usually debugging or slight improvements in the version of the software that you purchased.

Major changes are called "revisions" and are known as new versions. Decisions will need to be made when new versions not covered under the contract are available. Often vendors will provide their customers with significant discounts for installing or pilot-testing a new version of their software.

CONCLUSION

A successful installation and ongoing use of the staffing and scheduling system will significantly improve the image of the nursing management team. It will also provide managers with a powerful tool with which to control their human and financial resources. The chief nurse executive will be able to request resources during the budget process with data that is useful and credible. Patients will be provided with the budgeted level of care based upon their acuity level and budget parameters. A management team who is able to allocate its resources and stay within its budget will not only be able to retain its staff, but will provide better patient care.

REFERENCES

Denger, S., Cole, D., Walker, H. (1988). Implementing an integrated clinical information system. *Journal of Nursing Administration, 18* (12), 28–34.

Maylen, N. (1990). In *Choosing a clinical information system* 5952–1795, Hewlett-Packard, 35, Waltham, MA.

18

Evaluating the Effects of Computers in Acute-Care Settings

Judy L. Brett
Maureen McCormac

As health care systems have become more complex, expensive, and controlled by external regulating agencies, their management has become increasingly dependent on high quality, timely information available through fully integrated and automated information systems. Most contemporary institutions have already automated their financial systems, but few have implemented fully developed integrated systems that include clinical as well as financial data. The cost of such automation remains considerable. Conclusive data on the cost effectiveness of automated nursing information systems are sparse if not controversial. While it is important that all potential purchasers of hospital and nursing information systems carefully evaluate their system's performance and cost benefit standards before making final purchase decisions, it is also important to carefully plan to evaluate the effectiveness of such systems once installed and working. Only with careful evaluation can determinations about the ability of the system to satisfy the standards be determined. This determination becomes the basis for corrective actions that will ensure that the potential of the system will be fulfilled and the original project objectives will be met. The purpose of this chapter is to provide guidelines for the evaluation of a nursing computerization project. It presents a theoretical framework for evaluation as well as a model for the evaluation of computerized nursing systems. In addition, it describes variables included in the model and discusses common means for their measurement.

EVALUATION RESEARCH MODEL

According to Polit and Hungler (1991), evaluative research is an applied form of research which has as a goal the assessment or evaluation of the success of a program. The focus of this type of research is on identifying how well a program meets objectives rather than understanding why a program succeeds.

A Context–Input–Process–Product (CIPP) model was developed by the Phi Delta Kappa National Study Committee on Evaluation and has been described by Issac and Michael (1981) as the best known evaluation model. The CIPP model is intended to provide a basis for decision making within a systems framework of planned change. Product evaluation, one part of the model, is a valuable tool used to make recycling decisions that determine whether a program or product should be continued, modified, or terminated. Recycling decisions are based on systematically gathered information about the extent to which objectives are being achieved. Derived from CIPP, the major components of the product evaluation of a computerization project would include: (1) identifying objectives underlying the program; (2) selection and design of the indicators and systems to measure the presence or absence of achievement of these objectives; (3) measuring the achievement of objectives; (4) interpreting the findings; and (5) constructing a feedback mechanism to allow program adjustment, continuation, or termination. While this chapter will focus on identification of objectives and measurement of objective achievement, activities in all components are essential to development of recycling decisions about computers (see Figure 18.1).

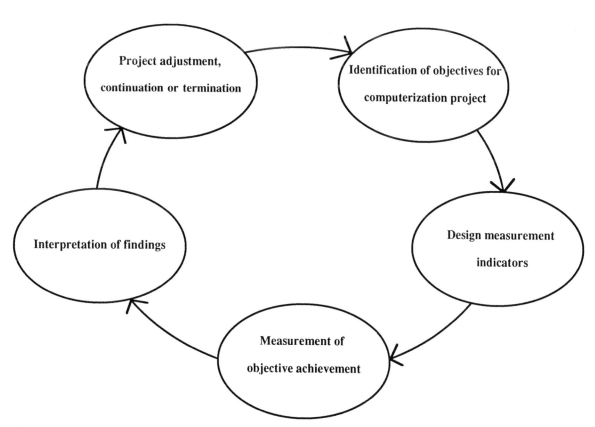

Figure 18.1.   Diagrammatic representation of the components of a computerization project evaluation.

IDENTIFICATION OF OBJECTIVES

A critical component of all evaluation projects is identification of the underlying objectives. While project leaders and managers have the responsibility for formulating these objectives, project evaluators must develop a clear understanding of their nature. Objectives typically involve a positive impact such as "Implementation of a computerized nursing information system will: (1) decrease the amount of time a nurse spends on documentation and (2) decrease the number of medication errors." They may also include some neutral impacts such as "Nurse job satisfaction will remain at current levels" or "Patient satisfaction will not decrease." Some objectives stipulate quantifiable goals, for example, "Computerization wiring and hardware will be installed on all nursing units by six months from the date of contract signing." Nevertheless, not all objectives need to be quantifiable. Some may necessitate categorical type answers such as "Yes, the objective was achieved."

The objectives should be outlined in the "request for proposal" form that was prepared for vendors to respond to or in any minutes of committees involved in developing the project. Other sources of information about the specific objectives of the project are project personnel and their supervisors.

SELECTION AND DESIGN
OF INDICATORS

Most computer implementation projects involve objectives about the time nurses spend on documentation and direct care activities, nurse job satisfaction, patient and physician satisfaction, nurse attitudes about computerization, automation costs, and quality of patient care. These objectives and examples of their conversion to measurable variables can be grouped into the following categories:

1. patterns of nurse time spent on indirect and direct care activities
2. employee satisfaction
3. patient satisfaction
4. nurse attitudes
5. cost considerations
6. quality of care
7. computer system factors

For the evaluation to be as objective as possible, a pre and postimplementation comparison of the variables is recommended. If possible, the experimental unit should be compared to a control unit. Since perfectly matched controls do not exist in the real world, the comparison unit should be randomly selected from the most similar units available.

MEASUREMENT OF OBJECTIVE
ACHIEVEMENT

Patterns of Nurse Time Spent on
Documentation and Direct Care Activities

Vendors' exhortations and project managers' expectations frequently include that computerization will reduce the time nurses spend on documentation and increase the time nurses spend with the patient. Measurement of changes in these two variables can be accomplished using a number of methods.

Activity logs can be used by nurses to record what they do throughout their workday as well as the amount of time they spend on each activity. Activities are then summarized and grouped according to predetermined categories. While this method is the least objective, it is also the least expensive, involving only the training time to explain the log to the nurses and the analysis time to compute the findings.

Work sampling techniques have been widely used to study changes in work patterns of employees and can be successfully used in computer studies. This method is based on sampling theory and has demonstrated that randomized brief periodic observations of an activity, in sufficient quantity, will enable the entire activity to be described with virtually the same accuracy as the continuous observation of the activity from start to finish (Abdellah & Levine, 1954). A variety of sampling techniques have been developed (Hoffman, Schafer, & Zuraikal, 1986a, 1986b). They typically involve a method similar to that of the San Joaquin study (U.S. Department of Health, Education and Welfare, 1978) in which observers make random rounds on a unit and record what the persons being studied are doing at the time of the round. More recent techniques involve alarms that are set to randomly notify subjects to record their activities (Brock, Scott, Pendergrass, & MacDonald, 1990). The object of the sampling is to determine what proportion of time a nurse spends in a variety of activities. It is essential to determine the level of detail required, as well as the form of clustering of activities that will ultimately be useful before the sampling begins. The greater the detail, the higher the number of observations that will be required to provide confidence in the findings. Table 18.1 provides a sample of categorization of activities that would be useful in determining the impact of a computerization project on nurse activities. If done correctly, the observed frequency of an activity will be proportionate to the magni-

Table 18.1 Categorization of Nursing Activities for Work Sampling

Code	Description of Activities

Direct Care Activities—Nursing activities done in the presence of the patient and/or family.
01 Nursing care activities such as treatments, medication administration, and teaching;
02 Charting activities in the patient's room;
03 Using a computer in the patient's room.

Indirect Activities—Activities done away from the patient to prepare for or complete patient care.
04 Actual writing or reviewing written communications in the chart such as nurses' notes or referral forms;
05 Other communication (generally verbal) regarding a specific patient with other personnel;
06 Preparing and cleaning up supplies or equipment for a specific patient such as medication or administration;
07 Transcribing orders or completing charge slips;
08 Report activities—giving or receiving.

Administration and Unit Support Activities—Activities that promote overall unit management.
09 Cleaning, housekeeping tasks;
10 Clerical or secretarial tasks such as stamping forms or assembling charts, answering the telephone for someone else;
11 Unit-related communication such as staff counseling, making assignments, and developing staffing schedules;
12 Errands off the unit, transport of equipment or specimens;
13 Checking and restocking supplies; narcotic counts;
14 Waiting time.

Personal
15 Any activity meeting personal needs of the employee.

tude of that activity if observation had been continuous. Therefore, analysis and comparison of the amount of time nurses spend on various documentation and communication activities can be calculated. The expectation that the nurse would spend less time in documentation or report activities and more time on direct patient care activities can be objectively tested.

Employee Satisfaction

Good managers continually strive to maintain high levels of employee satisfaction. Satisfaction is commonly measured before and after a change project is implemented in order to ascertain the effect of the change on nursing staff and to determine if alterations are needed to ensure a successful outcome. Increased nurse satisfaction is routinely expected and has been frequently reported as a result of computerization. For example, Baily (1988) reported an 18 percent increase in nurse satisfaction within four months of implementing a computerized nursing care planning system based on nursing diagnoses. Nevertheless, the majority of satisfaction literature related to computerization lacks rigorous evaluation using reliable and valid instruments.

Satisfaction instruments should be comprehensive, brief, easily scored, reliable, and valid. Several instruments are currently available for use, some of which include: (1) the Index of Job Satisfaction developed by Brayfield and Rothe (1951) and modified by Atwood and Hinshaw (1984); (2) the McCloskey/Mueller Satisfaction Scale (MMSS) developed by Mueller and McCloskey (1990); and (3) the Index of Work Satisfaction developed by Stamps, Piedmont, Slavitt, and Haase (1978). These scales typically assess factors such as pay, autonomy, task requirements, organizational requirements, inter-

action, job prestige or status, extrinsic rewards, and control. The installation of computers may or may not be expected to have an impact on these factors. For example, while computers may be expected to alter the task requirements of nursing personnel, they are not expected to alter satisfaction with pay. Since staff job satisfaction is important to an organization, and the relationship of computerization and nurse job satisfaction is unclear, it is important to include this variable in the evaluation design.

The measurement of satisfaction need not be limited to the registered professional nurse and licensed practical nurse, but should be expanded to include other nursing personnel (e.g., nursing assistants and unit clerks) and health care professionals. Since many hospital information systems are designed to encourage physician utilization (e.g., order entry and results retrieval), physicians should also be incorporated in the evaluation process. The inclusion of all types of users expands the scope of the evaluation and provides valuable and comprehensive data to determine if the project meets its objectives.

Patient Satisfaction

Risser (1975) describes patient satisfaction with nursing care as "the degree of congruency between a patient's expectations of ideal nursing care and his [sic] perception of the real nursing care he [sic] receives" (p. 46). It is perhaps the most commonly studied variable across change projects in health care settings and is thus an extremely important criterion of evaluation for computerization. While some studies report that computers increase the amount of time available for patient care (Staggers, 1988; Simborg, MacDonald, Liebman, & Musco,

1972), there is no evidence to support that this results in an increase in patient satisfaction.

A commonly used instrument to measure patient satisfaction is the Patient Satisfaction with Nursing Care Instrument developed by Risser (1975) and modified by Hinshaw and Atwood (1982). It incorporates three dimensions of satisfaction: (1) technical–professional, (2) interpersonal educational relationship, and (3) interpersonal trusting relationship. Computer implementation can potentially impact each of the dimensions through increased patient education, collaborative goal setting, and even discharge planning. Careful investigation is needed to provide concrete evidence of changes in patient satisfaction as a result of computerization. Existing hospital measures of patient satisfaction, such as discharge patient surveys and support service surveys, should also be incorporated into the evaluation process.

Nurses' Attitudes Toward Computerization

The installation of computers on nursing units results in a variety of changes in typical nursing functions. Computerized information systems automate medication administration records, intake and output records, vital signs, nursing notes, nursing care plans, physician orders, laboratory results, and many more functions which were originally performed manually. These vast changes ultimately impact the attitudes and behaviors of individuals involved in the change process (New & Couillard, 1981). While positive attitudes are preferred, negative attitudes are possible and may affect the success of computerization. According to Stronge and Brodt (1985), "it is imperative that the attitudes of the affected employees

be assessed adequately if the change is to be implemented successfully" (p. 154).

The measurement of attitudes toward computerization in health care is focused on six common themes: (1) job security, (2) legal ramifications, (3) quality of patient care, (4) computer capabilities, (5) employee willingness to use computers, and (6) benefit to the institution (Brodt & Stronge, 1986; Stronge & Brodt, 1985). The assessment of attitudes before and after computerization provides insight into both positive and negative views. While some users believe computers in the workplace take the nurse away from his or her patients and increase the potential for lawsuits, others believe they increase time for providing quality care while maintaining patient privacy (Bongartz, 1988). Attitudes change over time with the changing environment. For instance, nurses commonly experience insecurity before computerization, but develop job security when they realize computers support them in their positions.

Numerous authors suggest that a variety of factors potentially impact attitude development. These should be considered when assessing attitudes toward computerization. They include: (1) length of service in the nursing profession, (2) educational preparation, (3) age, (4) type of nursing unit, (5) years employed at the hospital, and (6) experience with computers. (Bongartz, 1988; Brodt & Stronge, 1986; Gibson & Rose, 1986; Krampf & Robinson, 1984; McConnell, O'Shea, & Kirchhoff, 1989). While it is commonly supported that experience with personal computers produces positive attitudes toward computerization on a nursing unit, the impact of other factors, such as length of service, age, and educational preparation is not conclusive. Additional investigation will assist evaluators to provide a basis for intervention when negative attitudes develop.

Knowledge which results from the assessment of attitudes and related factors is vital for understanding the training and support needs of users. Nurses without computer experience might require particular attention when learning computer functions in order to promote positive attitudes and reduce potential restraining forces, such as computer resistance. Restraining forces must be identified and avoided so they do not interfere with the planned change (Welch, 1979). Nurses who display signs of computer resistance, such as avoiding the computer and clinging to manual systems, require additional support to manage the change in workflow.

In order to support a smooth transition from a manual to a computerized environment, it is essential to assess the attitudes, encourage involvement in the design, implementation, and evaluation of the system, identify individuals who may need special attention during training and implementation, and reassess the attitudes of users to determine if additional intervention is needed.

Cost Factors

Workload on a nursing unit is typically subject to daily variations. While minor fluctuations should not impact the outcomes of a computerization project, major changes could have an impact. A decrease in workload might enable nurses to spend more time with patients while an increase in workload might decrease the time spent with patients even when a computer system saves the nurse time. For this reason it is necessary to control for any changes in workload. This can be easily accomplished by comparing the workload before and after implementation.

Workload is generally measured by a combination of census and acuity. Census is calculated from the official hospital admission statistics, for example, the number of patients in the hospital at midnight plus the number of patients who were admitted and discharged in the same day. Acuity should be measured with a patient classification system. In order to obtain dependable results, the system should be adequately tested for reliability and validity.

Computer project costs should be monitored and compared with budgeted expenses as part of the process of conducting cost effectiveness evaluation. Costs associated with the project include the cost of acquiring the hardware and software, the installation costs associated with wiring or additional equipment, and other related equipment and supplies. Personnel time spent on the project, including information system staff support, should be converted to dollars and incorporated in the costs.

The final cost analysis should examine the impact of the computerization project on the costs of unit operations. Incidental overtime (associated with end of shift charting) may be eliminated or decreased by implementation of bedside computers. System efficiencies predicted by the computerization should be tracked. For example, implementation of an integrated physician order, pharmacy, and nursing system may decrease the waste of expensive medications as the response time between the input of a physician order and execution of the order is decreased. Integrated radiology and results reporting systems may decrease the time required to return results to the attending physician. A quicker turnaround time could have potential for decreasing length of the patient's stay. Automation might be expected to facilitate nurses' completion of nursing care plans. Nevertheless, if as a result of the computer, nurses' compliance with the standard that every patient have a care plan is increased, the evaluator may find that nurses now spend more time doing care plans. The cost per patient of nursing care plan development would be expected to increase in this case. Hopefully that cost increase would be associated with enhanced quality of care. What to evaluate should be determined by expectations associated with the specific computerization project being implemented.

QUALITY OF CARE

An ongoing challenge of nurses in acute-care settings is to maintain or improve quality nursing care within a high-tech environment. Nursing station and bedside terminal systems are promising technologies which can contribute to improvements in quality care (Herring, 1989, Winter). Brett (1989) defines quality nursing care as "the achievement of explicit standards or criteria that have been formulated by authorities, norms, or scientific testing, after consideration of the values or variables unique to a specific situation of nursing care" (p. 355). Quality variables which are appropriate to computerization and require evaluation include: (1) accuracy and timeliness of medication administration, (2) timeliness of tests and procedures, and (3) legibility, timeliness, and completeness of nursing documentation (e.g., progress notes or care plans).

A major benefit of computerized information systems is the reduction of medication errors. In a manual system, medication errors commonly occur because of incorrect transcription that may result from illegible handwriting, errors of omission, failure to discontinue a medication when necessary, and errors during the preparation of medications from a written Kardex. A major advantage of using computers is the increased legibility of patient records (Beckman, Cammack, & Harris, 1981; Hammond, Johnson, Varas, & Ward, 1991). Computerized medication Kardexes, for example, aid in the re-

duction of medication errors. Additional reduction occurs "in those systems where physicians enter their own orders, thereby eliminating the transcription step" (Hendrickson & Kovner, 1990, p. 20). Evaluative research supports that medication errors are reduced. For example, a study of bedside terminals at three hospital locations in conjunction with a major health care information systems vendor found that medication errors were reduced by 34 percent (Herring, 1989).

While it is likely that a significant improvement in quality of care can be evidenced through greater timeliness of tests and procedures, there is a need for supportive empirical evidence. The ability to order laboratory and radiology tests and obtain online results undoubtedly enables the practitioner to act on the results more quickly than if the tests were ordered using manual requisitions. Although timeliness does not ensure quality, the potential exists for marked improvements in patient outcomes.

Significant improvements have been reported in nursing documentation as a result of computerization. For instance, Baily (1988) reported a 25 percent improvement in compliance with criteria for nursing documentation and a reduction in the rate of peer review organization (PRO) denials related to nursing interventions as a result of computerized care planning. Another study reported improvements in discharge teaching documentation (14 percent), increased accountability for charting and scheduling intravenous (IV) fluids, improved IV site assessment and documentation (4 percent), and more accurage and up-to-date care plans (Herring, 1989).

Standards for nursing provide the foundation for quality assurance indicators which are "measurable variables related to a structure, process, or outcome of care" (Tonges, Bradley, & Brett, 1990). Table 18.2 provides sample items of a documentation indicator

Table 18.2 Sample Items of Nursing Quality Indicators

1) Medication administration record includes:
   a) patient diagnosis;
   b) allergies;
   c) nurses' full name;
   d) nurses' status.
2) Physician order includes:
   a) name of medication;
   b) dosage;
   c) route of administration;
   d) frequency.
3) Nursing documentation includes:
   a) reason for administering prn medications;
   b) effect of prn medications;
   c) any unusual reaction to medication.

based on standards that can be used to evaluate the effect of computers on nursing documentation.

Computer System Factors

While it is ideal to avoid introducing any change to a nursing unit between the pre and postevaluation periods, it is not always possible to do so. It is, therefore, essential to monitor all factors which can impact the findings and conclusions of the computer evaluation. System factors include operational changes or physical modifications to the nursing unit. It is quite possible that a change in the physical structure and/or nursing model after the preevaluation survey might result in increased nurse and patient satisfaction in the postevaluation period. When this occurs, it becomes difficult if not impossible to determine if the improvement in satisfaction occurred as a result of the computer system or because other changes which coincided with the computer project occurred.

Computer factors which should be monitored due to their potential impact on satisfaction, quality, and cost include: (1)

system downtime, (2) interface communication problems, (3) equipment problems, (4) trips to the nursing station to use the computer if a bedside terminal system is not installed, (5) amount of time spent waiting to use a terminal, and (6) the amount of time spent by the user on the terminal. System downtime, interface communication problems, and computer usage can usually be obtained from reports which are generated by operations personnel in the hospital's information systems department. Logs can capture the number of trips to the nursing station and the amount of time spent waiting to use a computer. The information recorded in logs may be used to justify additional terminals at the nursing station, or even the installation of bedside terminals.

INTERPRETING THE FINDINGS AND CONSTRUCTING A FEEDBACK MECHANISM

As in all evaluation projects, the evaluation is never completed until the data gathered are organized in a way that facilitates interpretation. All data presentation techniques, including graphs, tables, or charts, that succinctly summarize data should be incorporated into a detailed report that carefully documents the study's design and results. While it is the responsibility of the evaluator to develop result reporting that is as objective as possible, the decision to act upon the results often rests with someone other than the evaluator.

Adjustments in the structure, process, or outcomes of a computer project may be indicated by the results. Project decision makers are expected to act upon the implications of the results. All evaluators need to bear in mind that decision making is not a completely objective process as our recycling decision-making model implies. Decisions regarding the computer project will also depend greatly on other factors such as availability of economic resources, time or expertise required to implement changes, and even political processes.

CONCLUSION

Although requiring large expenditures of capital dollars, computerization has been suggested as a valuable means to save nurses' time and increase the qualitiy of care that patients receive. Objective evaluation of nursing computerization projects is essential in order to verify the desirable benefit that vendors propose. Evaluation based on clearly identified project objectives is proposed as a way to not only measure achievement of objectives, but also to contribute to the success of the project.

REFERENCES

Abdellah, F. G., & Levine, E. (1954). Work sampling applied to the study of nursing personnel. *Nursing Research, 3* (3), 11–16.

Atwood, J., & Hinshaw, A. (1984). *Anticipated turnover among nursing staff* (DHHS Publication No. R01 N6 00908). Tucson, University Medical Center Corporation, Nursing Department.

Baily, D. B. (1988). Computer applications in nursing: A prototypical model for planning nursing care. *Computers in Nursing, 6* (5), 199–203.

Beckman, E., Cammack, B. F., & Harris, B. (1981). Observation on computers in an intensive care unit. *Heart & Lung, 10* (6), 1055–1057.

Bongartz, C. (1988). Computer-oriented patient care. *Computers in Nursing, 35* (5), 204–209.

Brayfield, A. H., & Rothe, H. F. (1951). An index of job satisfaction. *Journal of Applied Psychology, 35* (5), 307–311.

Brett, J. L. (1989). Measure and validation of the practice of nursing and nursing administration: Outcome indicators of quality care. In B. Henry, C. Arndt, M. DiVincenti, A. Marriner (Eds.), *Dimensions and issues in nursing administration* (pp. 353–369). Boston: Blackwell Scientific Publications.

Brock, D., Scott, C., Pendergrass, T., & MacDonald, S. (1990). Sampling clinicians' activities using electronic pagers. *Evaluation and the Health Professions, 13* (3), 315–342.

Brodt, A., & Stronge, J. H. (1986). Nurses' attitudes toward computerization in a midwestern community hospital. *Computers in Nursing, 4* (2), 82–86.

Gibson, S. E., & Rose, M. D. (1986). Managing computer resistance. *Computers in Nursing, 4* (5), 201–204.

Hammond, J., Johnson, H. M., Varas, R., & Ward, C. G. (1991). A qualitative comparison of paper flowsheets vs. a computer-based clinical information system. *Chest, 99* (1), 155–157.

Hendrickson, G., & Kovner, C. T. (1990). Effects of computers on nursing resource use: Do computers save nurses time? *Computers in Nursing, 8* (1), 16–22.

Herring, D. J. (1989, Winter). Bedside terminal systems. *Health Care Information Systems*, p. 1–4.

Hinshaw, A. S., & Atwood, J. R. (1982). A patient satisfaction instrument: Precision by replication. *Nursing Research, 31* (3), 170–175.

Hoffman, F., Schafer, T., & Zuraikal, N. (1986a). Setting nursing hours standards, Part I. *Journal of Nursing Administration, 16* (1), 13–16.

Hoffman, F., Schaefer, T., & Zuraikal, N. (1986b). Setting nursing hours standards, Part II. *Journal of Nursing Administration, 16* (2), 17–19.

Issac, S., & Michael, W. (1981). *Handbook in*

research and evaluation (2nd ed.). San Diego: EDITS.

Krampf, S., & Robinson, S. (1984). Managing nurses' attitudes toward computers. *Nursing Management, 15* (7), 29–34.

McConnell, E. A., O'Shea, S. S., & Kirchhoff, K. T. (1989). RN Attitudes toward computers. *Nursing Management, 20* (7), 36–40.

Mueller, C. W., & McCloskey, J. C. (1990). Nurses' job satisfaction: A proposed measure. *Nursing Research, 39* (2), 113–117.

New, J. R., & Couillard, N. A. (1981). Guidelines for introducing change. *The Journal of Nursing Administration, 2* (3), 17–21.

Polit, D. F., & Hungler, B. (1991). *Nursing research: Principles and methods.* Philadelphia: Lippincott.

Risser, N. J. (1975). Development of an instrument to measure patient satisfaction with nurses and nursing care in primary care settings. *Nursing Research, 24* (1), 45–52.

Simborg, D. W., MacDonald, L. K., Liebman, J. S., & Musco, P. (1972). Ward information management system—an evaluation. *Computers and Biomedical Research, 5* (5), 484–497.

Staggers, N. (1988). Using computers in nursing: Documented benefits and needed studies. *Computers in Nursing, 6* (4), 164–170.

Stamps, P. L., Piedmont, E. B., Slavitt, D. B., & Haase, A. M. (1978). Measurement of work satisfaction among health professionals. *Medical Care, 16* (4), 337–352.

Stronge, J. H., & Brodt, A. (1985). Assessment of nurses' attitudes toward computerization. *Computers in Nursing, 4,* 154–158.

Tonges, M. C., Bradley, M. J., & Brett, J. L. (1990). Implementing the ten-step monitoring and evaluation process in nursing practice. *Quality Review Bulletin, 16* (7), 264–269.

U.S. Department of Health, Education and Welfare (1978). Methods for studying nurse staffing in a patient unit. Washington, DC: Author.

Welch, L. B. (1979). Planned change in nursing: The theory. *Nursing Clinics of North America, 14* (2), 307–321.

Section Five
Computer Applications
in Nursing Education

Computers can be used to provide and evaluate instruction. In this section the computer applications described focus on innovative ways to use computers to deliver and evaluate nursing instruction. Arnold urges the reader to re-examine the meaning of computer-assisted instruction by using both the teacher and computerized simulations as a team in the classroom setting to teach problem solving behavior.

The use of computers in education has not always been successful. Mikan provides twelve strategies for integration of computers on an organization-wide basis. This model of implementation has been effective in other collegiate settings with nursing education programs.

In Chapter 21, three nurse educators explain how they used word processing and statistical software to teach nursing research. This methodology has been effective at both undergraduate and graduate levels of nursing education.

Lerner and Cohen describe how they used computer-assisted instruction with high risk baccalaureate nursing students to increase academic success. These authors state that nurse educators need to provide a supportive environment for computer usage. Both successful and unsuccessful interventions are shared with the reader.

Computers can greatly reduce the time required for the creation, administration, and grading of tests. Lombardi and Blume discuss how test management software works beginning with item entry and concluding with interpretation of test results.

The curriculum, selection process, and evaluation of the Healthquest/HBO Nurse Scholars Program are described by Skiba, Ronald, and Simpson. This chapter illustrates how nursing education and vendors can collaborate to educate nursing faculty about health care information systems.

19

How to Use Microcomputer Simulations in Academic and Staff Development Settings

Jean M. Arnold

INTRODUCTION

Computer simulations, formerly known as "case studies" in paper format, are increasingly being used in nursing education. Thomas's Survey of baccalaureate nursing schools indicated that the use of microcomputer simulations increased from 49 percent to 72 percent between 1983 and 1990 (Bolwell, 1991a). Microcomputer simulations offer text-only screens as well as sophisticated graphics and video screens. When asked about microcomputer simulations, nursing students consistently say, "I like them and want more because they prepare me for 'clinical.'" In spite of the heavy demand by students for computer simulations, nurse educators have only used this innovative teaching method as an adjunct to classroom instruction.

Tutorials and drill and practice computer-assisted instruction (CAI) are quite different and represent a totally new learning experience. Tutorials provide information and reinforce it through questioning and immediate feedback to learner's responses. Previous learning is validated through questioning and feedback with drill and practice CAI. Simulations portray a situation and require the learner to respond to it.

Purpose

The purpose of this chapter is to provide the nurse educator with guidelines for using microcomputer simulations with learners both in classroom and laboratory settings.

Redefining CAI

Computer-assisted instruction is a misnomer. The computer itself is a powerful and effective instructor–teacher which is under-utilized when treated only as an adjunct to classroom instruction. It is helpful to expand the limited use of CAI by altering the definition of computer-assisted instruction to mean the use of the computer to teach.

Phases of Instruction

A microcomputer may be used by the teacher and learner in either classroom or laboratory settings. Both authors of CAI and teachers must consider all four stages of instruction. Instruction begins with (1) presentation of information, (2) responses by the learner to the teacher's input (3) provision of practice opportunities by the teacher, and (4) assessment of learning achieved by the learner (Alessi & Trollip, 1985).

Definition of Computer Simulation

A computer simulation is a realistic representation (model) of the structure or dynamics of a real object or process with which the participant actively interacts. The participant applies previously learned knowledge to respond (decisions and actions) to a problem or situation and receives feedback about responses without having to be concerned with real life consequences (de Tornyay & Thompson, 1987, p. 25). In addition, the computer allows the learner to respond to the situation in a variety of ways. Simulations provide an opportunity for the learner to assume a role and see the consequences of his or her actions. The simulation itself is therefore a model of reality.

SIMULATIONS AND INSTRUCTION

Simulations and Social Learning Theory

Computer simulations are similar to observational learning experiences. According to social learning theory most human behavior is learned observationally through modeling; from observing others, one forms an ideal of how new behaviors are performed, and on later occasions this coded informa-

tion serves as a guide for action. Because people can learn from example at least in approximate form before performing any behavior, they are spared needless errors (Bandura, 1977, p. 22). Both computer simulations and observational learning experiences provide the learner with the opportunity to interact with a model and receive feedback regarding one's choices. The difference is that with the computer simulation, the learner controls the situation and may take different paths without anyone knowing his or her decisions. Some microcomputer simulations track and report paths taken by learners. The purposes of simulations are to: (1) develop problem-solving skills; (2) foster hypothesis formation, and (3) engage in discovery learning (Gagne, Wagner, & Rojas, 1981). These behaviors can occur with the use of microcomputer simulations. The teaching role of simulations has been further described by Steinberg (1984), who believes simulations teach content and processes. The focus of nursing simulations include clinical situations, rationale for actions, and nursing process.

Review of Literature

In the nursing literature there are many examples of use of computer simulations to teach problem-solving processes. In one study, a sample of practicing and student rehabilitation counselors were asked to complete a case management computer simulation. The simulations were used to measure counselling skills. As opposed to the students, practicing counselors took more appropriate action and avoided unnecessary steps when making eligibility decisions (Mecaskey, Chan, Wong, Parker, Carter & Lam, 1989).

In another study, computer simulations were used to examine diagnostic abilities of nurses and nursing students. The sample comprised four groups including 752 junior and senior nursing students, nursing students who were parents, and pediatric nurses. The objective of the simulation was to determine why an infant was crying. The pediatric nurses and parents differed from the student nurses by using less information and selecting different information, such as infant's age, earlier in the assessment (Holden & Klinger, 1988).

In a third study, eight computer simulations were used as a formative evaluation tool at the conclusion of a seminar on child abuse. The sample consisted of a control group (n = 43) and an experimental group (n = 38). Both groups were given reference material about child abuse, but only the experimental group attended a seminar. Both groups performed similarly on a classic case of child abuse. Nevertheless, different results occurred when both groups confronted the more difficult case of a shaken baby. The experimental group obtained higher total scores and achieved greater percentage of correct scores. It is possible to conclude that computer simulations were an effective measure of the success of the seminar as a teaching strategy (Kost and Schwartz, 1989).

Another investigation explored whether simulations could present and guide practice in decision-making theory. Junior and senior nursing students were taught cue recognition using a variety of computerized clinical situations. The major outcome of this study was that cue recognition and linking could be taught by using a computer simulation and improved accuracy of clinical decisions. Furthermore, the role of computer simulations in the first phase of instruction, as presenter of information, and third phase of instruction, as guide for practice, appeared to be effective in this study (Thiele, Baldwin, Hyde, Sloan, & Strandquist, 1986).

In a fifth study, researchers examined the use of simulations to evaluate students' reasoning process for pediatric clinical situations. The performance of students (n = 111) for the sample simulation differed widely from faculty observations of their clinical performance. Sixteen percent of this sample, who were judged to be very good or excellent in problem solving by the faculty, performed at least one standard deviation below the class average on the simulations (Schwartz, 1989).

Goldman (1988) discusses how computer simulations can serve as an objective measure of a learner's performance. Medical education provides some experience in this respect. Forty-two medical schools were using computer-based examinations (CBX) developed by the National Board of Medical Examiners for certification and licensure of physicians. The structure of CBX is a brief vignette with options for the learner to ask for more information, including history, physical examination, and laboratory tests or write treatment orders immediately. No specific questions about the case were asked to avoid cues or prompts. A clock kept track of the student's time. At one location, third-year medical students were scheduled to view case studies in preparation for class discussion or an examination. At another site, printouts of learners' responses to CBX were made available to faculty. Six of 50 senior students took highly inappropriate actions that raised questions about problem-solving skills; this information had not been discovered from clinical evaluations. Faculty reported the greatest value was in learning problem solving, establishing priorities, and patient management.

Arnold (1991) reports that similar findings in diagnostic reasoning were attained with nursing students. The use of an acute-care simulation with 49 junior nursing students provided evidence regarding correct and incorrect nursing problem choices. A graph of the group's performance was helpful to both students and faculty.

These studies provided evidence that simulations can be used to teach all phases of instruction including presentation of information, feedback to learner, practice, and evaluation of problem-solving abilities.

ROLES OF EDUCATOR AND TEACHING STRATEGIES WITH COMPUTER SIMULATIONS

Roles of Nurse Educator

The nurse educator should use microcomputer simulations in a variety of teaching roles. As a *prescriber*, selection of microcomputer simulations depends on a match with specific goals within a unit of instruction. Microcomputer simulations should be chosen carefully in accordance with course content and desired knowledge-acquisition processes. As a *discussion leader*, the nurse educator may plan follow-up sessions, with specific questions regarding the content of the simulation, immediately following the scheduled student viewing period in the laboratory. The microcomputer simulation itself may become the focal point in the classroom with the educator modelling problem-solving skills while interacting with it. As a *monitor*, the nurse educator can examine the feedback sheets students obtain from microcomputer simulations. There are two ways of achieving this. One is to request that students submit the printout received from the computer program, if it is available. Another method is to develop decision records which articulate with major judgments made in the software and to ask students to complete sheets while they use a given microcomputer simulation (see Table 19.1). The instructor can then analyze the students' problem-solving behavior as (1) an individual profile of a learner's problem-solving behavior and (2) as a group to assess class achievement. The nurse educator can also act as a *diagnostician* by reviewing the students' diagnostic profiles for individual and class strengths and weaknesses (see Figure 19.1). Finally, the educator should reteach weak areas and make course changes.

Teaching Strategies and Simulations

Three teaching strategies are recommended when using computer simulations: (1) presessions, (2) modeling sessions, and (3) postsessions.

Ideally, before the learner is asked to view a simulation he or she is provided with instructions as to what to do with a simulation. It is not enough to give the learner the

Table 19.1   Decision Record for Microcomputer Simulations

Problem	Decision Choice
1.	
2.	
3.	
4.	
5.	

PRESCRIBER — selects computer simulations in accord with specific goal

DISCUSSION LEADER — models the use of the model

MONITOR — feedback from computer simulations

DIAGNOSTICIAN — students' strengths and weaknesses

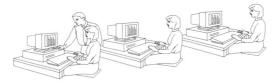

Figure 19.1. Roles of educator using computer simulations.

name of a simulation and a place to view it. One should provide information in software documentation that otherwise may not be available to the learner, for example, content overview, objectives and special booting instructions. The relationship of the simulation to clinical practice should be emphasized. Inform the student of the purpose for viewing the simulation and state the relationship of it to course content. Figure 19.2 illustrates this method.

Modeling involves identifying and describing the role of the learner, the role of the computer as a teacher, and the nature of

WHAT: Goals for using simulation within a given course

HOW: Directions for use — how many times to view it, what to look for, view it alone or with group, view it for process or content

WHERE: Laboratory or classroom use

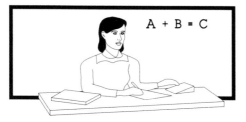

$A + B = C$

Figure 19.2. Instructions from teacher for using computer simulation.

simulation. Will the learner be assuming the role of the nurse as a practitioner or teacher? Will there be a time limit imposed within the simulation? How long will it take the learner to complete the simulation? Motivate the learner to take the time to view the simulation by describing its special features and benefits. Identify special features, such as color, crossword puzzle, diagnostic profile, and graphics. If the student has to type in responses and spelling errors are not tolerated, advise the learner to view it with a peer and a medical dictionary to decrease the frustration associated with this problem. In a classroom setting, a modeling session could be enhanced if the instructor uses a portable computer with a liquid crystal display overhead and verbalizes the responses to a simulation.

Postsession would include discussion of students' reactions to a given simulation. Decision records and printouts related to software-used scores could be reviewed. Also students' comments about software could be tallied using a brief evaluation. An example of a software evaluation form is presented in Chapter 38.

HOW TO USE MICROCOMPUTER SIMULATIONS: THREE EXAMPLES

The Thiele–Holloway Decision Making Taxonomy will be used as a framework for this discussion. This taxonomy classifies decision-making levels of computer simulations into four levels. Level I (novice) is primarily drill and practice with a series of problems with instructive feedback. Level II (advanced beginner) is a more complex simulation which focuses on applying facts to a new situation. The focus of Level III (complex) is priority setting and interpretation of multiple concurrent events. Level IV (proficient) builds on level three, requiring the learner to be accountable for decisions made. (Bolwell, 1991b). This rating system can also be used to select computer simulations for instruction. A detailed discussion of this Thiele–Holloway Taxonomy is provided by these authors in the appendix of Chapter 37.

Examples of these teaching strategies will be presented with three existing computer software programs. The first computer software is *Therapeutic Communication* (Fuld Institute for Technology in Nursing Education, 1990). This is an interactive video program which can be used by beginning nursing students to learn communication techniques. Instructions for *Therapeutic Communication* include (1) scheduled viewing time for each learner, (2) provision of course map, (3) decision record for assigned case study (see Table 19.2), and (4) specified time periods to complete quizzes. Modeling includes assuming the role of a nurse in client interactions and nurse-to-nurse interactions. Motivation results from the client situations and the use of color and graphics within the software program. Postsession incorporates a rationale for decision choices associated with communication techniques. *Therapeutic Communication* represents Level I (novice) decision-making computer-assisted instruction.

The second example is *Medication Administration I within Pharmacodynamics and Administration of Medications: Clinical Nursing Concepts* (Brown & Brown, 1990). This is a Level II (advanced beginner) decision-making microcomputer simulation which assists the learner in performing drug calculations. Instructions for use of this simulation would include objectives and overview of content including two case studies and a game on medication abbreviations. Students should be advised to review drug calculation rules for intramuscular and intravenous medication prior to viewing the program. Furthermore, students should be informed that maximum viewing time would be two hours and that a second disk is an optional assignment. Learner interaction would be encouraged by advising the learner to view the situation alone and then with others. Graphics provide motivation during the viewing of the simulation. For example, the learner's drug calculations are depicted on a syringe

Table 19.2   *Therapeutic Communication* Decision Record

Nurse's Statement	Technique	Facilitator or Blocker
I tried to get back as soon as I could. I didn't think I was gone that long.	Being defensive	Blocker
No, nothing special happened. The other nurse said you were asking for me.	Open-ended	Facilitator
He hasn't been here for two days. You seem a little nervous about his visit.	Sharing your observations	Facilitator
If it's nothing important, why are you so nervous?	Asking questions	Blocker
You had an argument	Reflecting	Facilitator

Fuld Institute for Technology in Nursing Education (1990).

which fills on-screen and also simulates an intravenous drip. Students can be advised to save their answer on disk and to print their results. Figure 19.3 illustrates teaching strategies for *Medication Administration I Software.*

U-Diagnose® offers a number of *teaching strategies.* Miss G. U-Diagnose Situation represents Levels III and IV of microcomputer simulations taxonomy (Patterson, Arnold, & Bower, 1989). A student should view the simulation twice; the first time he or she should use it as a teaching tool and the second time as a test of thinking skills for acute gerontological care. Teachers can model identification of a nursing diagnosis with supporting data and then develop a related action plan. The learner is advised to read

INSTRUCTIONS —Go through each situation twice within designated two week time period and submit individual diagnostic profile

INTERACTION —Go through situation alone and then with a peer

MOTIVATION — Simulated administration of intramuscular and IV meds using syringe and IV bottle with drip chamber

Figure 19.3. Teaching strategies for medication administration software.

```
                    U-DIAGNOSE

 Possible Problem Choices    |   Problem Identification

 PROBLEM CHOICES             |   PROBLEM

 1. Mobility, impaired,      |
    physical                 |
 2. Home maintenance         |
    management, impaired     |
 3. Cardiac status           |
 4. Sensory perception       |   Supporting Data
    alterations              |
 5. Body image disturbance   |   1:      3:
 6. Nutrition, altered       |
 7. Metabolism, altered      |   2:      4:
 8. Gas exchange, impaired   |

 PgUp, PgDn, or ESC to exit  |
```

Figure 19.4. U-Diagnose® problem identification screen.

the situation on-screen and then enter data on a test disk. Figure 19.4 illustrates the problem choices for one U-Diagnose® Situation Test (Arnold & Greenhalgh, 1989). The learner is advised to assume the role of a nurse for a specific day in a client's care and to plan care accordingly. No feedback is provided during the learner's interaction with this microcomputer simulation. Postsession would consist of interpretation of students' printouts. A detailed printout comparing learners' responses with experts is provided with this software.

WHY USE SIMULATIONS?

Nurse educators should remember that simulations model reality and because of that, they foster a transfer between theory and practice in a safe environment. The learner becomes more involved due to the presentation of a realistic situation and the opportunity to take action and receive individualized feedback. These problem-solving opportunities are of value to the educator as well as the learner. Both players benefit because information is not simply passively presented as in a lecture, instead the learner must respond and process his or her knowledge in doing so.

Most importantly, the nurse educator should model the model to teach information processing and clinical decision making. The use of simulations in a social environment such as the classroom may augment higher-order learning such as application and synthesis of knowledge. This means that the development of problem-solving skills cannot be left to chance. The writer strongly recommends that nurse educators use computer simulations to teach problem-solving skills within the classroom environment and to reinforce students' skills in the computer laboratory independently. The nurse educator cannot lose sight of the importance of modeling the model.

REFERENCES

Alessi, S. M., & Trollip, S. R. (1985). *Computer-based instruction: Methods and development.* Englewood Cliffs: Prentice-Hall.

Arnold, J. M. (1991). Custom item analysis interface with a U-Diagnose® gerontological nursing simulation. In E. J. S. Hovenga and K. J. Hannah (Eds.), *Lecture notes in medical informatics: Nursing informatics '91 (pp. 541–544).* New York: Springer-Verlag.

Arnold, J. M., & Greenhalgh, W. (1989). U-Diagnose® [Computer program]. Newark: Rutgers, The State University of New Jersey.

Bandura, A. (1977). *Social learning theory.* Englewood Cliffs: Prentice-Hall.

Bolwell, C. (1991a). 1990: 91% of US schools of nursing have microcomputers. *Nursing Educators Microworld, 5* (4), 27.

Bolwell, C. (1991b). Identifying decision-making levels of simulations. *Nursing Educators Microworld, 5* (4), 30.

Brown, P., & Brown, E. D. (1990). *Pharmacodynamics and administration of medications: Clinical nursing concepts: Medication administration I* [Computer program]. Chapel Hill: Professional Development Software, Inc.

de Tornyay, R., & Thompson, M. A. (1987). *Strategies for teaching nursing.* New York: Wiley.

Fuld Institute for Technology in Nursing Education. (1990). *Therapeutic communication* [Interactive video computer program]. Athens, OH: Author.

Gagne, R., Wagner, W., & Rojas, A. (1981). Planning and authoring computer assisted instruction lessons. *Educational Technology, 21,* 17–26.

Goldman, B. (1988). Computer simulations may change way medical students are taught. *Canadian Medical Association Journal, 138* (12), 1144–1145.

Holden, G., & Klinger A. (1988). Learning from experience: Differences in how novice vs. expert nurses diagnose why an infant is crying. *Journal of Nursing Education, 27* (1), 23–29.

Kost, S., & Schwartz, W. (1989). Use of a computer simulation to evaluate a seminar on child abuse. *Pediatric Emergency Care, 5* (3), 202–203.

Mecaskey, C., Chan, F., Wong, D. W., Parker, H. J., Carter, H.S., & Lam, C. S. (1989). Evaluating clinical problem-solving skills through computer simulations. *Journal of Rehabilitation, 55* (3), 34–39.

Patterson, J., Arnold J., & Bower, F. (1989). Acute gerontological care: Miss G U-Diagnose® situation. In *U-Diagnose gerontological situations.* Newark: Rutgers, The State University.

Schwartz, W. (1989). Documentation of students' clinical reasoning using a computer simulation. *American Journal of Disabled Children, 143* (5), 575–579.

Steinberg, E. R. (1984). *Teaching computers to teach.* Hillsdale: Lawrence Erlbaum.

Thiele, J., Baldwin, N., Hyde, R. S., Sloan, B., & Strandquist, G. (1986). What are the effects of teaching cue recognition? *Journal of Nursing Education, 25* (8), 319–24.

20

Implementation Process for Computer-Supported Education

Kathleen J. Mikan

NEED FOR ORGANIZATIONAL PLANNING

Institutional planning for computers has become more important in the past ten years. While the use of computers in education is not new, what is new is the diversity of microcomputer applications that are within the reach of individual educational units in higher education. Nursing schools no longer have to depend upon central administration for computer power. Along with the decentralization of computer power have come departmental obligations and responsibilities for planning computer implementation and evaluation. Thus, educational planning for computer implementation has become necessary not only at the higher administration levels, but also as a responsibility and expectation, within individual departments.

The nursing literature contains many articles describing examples of administrative, instructional, and research applications of computers within educational programs. Many of these applications are self-con-

tained, stand-alone uses rather than part of an overall nursing schoolwide plan for computer integration. While the development, implementation, and evaluation of stand-alone applications are important and essential, so too is organizational planning. Organizational planning for computer implementation considers the full range of computer applications as they relate to the mission, goals, and functions of the nursing education unit.

Regardless of the extent to which a nursing school is presently using computers, newer computer applications that are faster, easier to use, and more sophisticated, are becoming available regularly. While ten years ago only a few computer choices were available, now educational units have multiple options from which to choose. Educators are continually challenged by these rapid advances when determining computer technology's usefulness to nursing and planning for orderly, purposeful integration of computers in the organization.

The purpose of this chapter is to present the significant components of an implementation process which can be used as a guide for establishing or enhancing computer-supported education within a school of nursing. Computer-supported education refers to the use of computers within an educational setting to facilitate the achievement of the organization's educational goals, purposes, and functions.

The implementation process is comprised of 12 activity-based components that need to be considered during organizationwide planning. The 12 components contained in the process are presented below with a rationale as to their individual importance. Although the components are listed in a sequential fashion, they may or may not be performed in the sequence given. Depending on the educational setting, some activities may occur before others or some activities, such as the purchase of hardware, may already have been partially completed.

IMPLEMENTATION PROCESS

Establish Need

Initially, the need to implement the use of computers within nursing education may not be readily apparent or documented. Some schools have already discovered that having computers available does not mean they will be used or used appropriately, efficiently, or effectively. Administrators and faculty may be comfortable with the way things are being done and may not perceive a need to change. Faculty may not have thought about increasing the utilization of computers or expanding the usage of computers to new applications. Sometimes, nursing education units have been given access to computer resources but have never developed a plan for their use or considered the possibility of expanding computer uses

beyond those for which they were originally purchased. Besides, any department plan for computer utilization should be consistent with and supportive of the parent institution's master computer plan, should one exist.

Basic knowledge of computers and their potential is essential for understanding computer applications in nursing and nursing education. Faculty and administrators may have limited knowledge about the range of possible computer applications or how they can broaden their use of computers beyond what they are currently doing. Faculty may think that the learning opportunities provided by computer-assisted instruction or word processing are adequate to prepare students for a computerized workplace. Faculty may need to gain a more realistic vision of the current use of computers in health care agencies as well as potential future uses of computers in the agencies.

Documentation of the need for computer-supported education may come from a variety of sources. Minutes of meetings, annual reports, evaluations, and task force recommendations are all sources of documentation of existing conditions that could possibly be improved by the use of computers. If educational needs are not readily apparent, faculty may need to become better informed about the range of computer possibilities. Faculty educational opportunities in the form of presentations at faculty meetings, computer demonstrations, attendance at computer workshops, enrollment in computer courses, or previews of software can be effective in helping faculty become more knowledgeable about additional uses of computers within their particular educational programs. The need for computer-supported nursing education will become evident when the use of computers meets local needs and provides educational (teaching and learning) opportunities beyond those currently available.

Organize Early Adopters

The establishment of a planning committee to explore potential computer usage within the school is an ideal way to get the implementation of computers underway. Planning requires that those doing the planning understand and can predict future uses for computers within a nursing education organization. The implementation process will be greatly facilitated by the early involvement of individuals who have demonstrated an interest in computers. Individuals who have enrolled in computer courses, attended computer workshops and conferences, or have some computer skills are good candidates for membership on this planning committee. Membership of this committee would not necessarily have to be limited to faculty, but could also entail others in the nursing organization such as secretaries and staff. While each committee member will have vested interests in specific applications, such as research or word processing, the final plan should have a broad, organizational focus rather than a narrow departmental one.

While the planning committee needs to be formally organized, assigning computer planning responsibilities to an existing faculty committee may or may not be appropriate. Standing faculty committees already have other assigned tasks and responsibilities and may be too busy to take on an additional task such as organizational planning. Also, it is highly unlikely that the membership of any existing committee would be primarily composed of individuals who are interested in computers.

Although the organization of early computer adopters may fall outside of the formal faculty organizational structure, this group should be given the official power and responsibility for planning, implementing, and evaluating the computer implementation process. If the committee has less power, the chances for successful implementation of computer-supported education are reduced.

The planning committee coordinates the implementation efforts and communicates the implementation progress to faculty on a regular basis. Given the continuing emergence of new computer technology, this planning group may eventually become a standing or special technology committee of the organization.

Survey and Utilize Local Computer Resources

Initially, the implementation of computer-supported education is difficult without assistance from outside the nursing profession. Most nursing faculty are neither trained nor educated in computer technology, nor do most schools of nursing have computer experts on their staffs. Although a nationally known nursing computer expert might be helpful as a consultant, initially, the continued use of this person to handle the day-by-day computer implementation problems would not be justified. Thus, a major priority when collecting information about local resources is to determine the extent to which these resources (campus or community) will be able to provide assistance for the types of computer implementation activities being planned. Even though multiple computer resources may be available on campus, heavy demands on these resources by other educational units may make these resources inaccessible for use by nursing. Good technical support is vital to successful computer implementation. If technical problems cannot be resolved quickly, faculty, students, and staff will soon lose faith in computers as effective and efficient time-saving tools.

Information gathering tours of other departments on campus may help the planning committee become better informed about how other educational departments are implementing the use of computers and about the types of computer literacy experiences students are getting in prenursing and non-nursing courses. This information will be valuable when planning for utilization of campus computer resources and for determining what computer experiences need to be offered within the nursing portion of the curriculum.

Visits to off-campus facilities can also be very beneficial and enriching. Local health agencies that are involved with computer implementation activities themselves are excellent places to visit. Learning from others' computer experiences can save time, money, and effort.

Ultimately, the nursing unit will need to work with central administration, and perhaps others, on the purchase and maintenance of software and hardware. Plans for how the nursing computer applications will articulate with those available through central administration will need to be discussed.

Establish Computer Support Groups

The ever-changing nature of computer technology and of educational applications demands the continual sharing of information. An effective way to keep abreast of technological changes is to organize local computer-user groups. Computer support groups are appropriate at all levels of the organization and across all types of users—faculty, staff, and students. Support groups provide opportunities for individuals with similar interests and concerns for sharing information and experiences. These groups can be beneficial in overcoming frustrations of users and in resolving problems through networking with other users of the same technology.

While the original computer user groups were established around a type of hardware (e.g., IBM® or Apple®), a more beneficial approach for educational organizations is to organize a user group around a piece of software, such as a statistical program or database. The user groups, in essence, serve as peer tutoring groups and greatly increase the user's confidence in the operation of the technology. These user support groups may meet regularly or irregularly depending on the needs of the individuals in the group.

User groups can be established both between or within departments. Campuswide user groups provide a mechanism for networking with other educators about what is happening across the entire campus. Within a department, support groups can be used for previewing and evaluating software. The fear of not being able to get a program to run often inhibits an inexperienced computer user from volunteering to preview new computer programs or from using the computer in the classroom.

Conduct Faculty Development Sessions

Faculty development is a high priority. Most faculty are fearful of computers, at least to some extent. Attention needs to be given to alleviating faculty anxieties, fears, and frustrations about computers, and one way to do this is through education. The more knowledgeable faculty are about computers the less threatened they will be. As the faculty's computer knowledge, confidence, and comfort increase, so will the probability of use.

Faculty need to be educated and convinced that computers are essential for the advancement of the organization, the profession, and themselves as individuals. As many faculty as possible should be involved in these developmental sessions even though not all faculty need to learn the same things. Occasionally, faculty members will need to be sent to regional and national computer workshops, especially those offered by nursing educators, to get new ideas, to share learning experiences, and to keep abreast of changes that are occurring in the field.

All faculty need to be given time to develop their own computer knowledge and skills. Some faculty may want to limit their computer expertise to only a few selected programs, such as a statistical program. Nevertheless, once a faculty member becomes skilled with a particular program, he or she should be expected to teach and assist others to learn this program as well. Faculty will need to learn how to be a computer tutor to other faculty.

Implementing the use of computers takes time—time to learn and time to keep on learning. Generally, the more complex the computer program, the longer it takes to learn. Given the changing nature of the field, faculty development in the area of computer technology will never be complete. There will always be something more to learn; there will always be something new to apply to nursing.

Determine Administrative and Faculty Commitment and Support

Successful computer integration throughout the educational organization and curriculum requires administrative and faculty support and commitment. The lack of support or commitment on either party's part will yield minimum results.

Administrators. Administrative leadership, good communication, and adequate resources are fundamental to successful uses of computers within an organization. Equally as important are the commitment of time and effort, faculty development, and people to plan and implement the change.

By virtue of budget control, resource allocation, and personnel assignments, administrators strongly influence the degree to which computer implementation will be successful within an organization. The extent of the administration's commitment is reflected in the organization's budget, not only initially, but also annually. Funding to support the integration of computer technology must be allocated annually. Without stable funding and resources allocated to the implementation process, successful computer-supported education is highly unlikely.

Administrative commitment in terms of incentives and staff resources is also paramount to the successful utilization of computers within a nursing organization. Incentives (extra money, extra assistance, decreased workload, release time) that encourage teachers to grow and to develop innovative applications of computers need to be offered and made public. The development of computer-based learning experiences need to be included as part of the criteria for merit, promotion, and tenure. Only then will the administrators' commitment to implementing computer-supported education become real to the faculty.

Faculty. Not all faculty will embrace the use of computers. Initially, the use of computer technology in education will create more work for the faculty. Faculty will need to unlearn some of their old habits and learn new ways of doing things. Faculty will need to spend additional time previewing and selecting computer programs and deciding how to modify these programs to fit their particular courses. Asking instructors to change their teaching habits can be very stressful and make the teaching job, to them, seem harder, not easier. This may cause faculty to resist the use of computers.

Facutly may also be reluctant to use new technology on their own, especially without the assistance of a knowledgeable person they can call on for help (Cambre & Castner, 1991). Because faculty are in a position to either facilitate or sabotage the best laid plans, these barriers to faculty use of computers must be overcome. One way to overcome some of this reluctance is to hire computer support personnel to assist with the implementation process.

Finally, both the faculty and the administration must be open to change and to the possibility that the organization may need to be restructured and undergo power shifts in order to achieve full computer integration. Administrative and faculty involvement, support, and commitment will need to be continuously cultivated throughout the implementation process in order to achieve success.

Prioritize Computer Applications

Computer applications within any given institution can take different approaches depending on the interests, values, resources, talents, and creativity of the decision makers and implementors. Multiple educational applications are possible; it is not feasible to computerize everything at once.

Different components of the organization will computerize at different rates depending on the leadership, creativity, and resourcefulness of individuals within the organization. Individuals who are creative and enthusiastic about computer innovations should be encouraged to lead the way even though their areas of interest might not be the top priority on the list. Often getting something going is better than waiting until there is organizational consensus about the priorities.

A major area where faculty should have input into the implementation plan is in determining how computer applications will be integrated in the curriculum. The role and place of computer technology within each education program needs to be articulated so that progressive development of computer skills occurs across the curriculum.

Although many computer implementation decisions are based on expediency, the overall implementation plan should be flexible enough to allow for the delays that are sure to occur.

Select Hardware and Software

Computer equipment and software are critical to computer implementation. The types of hardware and software needed should be determined by the purposes for which the computers will be used. Decisions about hardware and software should be based on pre-identified selection criteria which are based on the planned uses for the technology. While the selection and purchase of hardware is usually an administrative, not faculty decision, a well-informed planning committee can be a valuable resource in helping the administrator make that decision.

Every effort should be made to ensure that the hardware purchased is compatible with the type of software programs available for nursing education. Typically, computer software programs are designed to work on specific types of computers, i.e., IBM® or Apple®. Thus, commercially produced nursing software will not necessarily work on all types of computer hardware without modifications to either the software or hardware. Hardware–software incompatibility problems inhibit rather than facilitate faculty and student use of computers.

Users should be involved in the selection of software whenever possible. The use of software evaluation tools can facilitate the selection process. While student input would be useful when making purchase decisions about instructional software, the final selection of instructional software is the responsibility of the faculty. All computer programs should be previewed before purchase by individuals who are likely to use them as part of their course assignments. Only those programs that are of high quality and "fit" the curriculum should be purchased. Developing one's own software is a costly, time-consuming process, and therefore, the availability of the organization's resources to support this type of creative endeavor needs to be determined before allocating resources to it. Involving faculty in the selection of software greatly enhances their commitment to using computers with students.

Plan for Computer–User Interface

Where and how computer resources will be made accessible to nursing users must be determined. Consideration needs to be given to locating the computers in places that are convenient to the intended users. Individual as well as group uses of the computers need to be addressed in the planning. Computers should also be available in the classroom for use by faculty, and if possible by students, during class. The more convenient and accessible computers are, the more likely they will be used.

Once the physical arrangements have been determined, operational policies and procedures about such things as software access, data security, loading and copying programs, virus control, and ownership of data need to be developed. Computer holdings need to be organized and inventoried to facilitate efficient and effective retrieval, utilization, and updating. Sufficient copies of each program, based on anticipated use, need to be secured in ways that comply with the copyright law.

Users should receive orientation and be held accountable for subsequent usage. Locally prepared user guides which are specifically designed for each instructional program can greatly expedite the novice computer user's interaction with the computer program. Immediate assistance from support staff needs to be available to the users to ensure proper and effective use of the equipment and programs.

Provide Computer Support Services

Efficient and effective computer systems need organizational resources. Not only do computers require servicing during their installation, but they require ongoing maintenance and repairs. Equipment needs to be repaired promptly to minimize any disruption to user productivity. Depending on the number of computer units being serviced and the extent of use, computer systems maintenance may require the expertise of more than one person. When this happens, consideration needs to be given to hiring an in-house technician to perform the routine maintenance and repairs and allow central administration or off-campus computer technicians to service the more complex ones.

Support personnel are needed to assist computer users while they are interacting with the computer. The types and number of personnel needed will depend on the staffing practices, the diversity of services provided (instruction, research, graphics, printing, publishing, testing, scanning, and so on), and the demand for each of these services. As the organization's use of computers expands, so too will the need for more people trained in the computer's use, operation, and support.

Funds must be budgeted annually for computer personnel, supplies, software, equipment, and maintenance. Periodically, money will need to be allocated for the modernization of the computer equipment and the purchase of computer peripherals to enhance the capabilities and operation of the basic computer equipment.

Evaluate Benefits and Effectiveness

All planning should have an evaluation component, and the implementation of computer supported education is no exception. The major difficulty in evaluating the implementation of computers is determining what outcomes to measure, how to measure them, and when to measure them. Without experience, it is not easy to forecast at the beginning of the computer implementation process where one will be at any future point in time. Therefore, precise planning for evaluation of the process is difficult at best.

A common way of evaluating computer implementation is to examine its cost effectiveness. This, however, is also difficult to measure since the cost of computer implementation entails more than the dollar amounts listed on budget documents. Also, implementation costs vary according to when the cost data were collected. Normally start-up costs will be high in both time and money while these same costs amortized over a long period might be interpreted as being low in cost.

Another way to evaluate computer implementation is to measure the computer's effectiveness. Typically, this kind of evaluation consists in the comparison of a computer approach to some other kind of approach, and the results are then reported in terms of which approach was better. Nevertheless, the generalization of the results from one setting to another is limited. A change in one setting may not be considered a success in another setting with different organizational characteristics.

Still another way to evaluate computer implementation is to measure the organizational benefits that have occurred such as time saved, changes in levels of productivity, learning achievements, better utilization of resources, or ability to do things which the organization was not able to do before implementation. Ways of identifying, defining,

and measuring these benefits need to be determined as soon as possible so that the data to document these benefits can be systematically collected along the way.

When determining the what, how, and when of evaluation, data need to be collected about both the intended and unintended outcomes. In the final analysis, the unintended outcomes may be more significant to the organization than the intended ones. Although process evaluation is difficult, documenting the need for continued computer growth and utilization is vital.

Expand Computer Applications

Computer-supported education will continue to grow, primarily due to societal demands for better and more efficiently managed education. Not only will the capabilities of computers expand, but so too will their uses with other technologies, many of which have yet to be developed. As more complex uses of computers emerge, they dramatically will change how learners learn; how teachers teach; and how nurses nurse. Nursing education organizations need to be open to newer and different ways of doing things and allow computers to shape and reshape our organizational practices.

USE OF IMPLEMENTATION PROCESS

The process for implementing computer-supported education presented here was first used as a framework to conduct a series of continuing education workshops about computer technology. The workshops were designed for faculty in undergraduate nursing programs in the South (Aiken, 1988). The components of the process guided the design of those workshops and were also used to plan faculty-directed computer implementation activities between workshops. Between 1985 and 1990, faculty in over 300 collegiate schools of nursing in the South used the process described in this chapter for establishing or enhancing computer-supported education within a school of nursing. Users found the process to be useful, flexible, relevant, and applicable to a wide variety of nursing programs.

for computer supported education have been presented in this chapter. Each component addressed particular planning activities that facilitate the use of computers within a nursing education organization. Users have found the implementation process to be useful and effective in establishing and enhancing computer-supported education in multiple and diverse collegiate nursing education organizations.

SUMMARY

The implementation of computer-supported education demands increased organizational planning in this age of rapidly expanding computers applications. Successful computer implementation entails many organizational activities beyond those commonly associated with the purchase of hardware and software. Twelve significant components of an implementation process

REFERENCES

Aiken, E. (1988). *Moving into the age of computer-supported education: A regional experience in nursing education.* Atlanta: Southern Regional Education Board.

Cambre, M. A., & Castner, L. J. (1991). *The status of interactive video technology in nursing education environments.* Athens, OH: Fuld Institute for Technology in Nursing Education.

21

Integrating Microcomputer Exercises into an Undergraduate Nursing Research Course

Ann L. Sedore
Jocelyne VanNeste-Kenny
Linda Beeber

INTRODUCTION

Few people would question the central role computers have assumed in the research process in nursing. Computer applications have contributed to efficient and effective information retrieval, data processing, statistical analysis, graphic development, database management, and text editing (Saba & McCormick, 1986). The increasing importance of computer applications to modern research efforts has required the development of new attitudes and skills among nurse researchers. This, in turn, has required that the basic competencies necessary for effective use of computers in nursing research be integrated into graduate nursing education (Heller, Romano, Damrosch, & Parks, 1985). There is increasing evidence of both mainframe and microcomputer use in teaching statistics to graduate students (Jacobsen, Tulman, Lowery, & Garson, 1988; Ludeman, 1982).

Faculty teaching undergraduate nursing students find less guidance in literature regarding teaching research-related computer applications. Broad guidelines urge that new graduates have the skills needed to evaluate and use clinical data and research findings as a basis for practice (American Association of Colleges of Nursing, 1986). General guidelines for computer education suggest that undergraduate students should be prepared with the knowledge, skills, and values necessary for roles as users of information technology (Romano et al., 1989). Translating these broad recommendations into specific learning activities and outcomes presents a challenge to baccalaureate faculty. Faculty at Syracuse University College of Nursing decided to accept the challenge and to introduce microcomputer use into an undergraduate nursing research course. After investigating both computer-assisted instruction and commercially prepared applications packages, faculty chose application software to introduce and illustrate the computer's contribution to the research process. The development of the first set of computer-related activities which focused on basic statistical analysis and text editing is described here.

PLANNING PHASE

Philosophical Basis

A team of two faculty members and a teaching assistant worked together to plan a set of learning activities which guided students through the use of computer technology to analyze data and develop and edit text. Because the seniors scheduled for the course had little computer experience, activities were included to ensure basic computer literacy as well. The learning activities were developed to support active, experiential learning (Bevis, 1989; Reilly & Oermann, 1985). Data, questions, and activities were integrated into a set of exercises which required active participation of the student and which allowed application of facts gained in classes and reading. Data for the exercises related directly to student experience and therefore sustained ongoing student interest. The activities were designed to encourage students to use the faculty members and teaching assistant as resources for individualized learning. In addition, exercises were developed with the objective of changing student attitudes about the value of statistical analysis. Real life questions were posed to demonstrate both the summary function of statistics and the use of simple data sets. The planning team hoped to create a sense of excitement, curiosity, and discovery about the use of computers in research as well as in all phases of nursing work.

Hardware

The college of nursing computer laboratory was used as the primary setting for this project. The laboratory has four Zenith 500 IBM compatible microcomputers with 640 Kb of memory. Each of these computers is equipped with a 20 Mb hard disk and a single 5¼-inch disk drive. All are connected to an Epson dot matrix printer. Standardized menus provide access to programs and files stored in the hard disks. Necessary programs could also be provided through a local area network.

Software

The choice of software was influenced by several factors. Three primary factors were quality of the program, cost, and ease of use. The software had to offer essential capabilities and accuracy. Programs had to be reasonable for the college budget and, if possible, reasonably priced for student purchase. Finally, programs selected had to be user friendly and had to provide some basic tutorial which explained basic functions and use. For this project, the software programs chosen were MYSTAT and WordPerfect 5.1.

MYSTAT is an inexpensive, interactive statistics and graphics package for the microcomputer (Wilkinson, 1988). It is described as a personal version of SYSTAT, a powerful, multifaceted statistical program (Wilkinson, 1987). MYSTAT allows rapid calculation of a range of descriptive and inferential statistics. (See Table 21.1 for available tests.) It is an interactive package available for both IBM PCs and the Macintosh. It requires 256 Kb of memory and a floppy or hard disk drive. With adequate disk space it can handle up to 50 variables and 32,000 cases. For this project, MYSTAT was loaded on the hard disk and used in the interactive analyses mode (default) which is menu driven.

WordPerfect 5.1 is a comprehensive word processing package which allows the user to create professional looking documents. Some of the capabilities of this program include the ability to create columns, tables,

Table 21.1 Types of Statistics and Available Functions in MYSTAT

Descriptive Statistics
Sum, mean, standard error of the mean, minimum, maximum, range, standard deviation, variance, skewness, and kurtosis

Graphical Data Analysis
Scatter plots, histograms, box plot, stem and leaf diagram, and T plots

Frequencies and Contingency Table Analysis
N-way cross tabulation tables and frequency, two-way tables chi square test statistics, association coefficients, frequencies, row percents, column percents or cell percents

Correlations
Pearson product moment correlations and Spearman rank-order correlations

Dependent and Independent Group Tests
Dependent (paired) or independent T-tests, Wilcoxon signed rank test, Friedman nonparametric analysis of variance

Linear Models
Regression analysis, ANOVA, and ANOCOVA

---

footnotes, endnotes, and macros.[1] The program also provides a spell checker and a thesaurus. The MS-DOS version of WordPerfect 5.1 runs on any PC. The program requires DOS 2.0 or higher and 384 Kb of free memory, and at least two floppy disk drives; a hard disk drive is recommended. WordPerfect was selected for the project because it is available in the college laboratory and on local area networks across campus. Nevertheless, any text editor could be used for this project.

Development of Structured Learning Activities

The team constructed a set of structured learning activities which had two primary focuses: enhancing computer literacy skills and developing statistical analysis and interpretation skills. Exercises guided and facili-

---

[1] WordPerfect includes a programming language that allows users to create macros, "sets of stored keystrokes that allow you to perform the same task over and over again with the push of a key" (Salkind, 1991, p. 279).

tated the development of essential computer skills such as floppy disk management, file manipulation, word processing, and printing statistical output and written documents.

Other learning activities focused on moving students beyond memorization of facts about statistics to the development of skills in manipulation of data and interpretation of results. Students were provided with exercises in data manipulation using MYSTAT. Real and hypothetical data were provided to the students on a floppy disk. The data were linked to simulated research problems involving student characteristics and performance on class and the National Council Licensure Examination (NCLEX). Step-by-step guidelines led the student through the generation of descriptive statistics, histograms and scatter plots, correlation coefficients, and multiple regression statistics. At the completion of this work, each student had a set of printed outputs from the statistical package.

Two interpretation exercises followed. Students were asked to respond to two sets of questions which forced systematic examination of the meaning of the statistical results (see Tables 21.2 and 21.3). The

Table 21.2 Exercise Set #1—Comparison of Class Performance: Interpretation of Descriptive Statistics, Histograms, and T-tests

Instructions: Your professors believe that class of 1990 students in the research course are more hard working and more intelligent than those of previous years. Despite this, the professors are worried that the class is not doing as well as previous students. To answer this, professors compare this year's test scores (CLASS 90) with last year's (CLASS 89). Using your output of both classes' test scores, answer the following questions:

1. What is the range of scores for each class?
2. What is the mean of the scores for each class?
3. What do the standard deviations tell you about the distribution?
4. Describe each distribution in terms of its shape (modality, skew).
5. Based on the shape of each curve, which class had a larger proportion of scores at the lower end of the scale?
6. Based on the shape of the curve, which class was more homogeneous? Explain your reasoning.
7. What is the t-value of the difference in the class means?
8. Explain what the term "DF" means in the output.
9. Were the means of the two classes significantly different? Support your answer with data from your output. Explain the meaning of the output data.

Table 21.3 Exercise Set #2—Examining the Relationship between Student Characteristics and NCLEX Scores: Correlations and Scatter Plots

Instructions: Your professors would like to know which characteristics of students predict their success on the state board examination. They considered the following variables:

TESTSC1 —NUR 451 test score
TESTSC2 —NCLEX Score
SAT —Scholastic Aptitude Test Score
FAMINC —Family Income
GPA —Grade Point Average
CONSTANT—Statistical constant (Not needed to answer questions.)

Using your output of the variables in file:a:sample, answer the following questions:

1. Describe the scatter plot of TESTSC2 and SAT. Is there any relationship? Is it a direct or indirect relationship?
2. What is the correlation of TESTSC2 and SAT scores? Explain the meaning of the correlation in layperson/nonstatistical terminology.
3. What is the correlation of family income and SAT scores? Explain it in layperson/nonstatistical terminology.
4. List any variables that were significant predictors of scores on the NCLEX. Support your answer with data from your output.
5. What percentage of the variance in NCLEX scores was associated with the variables of TESTSC1, SAT scores, FAMINC, and GPA? Support your answer with data from your output.

questions were given to the students on a floppy disk as word files and the student was asked to respond and return the answers on the disk and as hard copy. Questions led the students to interpret statistics, histograms, and scatter plots in light of simulated variables and group performance.

Development of a Study Packet

The team designed a study packet which described the purposes and activities and clearly identified the learning goals involved. Included in the packet were relevant vocabulary words to be defined, hardware information, tips on handling and working with diskettes, samples of screens and output, and step-by-step directions for all exercises.

To check for clarity and effectiveness, two faculty who had no experience with the software packages were asked to use the packet to complete the required activities. Each was able to generate the statistics required, access the questions sets, save the required data, print outputs and reports, and exit with no difficulty. The exercises were completed in a reasonable amount of time.

IMPLEMENTATION

Following completion of didactic instruction related to statistical analyses, the students were introduced to the computer-related activities. Each was assigned a two-hour computer laboratory time for guided group activity. The teaching assistant conducted four separate laboratory sessions to accommodate 34 seniors. The computer laboratory replaced regularly scheduled class time.

During the computer laboratory period, students worked in pairs. The students were given the module and a formatted diskette containing three files: two data files and one containing questions to be answered on WordPerfect. Following an explanation of the assignment, the students worked through the statistical analysis with assistance, as necessary, from a teaching assistant. In the first portion of the laboratory period, one of the two students in a pair used the files stored on the data disk to generate and print statistical results about the data while the other gave directions from the packet. In the second portion of the laboratory period, the students changed places and ran through the statistical analysis again. The teaching assistant was available throughout this period to answer questions, solve technical problems, and stimulate problem solving. In particular, she dealt with problems of using one printer to generate hard copy from four computers.

The students were initially very anxious about the experience. They appeared uneasy and commented about their dislike of computers, their feelings of powerlessness and ignorance about the technology, and their lack of typing skills. Despite this, almost all of them completed the laboratory assignment on a timely basis and, upon completing the class, commented on the ease with which the data was generated.

Students were required to complete the interpretation exercises on an independent basis. They were told that they could complete the assignment at their convenience in the college laboratory or at university clusters. The majority of the students completed the work with no difficulties. A small group of students were more anxious about the technology and made individual appointments to obtain technical assistance from the teaching assistant. In these cases the mere presence of the teaching assistant was sufficient to enable them to complete their assignment.

EVALUATION

The effectiveness of the new computer-related exercises in statistical analysis and interpretation was evaluated in three ways. First, the course instructor was asked to comment on students' classroom behaviors after the computer activities. Second, the course instructor evaluated required written assignments. Third, students were asked to submit written evaluations of the experience.

Student performance in class-related behaviors did change positively as a result of these learning activities. In classroom discussions of research reports, students demonstrated an increased ability to discuss and critique data analysis techniques after the exercises. Student laboratory behaviors indicated an increase in computer skill and comfort. The course instructor also reported that students were able to transfer statistical concepts learned through MYSTAT work into a final poster project.

In addition to changes in classroom behavior, faculty observed expanded computer use by the student group. Many of the students came back for more instructions and several developed the computer skills necessary to produce scholarly papers and resumes. Many students used computer-generated text in their final poster presentations and commented this was a result of their recent exposure to computer capabilities. One student with no previous computer experience purchased a PC. Despite a general lack of previous computer experience, all students were able to achieve a passing grade on the required computer assignments with minimal assistance.

Students' written evaluations were consistently positive. Two-thirds of the students indicated in the course evaluation that the computer exercises and poster sessions were the "best part of the course." They commented that the computer exercises were an interesting way of applying their knowledge about statistics. They felt that using real data which were specific to them as a group made the exercises more enjoyable. Interestingly, students reported that because of these learning activities, they had developed an appreciation for the role of the researcher in the research and analysis process.

Students' comments suggested some change in attitudes toward computer use. Students reported that they felt the project decreased their anxiety about using computers. Some had not dared to even sit at a computer console before, and this experience forced them to take that first step. Students indicated that they were pleased to learn some of the basics of computer operations such as manipulation of disks and retrieving and storing of files. For some students, the hardest part was selecting and purchasing the appropriate diskette. Most students were pleased that they had the opportunity to learn about word processing.

EXPANSION BEYOND THE UNDERGRADUATE PROGRAM

Since the success of the initial project with over 60 undergraduate students, computer exercises have been introduced into the research course in the baccalaureate and the master's nursing programs. Over the last year, results with 32 baccalaureate nursing students and 81 master's nursing students were slightly different, but equally positive. For the graduate students, the learning module was altered significantly to reflect their theoretical and methodological interests and to include an emphasis on more complex statistical analysis.

CONCLUSIONS

Overall, the initial integration of commercially prepared software into an undergraduate research course was a success. The exercises provided an experiential basis for students to understand the power and meaning of statistics and the vital role of the computer in statistical work. At the same time, the activities produced increased computer literacy and stimulated an interest in expanding personal use of computers.

Using commercially developed software packages to develop learning activities for nursing students is exciting and interesting. It provides an alternative and addition to the use of computer-assisted instruction and supports the development of computer skills that will contribute to personal and professional excellence and productivity.

REFERENCES

American Association of Colleges of Nursing. (1986). *Essentials of college and university education for professional nursing* (Final Report). Washington, DC: AACN.

Bevis, E. (1989). *Curriculum building in nursing: A process.* New York: National League for Nursing.

Heller, B., Romano, C., Damrosch, S., & Parks, P. (1985). Computer applications for nursing: Implications for the curriculum. *Computers in Nursing, 3,* 14–21.

Jacobsen, B., Tulman, L., Lowery, B., & Garson, C. (1988). Experiencing the research process by using statistical software on microcomputers. *Nursing Research, 37* (1), 56–59.

Ludeman, R. (1982). Strategies for teaching nursing research: Experiential learning in data analysis. *Western Journal of Nursing Research, 4* (1), 124–126.

Reilly, D., & Oermann, M. (1985). *The clinical field: Its use in nursing education.* Norwalk, CT: Appleton-Century-Crofts.

Romano, C., Damrosch, S., Heller, B., & Parks, P. (1989). Levels of computer education for professional nursing: Development of a prototype graduate course. *Computers in Nursing, 7* (1), 21–28.

Saba, V., & McCormick, K. (1986). *Essentials of computers for nurses.* Philadelphia: Lippincott.

Salkind, N. (1991). *WordPerfect™ 5.0/5.1: A self-teaching guide.* New York: Wiley.

Wilkinson, L. (1987). *SYSTAT: The system for statistics.* Evanston, IL: SYSTAT.

Wilkinson, L. (1988). *MYSTAT: The system for personal version of SYSTAT.* Evanston, IL: SYSTAT.

22

Computer Usage among High-Risk Baccalaureate Nursing Students

Helen Lerner
Barbara Cohen
Marcia Brown

INTRODUCTION AND BACKGROUND

This chapter focuses on the use of computer-assisted instruction (CAI) with baccalaureate nursing students at Lehman College who were at high risk for academic failure. High-risk students are those students who have received a grade of C or less in a previous nursing course. The desired outcome was increased academic success of students. In order to provide CAI, a computer laboratory with a library of CAI software was established. The process of these efforts is also discussed.

Lehman College is the only senior public college in the Bronx. The demographics of Lehman College students reflect the population of the geographical location it serves. Like other public universities, the students are older (their mean age is 31) and many are in need of educational and financial support services. Many students enter the college with academic deficiencies in basic skills such as reading and mathematics. Subsequently, they have difficulty with concepts taught in nursing courses.

The college obtained two grants that made the establishment of a nursing computer center possible. The first grant was awarded by the Department of Health and Human Services, Health Resources and Services Administration, Division of Nursing. The goal of this grant was to increase the retention rate of disadvantaged students through the use of CAI. Funding was used to identify students at risk of academic failure, purchase educational software, author computer-assisted instruction programs, and purchase the needed hardware and software to accomplish the goal of the grant. One year after federal funding, a Helene Fuld Foundation grant enabled the division of nursing to convert a nursing audiovisual room into a nursing computer laboratory. Two of the authors were grant coordinators.

Preparation of this article was supported in part by a grant from the Department of Health and Human Services, Health Resources and Services Administration, Division of Nursing D19 NU 22164 to Dr. Rosanne Wille.

SETTING AND HARDWARE AVAILABLE

Prior to the awarding of the two grants the only computer resource available to nursing students was at the Academic Computer Center (ACC). This facility is utilized by all Lehman College students. Although there were computers available at the ACC, only five computers had monitors with color and graphic capabilities, the attributes needed to run the CAI being purchased for nursing students. Currently there are twelve computers in the ACC that have these features.

In the nursing computer center, seven computer stations were established, each equipped with an IBM PS2 model 25 computer. An Epson FV 850/1050 printer was purchased for use with the seven computers. A local area network (LAN) was established using an IBM PS2 model 60 computer as a file server. This eliminated the need for personnel to distribute CAI program disks to students. Students could access the software via a menu established by the computer consultant.

DEVELOPMENT OF A SOFTWARE LIBRARY

In order to develop a software library that would be relevant to the nursing curriculum and students' learning needs, an evaluation plan was established. This included review of potential purchases of CAI by students and faculty. Technical personnel at the ACC were also consulted to ensure that CAI purchased could be used with the network and computers in the ACC.

Faculty were asked to consider CAI programs from the viewpoint of both strong and weak students. Faculty tended to evaluate programs as being too simple and basic.

These very attributes are the ones most often prized by students.

The authors established the following criteria for software purchase: (1) the hardware requirements of the authors or publishers of the CAI would be compatible with the hardware available at Lehman College; (2) the intended use of the program reflected the objectives of individual nursing courses; (3) the content should be correct and should facilitate learning.

Hardware requirements were considered when faculty identified programs in catalogs or other listings. It was necessary to confirm that the program was available for use with an IBM computer. Faculty were given information about the memory capabilities of the computers at the college and the possible CAI requirements of a color monitor and graphics package. Since the plan was to place CAI on local area networks in the ACC and in the nursing computer center, site licenses needed to be obtained. A site license from the publishers of software programs gives the college the right to use the programs anywhere on campus.

To ensure that CAI would foster the objectives of individual nursing courses, faculty were provided with a workshop addressing the various types of CAI available (e.g., tutorials, drill and practice, simulations) and their uses in the nursing curriculum. Faculty were encouraged to examine the congruence between CAI program objectives and course objectives. At first, faculty felt most at ease with tutorials and simulations. Later, faculty recognized the need for drill and practice, test construction, and games that taught concepts.

To address the third criterion for software purchase, faculty were asked to critique the feedback in the program and check for correctness of the content. Students were asked to comment about the effectiveness of the programs in facilitating learning. While reviewing programs, students often tended to get sidetracked when they did not do well in answering questions. They needed reassurance that this was not a test of their knowledge and that their comments were important.

The software evaluation checklist shown in Table 22.1 was constructed to evaluate CAI programs. Initially, the purchase of software was difficult because there were few appropriate software programs on the market. Fortunately, this situation changed and at the current time there are 50 CAI programs available for student use on our local area network. Purchases have been concen-

trated in tutorials and simulations. Difficulty has been encountered with finding appropriate drill and practice programs.

Intended Use of Software

Initially, the focus was on purchasing programs that could be used in courses with a high attrition rate (i.e., adult health nursing, pharmacology, and pathophysiology). Programs that would enhance the teaching of basic concepts such as medication administration and drug calculation were purchased. These included *Medication Admin-*

Table 22.1   Software Evaluation Checklist

A. Hardware Requirements of CAI	(Fill in the blanks)
brand of computer	_____
memory of computer	_____
graphics capability	_____
color monitor needed	_____

B. Intended Use of CAI	(Place a check if applicable)	
drill and practice	_____	
tutorial	_____	
simulation	_____	
test	_____	
other	(explain) _____	

C. Content	(Circle your response)	
accuracy	accurate	not accurate
timeliness	current	not current
presentation of material	enhances	does not enhance learning
reflects course objectives	yes	no

D. Miscellaneous Information	(Circle your response)	
accessing program	easy	difficult
exiting program	easy	difficult

E. Additional Comments:

istration I & II (Brown and Brown, 1988) and *Eliminating Medication Errors* (Willis, 1988a). The first program is a tutorial that gives students the opportunity to calculate drug dosages and intravenous solutions. Students can view syringes and IV bottles on the screen and calculate the medication dosage or the IV drip rate. Students are also given opportunities to carry out their calculations by filling a syringe and regulating an IV.

Eliminating Medication Errors is a game in which the student is asked to administer medications to patients. The student is presented with a series of questions regarding knowledge required for this skill. Immediate feedback and the total score obtained is provided at the end of the game. When a student completes the game within the allocated time and receives a high score, a reward of a coffee break is given.

Because understanding disease processes is often difficult for students, the CAI program *Type II Diabetes* (Willis, 1988b) was purchased to facilitate learning. This program makes liberal use of graphics and animation and uses the nursing process in caring for a person with diabetes. Students are assigned this program in the course Pathophysiology II.

The division of nursing also considered programs that would give instruction in basic principles of nursing care. The goal for purchasing this type of software was to free faculty from giving repetitive information that could be presented just as effectively in another format. Students were then responsible for learning specified content with CAI.

FM Tutor: Computer-aided instruction for fetal monitoring interpretation (Catanzarite, 1986) and *Nurs-Comps: The twelve point postpartal check* (Hill & O'Connor, 1989) were purchased to help students prepare for the clinical laboratory. Students were expected to learn fetal monitoring by using the assigned CAI before their clinical experiences in labor and delivery. Learning to

check patients postpartum was also expected of students prior to their clinical laboratory. Subsequent to the purchase of these programs, the content addressing fetal monitoring and postpartum assessments was eliminated from classroom instruction.

ASSISTING STUDENTS AT RISK OF ACADEMIC FAILURE

Through analysis of students' grades and selected demographics variables, the authors concluded that the best indicator for predicting student performance in a specific course was performance in previous nursing courses. One of the courses with the highest attrition rate was the junior level course, adult health nursing.

When documentation of the effectiveness of CAI as a learning strategy began, 79 students were enrolled in the adult health nursing course. Twenty-five of the students enrolled in this course were identified as being at risk of academic failure. Letters were mailed to all 25 students scheduling an appointment with one of the computer grant coordinators.

When the student met with the grant coordinator, the following areas were discussed: (1) personal problems, (2) study habits, and (3) previous nursing course grades. Students were given information about the academic computer center and the nursing computer center and provided with explicit directions about computer use. Software programs were selected for each student according to their appropriateness for the course and the student's particular learning needs. Students were provided with an individualized CAI listing. The students were asked to schedule appointments with the grant coordinator throughout the semester.

Fifteen students failed adult health nursing. Fourteen had been among the twenty-five students that the grant coordinator had counseled. Only three of the 15 students who had failed had used more than one CAI program. The other 12 students had used one CAI program or none at all. Determination of why nursing students who were unsuccessful in this course did not take advantage of CAI requires further analyses.

Description of Students at Risk of Academic Failure

The 15 students who failed the adult health nursing course were typical of the students who comprised the student body. Their ages ranged from 22 to 53 with a mean age of 33.8. Eight students were Black, three were Hispanic, and two were Caucasian. The grade point averages that the students had obtained when they entered the nursing program ranged from 2.21 to 3.5. All students were female.

All students were enrolled in at least two other courses at the time they failed the adult health nursing course. Six of the students reported being employed, working between eight hours to 35 hours per week. All students reported personal problems (e.g., a miscarriage, death of a family member, or a severe financial crisis). The most frequent reason cited for nonuse of the computer was lack of time.

Intervention

The 15 nursing students met with and were interviewed individually by the computer grant coordinator. The interview consisted of the following questions:

1. Did you use CAI during the adult health nursing course?
2. If you did not use the computer, can you tell me why?

3. What other courses did you take last semester?
4. Were you employed while you were taking the course in adult health nursing?
5. Can you tell me of any personal problems you experienced while taking this course?

After being interviewed, students were invited to sit down and turn on the computer. If necessary they were shown how to do this. They were then asked to use the computer to answer approximately 15 questions on the adult health nursing portion of one of the NURSESTAR tests (Lochaas & Miller, 1984). As the students responded to the questions, they were asked to give a rationale for their answers. If necessary, the grant coordinator provided suggestions that might help students to arrive at the correct answers. The computer provided students with immediate feedback.

Students were then directed to select a CAI program. As students used the program, the grant coordinator was available for help. Students were given information about each program available for their use. Encouragement was given to use the computer facilities. Information about the hours of both the ACC and the nursing computer center was provided.

OBSERVATIONS OF STUDENTS WITH COMPUTERS

A first observation was that most students were very fearful of the computer. Even students who had used computers previously were concerned with turning on the computer. They expressed fear that they would break something or do something wrong. Many students had never used a typewriter and were intimidated by the keyboard. They needed help in locating the space bar, the enter key, and keys for letters and numbers. When an unexpected response was made by the computer (due to student error or accident) the students expressed fear that they had damaged the machine and indicated they would never be "good with machines."

When students selected a CAI program, several of them were surprised at what the computer could do. Many students interpreted feedback from the computer such as "try again" or "incorrect" as negative. Comments that indicated students' insecurities included, "I don't think I know this," "I'll probably make a mistake," "I probably can't do this," "I'm not very good at answering questions . . . using the computer, . . . doing math." Students needed encouragement and personal reinforcement from the grant coordinator. Personal contact and instructor availability decreases frustration and increases the effectiveness of CAI (Paulanka, 1986).

Reading difficulties of students became apparent as they worked with the computer. Indications of this were students reading aloud or reading more slowly than one may anticipate of college students.

Follow-Up

The following year, the same 15 students were contacted after repeating the course in adult health nursing. All 15 students passed the course the second time. Thirteen of the 15 students who were contacted responded. The students were asked if their approach to the course in adult health nursing the second time was different. They were also questioned about changes in their use of software and which software programs they used. Information was again solicited regarding changes in their work hours and changes in their personal lives.

The second time students took the course, all students interviewed reported that their approach to the course had changed. They reported changes such as using of a tape recorder, reading more, studying in advance, and using the computer to a greater extent. Two students, however, still reported no computer use for the course in adult health nursing. These students stated that CAI was not required for the adult health nursing course. They also indicated that their personal and work schedules were too demanding and they had insufficient time to use the computer. The two students could not cite any factors that could make computer use easier for them. These same two students noted that in the course in psychiatric nursing, which they were currently taking, computer programs were required. They had used the required programs and found them helpful.

Students were asked what changes would make it easier for them to use the computer. All students reported lack of time as a problem. Other responses noted were: more computers (n=4); more flexible hours needed for both centers (n=4); more programs (n=2); more items on tests related to information given in computer programs (n=1); and computers required for papers in the course; and other course requirements (n=1).

Discussion

Most students who failed the course the first time seemed to be afraid of the computer and had low opinions of their abilities related to computer use. The students seemed to be very fearful of operating the computer and very concerned that they would do something wrong and harm the machine. Even the two students who said that they had used computers in the context of their jobs reported that they did not feel comfortable operating the computer and using the CAI programs. The importance of a supportive environment to foster computer use is clear. This is particularly important for students who are not well-motivated to use the computer and those with little experience with computers. An environment perceived as nonsupportive can easily discourage computer use (Bratt & Vockell, 1986). Even when the environment has adequate support, students can be easily discouraged by a minor mishap. They may be afraid to ask for help from those who appear much more knowledgeable about computers.

Negative feedback from CAI can be more destructive to students than faculty realize. Although the majority of programs try to keep the feedback as positive as possible, students may still feel intimidated.

RECOMMENDATIONS FOR THE FUTURE

The benefits of CAI cannot be fully realized unless students use the computers. After meeting with students who had failed adult health nursing, it was clear that the strategies being employed were not successful. It was decided that changes needed to be made in the approach to students and computers. These changes were divided into three categories: (1) making computers easier to use, (2) integrating CAI into the curriculum and (3) increasing student self-esteem.

Making Computer Use Easier

Now explicit instructions have been attached to each computer. This includes information on how to turn on the computer and access software programs. The computer consultant created a program so that when students turn on the computer, they are greeted by their first and last names. The network runs all software programs so that students do not have to handle disks. A cus-

tomized menu has been designed to facilitate accessing programs. The main menu lists: a computer tutorial, database programs, games, CAI, DOS utilities, and word processing programs. A computer technician is available for assistance during the hours that the nursing computer center is open. The first week of class, all students in the first nursing course are oriented by clinical groups to the computer center. They are shown how to log on and off the computer and to access CAI programs. All CAI programs on the network are briefly described. Other software programs are explained and the students are encouraged to come in and use the programs. Students are encouraged to use the word processing programs for required papers, individualized instruction is provided in learning this.

Integrating CAI into the Curriculum

CAI is integrated into every nursing course. See Table 22.2 for a listing of courses and software. Faculty have recognized that CAI is an important teaching strategy. Faculty need to address the questions of whether to require a CAI program, when to require the program, and how to determine if the students have fulfilled this requirement. There are some students who will not use CAI unless it is required.

Moreover, faculty need to determine how to incorporate CAI into course requirements and how students will demonstrate they have used assigned CAI. How to use the CAI in a course will depend on the availability of appropriate software and faculty's familiarity with the capabilities of CAI. It may take time for faculty to feel comfortable in allowing CAI to be the mode of instruction rather than classroom lectures and discussion.

The literature supports CAI being used in nursing curricula (Bratt & Vockell, 1986;

Table 22.2 CAI Assigned in Nursing Courses

Level of Nursing	Course Name	Software
Sophomore Year	Concepts of Professional Nursing	Introduction to Patient Problems (1) Documentation: Doing the "Write" Thing (2) Nursing Diagnoses (1) Universal Precautions (2)*
	Nursing Practice Laboratory	Handwashing (2) Introduction to Patient Problems (1) Therapeutic Patient Communications I&II (2)
	Health Assessment	The Heart & How It Works (2)
	Pathophysiology I	Inflammation, Infection, and Wound Healing (4) Fluid and Electrolyte Balance (4) Acid–Base Balance (4)
Junior Year	Pathophysiology II	Diabetes Type II (2)
	Adult Health Nursing	Calculating Tablets & Liquids (3) Parenteral Dosages (3) Medication Administration (4) Eliminating Medication Errors (2)
	Psychiatric Nursing	The Med Clinic (2) Nursing Care of Patients with Anxiety Disorders (3)
Senior Year	Parent Child Nursing	FM Tutor: Computer-Aided Instruction for Fetal Monitoring Interpretation (5) Pharmacological Interventions in Obstetric Care (2) The Twelve-Point Postpartal Check (1)
	Community Health	Neurology—Mr. Woody, A Gentleman With a Spinal Cord Injury (1) Neurology—Harvey, a Sixteen-Year-Old Boy With a Head Injury (1)

Code for Software Vendors
 1. J. B. Lippincott & Co., Philadelphia, PA
 2. Computerized Educational Systems, Orlando, FL
 3. Medi-Sim, Edwardsville, KS
 4. Professional Development Software, Manhasset, NY
 5. Williams & Wilkins Co., Baltimore, MD
* Universal Precautions is assigned every year to all nursing students

Goodman, Blake, & Lott, 1990; Belfry & Winne, 1988; Yoder & Heilman, 1985). CAI is considered most useful when it is used to supplement other forms of instruction. Students can learn material in less time and the learning can be adapted to their own pace and convenience (Belfry & Winne, 1988).

Increasing Student Self-Esteem

It is important to create an environment where CAI use will result in enabling students to feel positive about themselves as learners. Alerting computer staff to student needs and concerns relating to computers is essential as is providing positive feedback to the staff themselves. Some students have found that it is helpful to work on computer programs in groups to collaborate and work together. Other students prefer to work alone stating that the self-paced learning offered by CAI provides them with an opportunity for control over their learning experiences (Koch, Rankin, & Stewart, 1990). It is important to talk with students and determine which learning situation they feel is more beneficial.

Since computer feedback seemed to be intimidating in our experience with the students, it is important students be prepared for the type of feedback that computers use. They should be informed whether or not faculty will have access to scores and what will be done with this information.

It is useful to consider variables such as stress, personal problems, and change when introducing students to new instructional media (Paulanka, 1986). Students with visual or orthopedic problems may have difficulty working with CAI. Lighting and seating for computer laboratories need to be carefully selected.

By determining how CAI will be used to best meet the needs of the students and the course content, faculty can help ensure that the students will benefit from using CAI as a learning strategy. By facilitating the use of CAI for students, faculty will have provided an additional strategy that will assist students' learning.

REFERENCES

Belfry, M. J., & Winne, P. H. (1988). A review of the effectiveness of computer assisted instruction in nursing education. *Computers in Nursing, 6*, 77–85.

Bratt, E., & Vockell, E. (1986). Using computers to teach basic facts in the nursing curriculum. *Journal of Nursing Education, 25*, 247–251.

Brown, D., & Brown, P. (1988). *Medication administration I & II* [Computer program]. Manhasset, NY: Professional Development Software.

Catanzarite, V. A. (1986). *FM tutor: Computer-aided instruction for fetal monitoring interpretation* [Computer program]. Baltimore: Williams & Wilkins.

Goodman, J., Blake, J., & Lott, M. (1990). CAI: A strategy for retaining minority and academically disadvantaged students. *Nurse Educator, 15*, 37–41.

Hill, D. W., & O'Connor, M. (1989). *Nurs-Comps: The twelve point postpartal check* [Computer program]. Philadelphia: Lippincott.

Koch, E. W., Rankin, J. A., & Stewart, R. (1990). Nursing students' preferences in the use of computer assisted learning. *Journal of Nursing Education, 29*, 122–126.

Lochaas, T., & Miller, A. (Eds.). (1984). *NURSESTAR* [Computer program]. St. Louis, MO: The C. V. Mosby Company.

Paulanka, B. J. (1986). The learning characteristics of nursing students and computer assisted instruction: An exploratory study. *Computers in Nursing, 4*, 246–251.

Willis, M. A. (1988a). *Eliminating medication errors* [Computer program]. Orlando, FL: Computerized Educational Systems.

Willis, M. A. (1988b). *Type II diabetes* [Computer program]. Orlando, FL: Computerized Educational Systems.

Yoder, M. E., & Heilman, T. (1985). The use of computer assisted instruction to teach nursing diagnosis. *Computers in Nursing, 3*, 262–265.

23

Using Integrated Software for Test and Grade Management

Gloria Lombardi
Rosemarie Blume

INTRODUCTION

Traditionally, management of tests and grades is costly and time consuming. Often, tests are generated by the cut-and-paste method using old tests or from test questions on cards. Equipment used to manage and generate tests includes: pen and pencil, index cards, file folders, cabinets, typewriter, grade books, and loose leaf notebooks containing grids that evaluate course objectives. Because secretarial support is required, preparation time has increased.

Software programs available for the personal computer combine one or more of the above functions. Now, integrated software packages that handle all aspects of test management are available. These integrated software packages not only store items, but also generate, score, and analyze tests. The grade book section assigns a grade, posts the grade in a student roster, and calculates a final grade.

Description of an Integrated System

Test items are entered into a bank and a test is generated. The student takes the test either on the computer (online) or from a printout (offline). An optical scanner scores offline testing, whereas the program scores online test taking. Then the test is analyzed and scores recorded in a grade book. A printed copy of the grade book is available.

An integrated system manages all the details of producing a test in an interactive form. Changes in one part of the system will cause changes in other areas. For instance, grading the test will place the point value in the grade book and update the item analysis. If the answer key needs correction, the test is rescored automatically. Roster updating occurs within a few seconds.

AVAILABILITY OF SOFTWARE

Several software programs on the market are geared to manage test delivery and analysis. These include ParSYSTEM, Exam-SYSTEM, MicroPac, MicroTim, and the Examiner. These systems are user friendly and do not require sophisticated computer or programming skills. On-screen menus and online help prompt the user at every step. Besides the online help, written documentation is available. Software developers are usually available for consultation. Educators and staff training can be facilitated by use of software manuals and available consultants. The vendors (listed in Appendix A) will send demonstration disks on request.

This chapter focuses on features common to all integrated software packages especially the ParSYSTEM, the software package with which the authors have the greatest familiarity. There are also some features unique to specific systems. For further information on considerations for choosing a package refer to Lombardi (1990).

TEST PREPARATION

The most difficult task in the use of integrated software packages is having educators develop or contribute to item banks. Foremost is the time and skill required for the development and maintenance of an item bank. Another factor is the educator's degree of familiarity with computers. Based on the writers' experiences conducting workshops, educators appear more willing and enthusiastic to put in the time necessary to develop and maintain item banks after an orientation session.

Characteristics of an Item Bank

An item bank is a large collection of test items (questions) used in a test. The item bank must be larger than the number of items used in one test and must be classified in some way to simplify test assembly. The type of items that can be stored in an item bank includes multiple choice, true–false, fill-in, matching, and essay. Some systems include an item bank. MicroTim includes a biochemistry item bank of 7,000 questions.

Creating an Item Bank

The creation and classification of item banks in order to generate tests varies

greatly in each integrated system. A feature to take into consideration is the ability to create or add to an item bank independent of the total integrated system. An important software feature is a word processor which includes a speller checker option providing easy item entry and item editing.

Another feature to look for is the banking and inclusion of visual images on a test printout. Graphs or pictures drawn or scanned by an optical character scanning program gives more flexibility in test design. Users who do not have the hardware necessary for printing graphics need to see that the printed test allows the space necessary for the graphics to be pasted onto test printouts.

Classifying Item Banks and Items

Creating separate item banks enhances the grouping of items that refer to a specific course or content area. Separate item banks eliminate the cumbersome task of sorting or searching through hundreds of items for specific items. Item banks can be renamed, merged, moved, deleted, or subdivided later.

It is necessary to have a well-designed method for entering items into an item bank. A good item entry design enhances the ability to select items to be included on a test. This is accomplished by classifying each item. There are a number of ways an item can be classified. Some data are classified automatically each time a test using that item is scored. These data are referred to as fixed descriptors. The fixed descriptors include difficulty and discrimination evaluations, the last date the item was used or modified, and item analysis data.

The most important method of classifying items is for users to create their unique categories (user-defined categories). This will enable users to evaluate whether or not the test measures what it was designed to measure. These categories can be further defined for

Item Descriptors Screen

```
Item Bank: Multiple Injury                                    (edit items)
                          ITEM DESCRIPTORS

Lines before item:          ┌─Health Need:─┐   Discrimination: M
Lines after item:           │ Psychosocial │   Last used: 3-90
Health Need:                │ Elimination  │   Modified: 9-89
Nursing Process:            │ Rest & Activity│ Topic:
Objective:                  │ Safety       │   NCLEX Match:
     ----Item A             │ Oxygen       │   Cognitive Type:
  Last: N337  C.87          │ Nutrition    │   —Response Frequencies—
  Overall: N. 773  C.84     └──────────────┘   A.87 B.2 C.3 D.2 E.6
                                                A.84 B.4 C.4 D.4 E.5

              Press the (+) key to add a new descriptor.
```

Figure 23.1 Partial descriptor screen. Above is a partial descriptor screen from ParTEST that illustrates user-defined categories and descriptors. (Source: Economic Research 1988, release 2.0.)

clarity by entering descriptors within each category. For example, one category can be "health needs." The descriptors would be what the user defines as "health needs" (see Figure 23.1).

These categories and descriptors can provide an excellent instrument for periodic curriculum review and revision. Student outcomes and progression can be documented. It is important that the software has the flexibility for the educator to design categories that match a curriculum. In the ParSYSTEM, the user is able to create six user-defined categories and up to 250 descriptors for each category. Categories and descriptors can also be deleted, changed, or edited.

The Examiner software system, for example, can contain up to 99,000 items. Besides multiple choice questions, this program will support and correct open-ended questions. The items can be classified in an hierarchial structure.

Item Bank Printouts

Educators may obtain a hard copy of the entire item bank or a specific portion of the

bank. The educator can select the information to be included with each item for the printout. The selection options include: correct answer, question type, last used, data modified, answer explanation and answer reference, figures or graphs, categories and descriptors, difficulty and discrimination levels, and current cumulative item analysis. The printed copy enables the educator to select test items if there is restricted access to use of the computer.

GENERATION OF TESTS

Tests can be constructed from the item bank and stored as a test file. A test can be generated from more than one item bank. Multiple versions of the same test can be created with varying question order. Test key creation is automatic.

Item Selection

When developing tests, the educator can specify the characteristics (test blueprint) of the items desired. The program searches for and displays items that match these characteristics. These items can be added to the test file one-by-one or a specified number can be added at random.

The parameters of the item selection are completely at the discretion of the educator and are limited only by the way the item bank is classified. For example, one might choose to select an item that tests a specific objective, meets a cognitive level (for example, synthesis), and meets a certain level of difficulty and discrimination. The items that meet these criteria are displayed. The educator can then choose to include all or any of the items on the test.

Printout of a Test Blueprint

A test blueprint (cross reference table) is printed for each test. This replaces manual item recording in a grid (see Figure 23.2). Using the blueprint, a battery of tests can be evaluated before or after administration to assess and document a curriculum match.

Exam #3 - Spring 1991

Study Guide (Item Bank)	Multiple Injury	Premature	Crisis
# of items	21	32	22
Difficulty Level	14 Easy	13 Easy	9 Easy
Disc. Level	5 High	6 High	4 High
Objective	Goal 3	Goal 2	Goal 6
Topic	Law 1	RDS 2	Rape 6
Need	Oxygen 8	Oxygen 3	Oxygen 2
Nursing Process	Planning 4	Planning 5	Planning 2
Cognitive Level	Analysis 7	Analysis 4	Analysis 8

Figure 23.2 Test blueprint. Above is a partial test blueprint designed by the authors to record data obtained from the test analysis. (Numbers refer to the number of items.)

ADMINISTERING THE TEST

A test can be administered to the student via the computer (online testing) or in a printed form (offline testing). Options available for printing include the default or customized instructions for the entire test and instructions for individual item types. Several forms of the same test can be produced by altering the order of the test items or by altering the order of the alternative answers within test items.

Test Scoring

Printed tests may be scored manually or by using an optical mark reader commonly called an optical scanner. While scanning student answer cards, the program identifies problems such as incorrect identification number, incomplete erasures, multiple responses not required, or omitted responses. The program will not continue until the scorer addresses the problem encountered. The scorer can make a correction by keyboard or rescanning the student card. A printed error log identifies student answer cards that had problems during the scanning.

Multiple Testing

Some material demands mastery rather than relative performance levels. There are curricula that recognize that students learn at different rates because of individual learning styles and life experiences. The program generates and stores multiple tests with excellent evaluations.

Multiple testing with immediate feedback allows for diagnosis of specific learning problems. The educator can then prescribe learning activities that facilitate learning of content. The educator can create an individualized approach to the learning and evaluation process by using multiple testing.

TEST ANALYSIS

Once scored, the test is analyzed for reliability and validity, and an item analysis is done. The results of the item analysis are recorded on the items selected for the test file. Programs differ in statistical analysis packages provided.

ParSYSTEM has a very sophisticated item analysis package. Besides item difficulty and item discrimination ratio (IDR), a point biserial correlation coefficient (PBCC) measures the correlation between the correct answer on an item and the total test score of a student. ParSCORE automatically calculates the Kuder-Richardson Formula 20.

Difficulty and Discrimination Criteria for Item Banks

Each item bank can be assigned difficulty and discrimination levels. The educator enters the criteria for assigning difficulty levels and discrimination levels. After scoring a test, the program automatically transfers the difficulty and discrimination levels to the item bank. The criteria parameters can be revised and the program will reclassify the items within the bank according to the new criteria.

Item difficulty analysis identifies whether the item is too easy or too hard. In either case the item may add to the unreliability of a test because it does not aid in differentiating between students who know the information and those who do not. Item discrimination is the best measure of the effectiveness of an item in its ability to discriminate between students, who vary in their degree of knowledge about the content tested. The PBCC is the preferred method of measuring item discrimination because it identifies items which discriminate between high and low groups (generally the higher the PBCC, the better the item discrimination ratio, thus the better the item).

Item Difficulty should be between 30 and 90 percent; Item Discrimination by IDR should be 25 percent and above, and Item Discrimination by PBCC should be .20 or above (Lewis & Ortiz, 1988). If an item does not meet the above standards it is likely that it should be revised or discarded.

For norm-referenced tests that rank students for grading, the better the item discriminates, the more valid the test will be as a measure of relative achievement. Therefore, discrimination is the most important aspect of the test.

For criterion-referenced tests where a student's level of mastery of a subject is important, the discrimination power is of lesser importance. For instance, discrimination power is irrelevant where mastery of a particular skill is necessary before a more complex skill that builds upon a prior skill can be taught.

Test Validity

Validity refers to the extent to which a test measures what it is supposed to measure. Content or curriculum validity is generally used to assess whether a test parallels the material being taught and utilizes thinking skills that have been important in the course. Content validity is accomplished through a logical analysis of a test.

An educator creates a test blueprint to perform the analysis. The blueprint is based upon the categories determined in the item bank. With a well-designed test bank, the printed cross reference table (blueprint) for each test can be used in measuring test validity.

Test Reliability

Reliability refers to the consistency of test scores; it identifies how consistent one's test scores are from one test to another. It is important to measure test reliability as well as validity. Without reliability, it is not possible for a test to measure precisely. If the test does not have reliability it affects validity.

One of the best means of estimating the reliability of test scores on one test is by using the Kuder-Richardson Formula 20 (KR20). For good classroom tests, the reliability coefficients should be .70 or higher (Lewis & Ortiz, 1988). Multiple tests with good statistics document reliability.

GRADE MANAGEMENT

Once scored, the test grades are stored on a student roster. The cumulative and final grades are automatically calculated according to the weighing of tests established by the educator.

Adding Students to a Roster

Roster files are first created for the class sections of each course. Student data are then added to the files. Student data must include the individual identification number (social security number) and name. Optional student data include addresses and telephone numbers.

Student data can be entered manually by keyboard or scanned automatically with enrollment forms. The program will alphabetize student names and search for errors in the entry process. In ParSystem, student data can be imported from other databases or exported to other databases.

Multiple Grading Schemes

The software programs are flexible and allow multiple grading schemes within classes. Raw scores are converted into nu-

merous standardized scores such as percentiles, t-scores, stanines, or percents. In ParSCORE, gradebook features include "drop the lowest scores," "weight the roster by percentage," and "standard test scores." These features are interactive with each other.

Assigning Codes

Special codes can be assigned for grades that are not based on the results of written examinations. Examples of special codes are: W (withdrawal from class), I (incomplete), P or F (pass or fail), or U (unsatisfactory). This option is designed so that the code will override any letter grade that the student has received on tests while maintaining the record of the numerical average of test scores.

Roster Printout

Each class section can have a customized roster printout format that contains columns designed by the educator. When taking an online test or a test that is scored by the scanner, the test score is automatically posted in the appropriate column of the student roster. If a test is regraded, the new score is replaced by the revised score. When a test is scored manually, such as essay tests, the grade is entered by keyboard into the appropriate column.

Recording of Test Responses

Once scanned, student answer selections are recorded, and a printed copy (along with the error log) is available. This printed copy is the permanent, on file record of the students' test response. It is important to inform students in writing that the recorded copy of the answer responses replaces the hand written student answer card. This deters students from altering their answer cards during test reviews. Legally, the students cannot claim entrapment because they have been informed of this policy prior to the administration of the first exam.

Student Feedback

Detailed feedback reports for students may be generated. The report provides the correct answer, total score, reference, and detailed explanation for each question (see Figure 23.3). Feedback can be online if students took the test via the computer or printed if it was a pencil and paper test.

Subtests

In ParSYSTEM, items can be selected from a test and scored as a subtest. All statistical reports are available for a subtest. Any number of subtests can be generated and recorded. An advantage of subtest scoring is the ability to analyze specific areas of content within a test. This enables the educator to identify portions of a test that students had difficulty answering correctly. Thus students can focus on manageable portions of content area in which they are having difficulty.

SECURITY

Program security is an important consideration, especially when building a large pool of items. Programs differ in security methods. The *Examiner* software meets the most stringent requirements by using passwords and encrypting items when stored on disks. Another method of attaining security is to keep item banks stored on floppy disks.

Class rosters and test analysis data can be accessed only with the use of passwords. This option permits for multiple users of the program while maintaining the confidentiality and security of data contained within each class roster.

Test Feedback Report

```
Course #: 201
   Name: Jane Doe
   ID#: 134364528
 Score: 65 correct of 75 possible
 Test File: Exam 1
Items answered incorrectly:
   1. Correct Answer: B     Your answer: C
      Reference: Kneisl pg 265
      Answer Explanation:
      Immediately following the burn, the body releases massive amounts of vasoactive
      substances such as serotonin and histamine. These substances increase capillary
      permeability allowing water to escape into damaged and normal tissue.
   5. Correct Answer: D     Your Answer: C
      Reference: Math Text
      Answer Explanation:
      You appear to be having trouble with math. See your clinical instructor for help.
```

Figure 23.3 Feedback for students. Above is an example of a student feedback report from ParTEST. The contents of this report can be chosen by the instructor. It can contain as little information as a raw score or a detailed report of the items missed. (Source: Economic Research 1988, release 2.0.)

ORIENTATION SESSIONS

The authors recommend well-designed orientation sessions for the use of the software. Educators have to be introduced to the ease with which items are entered into an item bank and the amazingly short time in which tests can be generated and printed from item banks. It has been the authors' observation that educators need the most assistance in categorizing item banks and entering descriptors. The authors found that these sessions motivate the educator to use the features of the integrated system.

IMPLICATIONS FOR EDUCATORS

Decreased educational funding and less available secretarial support have forced educators to cope with the need for increasing lead time to compile tests for typing and printing. Make-up tests or a curriculum based on student self-pacing with interim testing compound the problem. Having the ability to generate online or offline tests with a valid method of selecting test items saves time and money and reduces stress.

The ability to classify and store items on floppy disk eliminates the need for large storage cabinets and boxes. The word processing feature simplifies the entry and editing of items. There is improved quality of developed items.

The ability to search for specific items using categories, descriptors, and difficulty and discrimination levels simplifies test construction. The creation of and addition to item banks and the generation of tests can be done at many sites including the office or home. This enhances the flexibility of managing time to complete education-related tasks.

The ability to obtain a profile of the test before administering it to the student enables the educator to evaluate test validity. Measurement of test reliability and validity is accomplished in a time and labor saving manner.

Grades are computed according to the grading scheme set up by the educator. There is a great deal of flexibility in setting up the grading criteria. Once the grading criteria are set up at the beginning of a course, they become the standard for each student. After the grading criteria is published for the course, it becomes an objective form of student evaluation.

Grading of tests and calculation of final grades can be done in a timely and efficient manner. Using ParSYSTEM, the scoring and analysis of the final exam and calculation of 80 student semester grades was done by the authors in less than one hour.

REFERENCES

Economic Research. (1988). *ParTEST* 3.01 [Computer program]. Costa Mesa, CA: Author.

Lewis, R. L., & Ortiz, K. K. (1988). *A guide to classroom testing and evaluation.* Costa Mesa, CA: Economic Research.

Lombardi, G. (1990). Integrated systems for testing and grading. *Computers in life science education, 7,* 65–67.

APPENDIX A: INTEGRATED EXAMINATION SOFTWARE VENDORS

Examiner
Mendota Heights, MN 55118

ExamSYSTEM
Minneapolis, MN 55440

MicroPac
Tempe, AZ 85281

MicroTim
Dallas, TX 75235

ParSYSTEM
Costa Mesa, CA 92626

24

HealthQuest/HBO Nurse Scholars Program: A Corporate Partnership With Nursing Education

Diane J. Skiba
Roy L. Simpson
Judith S. Ronald

INTRODUCTION

Dramatic changes in health care over the past decade—shifting populations, more acutely ill patients, staff shortages, expanding information needs, and crises in educational and institutional funding—compel the nursing profession to seek creative technological solutions. While some of these changes are limited by boundary conditions and thus are fixed, others are not.

Nursing care delivery can benefit from the information explosion through mastery of computer and information systems. Information systems can produce improvements through better and faster access to patient and clinical data, higher quality data, and faster communications between hospital or institution departments. Schools of nursing have been quick to realize the potential of information management and now need to incorporate the study of computers and their applications into basic core curricula. Practicing clinical nurses faced with the pressures of caring for more acutely ill patients

during a nursing shortage need assistance to master computer applications for which they may not have been adequately prepared.

Furthermore, many of the nurses who graduated even as recently as five years ago, as well as nurses currently in the work force, have had little or no exposure to nursing informatics. Informatics, in general, is the study of both computer and information science to facilitate the processing and management of data, information, and knowledge in the discipline of nursing (Grobe, 1988; Ball & Hannah, 1988; Graves & Corcoran, 1989). Graves and Corcoran (1989) have expanded the definition to include the "data-to-information-to-knowledge" continuum.

To move the use and management of nursing information systems in nursing education and training into the twenty-first century, HealthQuest/HBO & Company created a unique collaboration between corporate business interests and nursing education. This collaborative effort resulted in a program that can be used as a model by other disciplines in nursing to establish partnerships with business.

The purpose of this chapter is to describe the development of the HealthQuest/HBO & Company Nurse Scholars Program. The chapter provides information about the corporate sponsorship and their involvement in the hospital information system industry. The curriculum, selection process, and program evaluation techniques are also detailed in the chapter.

The Company, leaders in the development of hospital information systems, created the Nurse Scholars Program specifically to offer an educational forum for nursing school faculty to facilitate the integration of informatics into the curriculum at their schools. The short-term goal of the program was to put the structures in place to better prepare students for automated clinical practice. The long-term goal was to establish a means for future generations of health care clinicians to be educated in the use, design, implementation, and management of information systems in the clinical arena. Nursing school faculty need more venues to develop a level of system proficiency necessary to drive the process. These faculty, the future of nursing informatics, are the group HealthQuest/HBO & Company supported through the program.

The overall objective of the Nurse Scholars Program was to nurture a new generation of computer proficient nurses. This new generation of nurses and nurse administrators would not only embrace technology in the service of health care, but become part of the development process to ensure that future systems can more closely meet unique information needs of the nursing profession. Today, the systems used by nurses in clinical practice typically are selected by professionals outside of nursing—information system directors, financial executives, and operations executives. As a result, nurses are often left with a system that does not meet their needs and can add to already high levels of frustration, anxiety, and exhaustion in the profession.

Nursing is slowly realizing change. In 1991, the Joint Commission on Accreditation of Healthcare Organizations (JCAHO) mandated nursing's involvement in the system selection process. Nursing gained representation on the system review and selection committee, as well as a final vote on the system of choice (Simpson, 1991). This newly mandated participation requires that nurses come to the selection process educated on the many choices and options available, and knowledgeable on the basic concepts and principles driving hospital information systems and their activity cycles.

The unique collaboration between business and academia, the hallmark of the Nurse Scholars Program, should serve as a model to other nursing disciplines—it exemplifies how goals of nursing education can be achieved without sacrificing integrity to business/corporate interests. The Company achieved this level of integrity through the intense participation and involvement of several respected scholars of nursing and informatics who served as consultants to the project. Two of these consultants—Diane J. Skiba and Judith S. Ronald—have spent the last 15 years actively promoting the integration of informatics into the nursing curriculum. Both consultants served as original charter members of the National League for Nursing (NLN) Council for Nursing Informatics.

HealthQuest/HBO & Company, with the expertise of these two distinguished educators, created a program that would serve as the foundation for many curricula. The Company also worked under the guidance of its own director of nursing affairs, Roy L. Simpson, RN, who also served as an original charter member of the NLN Council for

Nursing Informatics. There was a widening gap between the preparation nursing students received in schools and the increasingly automated work environment in which they practiced. There are serious long-term consequences of such a gap not only to hospital information systems (HIS), which require highly educated buyers, but also to the nursing profession as a whole. In 1987, The Company's representatives began talking to academicians about the vision of uniting academia and business to move both parties forward with advancing technology.

In 1989, the Nurse Scholars Program was launched. Economic pressures have made such joint ventures not only desirable, but imperative. Few schools of nursing have the resources to provide their students with the massive hardware platforms and software programs required for research and orientation in clinical practice. HealthQuest^{SM} in particular, the mainframe division of The Company, always maintained close alliances with academic institutions. HealthQuest supports many university research programs by providing access to mainframe relational databases via Questnet, which gives users access to external clinical, financial, and government agency databases. As a result, close, mutually beneficial relationships emerged between the company and academic institutions. The universities provide HealthQuest with a "brain trust" and academic resources to develop and test new ideas, while the company provides universities with financial support and access to mainframe computing.

HealthQuest/HBO & Company of Georgia, a wholly owned subsidiary of HBO & Company, is a publicly held company listed on the NASDAQ as HBO. By 1990, The Company, formed in 1970 as a hospital information systems supplier, burgeoned into a highly regarded $200 million company. HealthQuest operates within an IBM mainframe environment. Its client base is comprised primarily of large (450 + beds) teaching university hospitals. HealthQuest product line includes: CliniPac (clinical management systems), MediPac (financial systems), Quantum (Executive Information System) and QuestNet (Healthcare Enterprise Information Network). HBO & Company of Georgia, on the other hand, operates on Data General and Digital minicomputer hardware platforms and is in the process of moving to a UNIX operating system platform. This Company's client base consists of largely midsized hospitals that operate in networked or minicomputer environments. HBO product line includes: ClinSTAR (clinical information systems), STAR Financials, TrendSTAR (cost accounting and budgeting) and Paragon (Executive Information System).

Both companies hosted the Nurse Scholars Program to: (1) expose nurses to hardware options in an interactive environment where hardware performance variables could be witnessed and examined and (2) demonstrate the functional similarities and differences of each platform. In addition, each company utilizes different software strategies, which reflect the depth of choices in the marketplace. HBO & Company of Georgia sells proprietary software, which means the company is sole owner of software that the buyer licenses for a fee. HealthQuest, on the other hand, sells "source code," the actual software program that the buyer or hospital can change and adapt according to its own needs.

The interactive environment helped Nurse Scholars understand the concepts of automation in a way theoretical discourse could not. Scholars received intensive hands-on practice and were educated in the basic concepts of automated health care information systems while observing how hospital technology may progress and change by the year 2000. This program graphically showed how nursing will have to adapt and benefit from this technology.

OVERVIEW OF PROGRAM

The Nurse Scholars Program is held in the corporate headquarters of HealthQuest/ HBO & Company in Atlanta, Georgia. All expenses for the program are assumed by The Company. Those individuals selected as Scholars receive an all expenses paid scholarship to study health care information systems for four days.

The program consists of intensive classroom study, with evening seminars and workshops. In addition to lectures and demonstrations, hands-on experiences with both the mainframe and minicomputer-based hospital information systems of HealthQuest and HBO are included. Part of each day is designated as "Journey to the Curriculum" when the day's learning experiences are reviewed and the scholars discuss how their newly acquired knowledge and skills can be shared with their students and nursing colleagues.

The program faculty, approximately 25 individuals, are selected by the program consultants for their level of expertise. Neither HBO nor the consultants want the program to be product specific or have a sales focus. Thus, nationally known leaders in nursing information systems from universities and health care institutions serve as faculty along with experts from HealthQuest/HBO & Company.

CURRICULUM

The goal of the Nurse Scholars Program is to provide nurse educators with the opportunity to learn concepts and methods of automated health care information systems and share this knowledge with the nursing community—students, faculty, practitioners, and administrators. It is anticipated that the dissemination and diffusion of this knowledge will help nurses at all levels to function as informed participants in the design, selection, implementation, and evaluation of automated information systems.

The curriculum is designed to use the life cycle of an information system, from determination of information requirements to evaluation of an installed system, as a framework. Program objectives reflect the belief that nurse educators need to have a broad perspective about health care information systems with an emphasis on nursing information systems and the issues related to their development. The specific objectives of the program are to:

1. Analyze health care information systems and how they assist nurses to provide quality patient care, increase efficiency, and manage shrinking resources.
2. Explore the issues of identifying information requirements for nursing.
3. Understand the principles of selection, implementation, and evaluation of health care information systems.
4. Examine strategies and issues related to integrating informatics into the nursing curriculum.
5. Interact with the HealthQuest and HBO hospital information systems.

The broad content areas included in the program to meet these objectives include definitions of nursing informatics, basic concepts of health care information systems, life cycle of an automated information system, emerging technological and human issues, curriculum integration, and research opportunities.

Discussion of nursing informatics as an evolving discipline pervades the program, and time is provided for formal discussion of various definitions (Grobe, 1988; Ball & Hannah, 1988; Graves & Corcoran, 1989). The scholars explore the emergence of nursing informatics as a discipline and the difference between the study of computer applications in nursing and nursing informatics. The faculty emphasize the interdisciplinary nature of nursing informatics along with what it means to manage and process nursing data, information, and knowledge as defined by Graves and Corcoran (1989). Scholars share their personal definitions of nursing informatics at the beginning and the end of the program. Many find their perspective has broadened considerably by the end of the program.

To gain an appreciation for how a nursing information system fits into the whole, time is devoted to discussions of the basic concepts of health care information systems. Faculty review the historical evolution of hospital information systems and, in particular, nursing information systems. To give scholars a comprehensive perspective, faculty review different approaches to system development such as mainframe versus distributed systems, turnkey versus in-house development, and others. Faculty present evaluation criteria related to functionality, system architecture, flexibility, time for implementation, and cost. The program covers technological dimensions such as work stations, point of care terminals, networks, and open architecture. The program also explores the benefits and constraints of the electronic medical record with several systems in use today as examples.

Nurse Scholars Program faculty extensively discuss nursing information systems including the computer design criteria for these systems (Zielstorff, McHugh, & Clinton, 1988). These include system capabilities, user–machine interfaces, hardware requirements, and data and security issues. Also discussed are different types of information systems that support the practice of nursing including acuity and classification, decision support (administrative and clinical), care planning, documentation, point of care, and others.

Throughout the program, faculty identify issues that serve as barriers to the development of information systems that meet the needs of nursing. Current research and development initiatives to resolve some of these issues are presented by various faculty members. For example, research efforts in relation to developing a nursing taxonomy and lexicon are discussed. In addition, as the issues are explored, the group generates challenges and opportunities for future research and development in nursing informatics.

After analyzing the basic concepts of information systems, the life cycle of a health care information system is reviewed by nursing systems analysts. The specific steps involved in the process of developing an information system and the nursing role in each of these steps are discussed. Knowledgeable use of consultants in any or all stages of the life cycle is presented as one alternative in this process.

The life cycle begins with a feasibility study to determine the need for an automated health care information system. It proceeds to identify the nursing requirements for the system through use of the principles of systems analysis and includes methods to develop request for information (RFI) and request for proposals (RFP) from vendors. Scholars review a request for proposal from the field and examine the nursing portion of it in detail. In addition, they suggest guidelines for evaluating vendor presentations and site visits. Strategies for organizing an automated information system are explored. These include techniques for gaining administrative support, forming and using steering committees, planning educational programs, and developing policies and procedures.

The latter stages of the information system life cycle—implementation and maintenance—are presented as they relate to the change process, need for administrative support, training, conversion, and installation. In this discussion, the human aspects of introducing and maintaining a significant change into the clinical work environment are emphasized. The final stage, evaluation, is discussed from multiple points of view. A general view of evaluation research is presented via several research models.

In addition to concentrated classroom experience, scholars receive considerable hands-on practice with both the HBO mini-computer hospital information system and the HealthQuest mainframe system. Each scholar has access to a terminal to work on case studies that focus on computer applications from patient admission through discharge. The applications include computer activities such as Admission-Discharge-Transfer (ADT), order entry, results reporting, nursing care planning, and documentation. The scholars also have an opportunity to view a demonstration of point-of-care technology.

The curricular implications of nursing information systems are incorporated throughout the program. They are the focus of daily discussions labeled "Journey to the Curriculum" that take place at scheduled times during the day or evening activities. Each day, scholars consider integration of their new knowledge of information systems into their curricula. A framework was established that views current computer course offerings in nursing on a continuum ranging from computer literacy to computer applications to nursing informatics. The scholars analyze their current curricula in relation to the continuum and explore how they might move their teaching toward the informatics end of the continuum.

In addition to the informatics content in the curricula, scholars analyze the impact of the computer on the nursing curriculum based on practice implications. They begin to rethink how to teach nursing content, given the capabilities of nursing information systems to access, retrieve, and record patient data. Questions about the skills nurses need in an information age lead to discussion of curricula that focus on critical thinking and information retrieval skills rather than memorization.

Each scholar receives teaching materials that include objectives, content outline, bibliography, a textbook, a monograph, a set of generic slides, and demonstration disks. These materials provide the scholars with materials to use as they share their new knowledge with students and nursing colleagues.

SELECTION PROCESS AND CRITERIA

Once the curriculum was developed, the process of selecting faculty for the Nurse Scholars Program was determined. The coordinators notified all schools of nursing to solicit nominations of faculty candidates. To notify all possible schools, mailing lists were requested from several organizations, but were not secured. Therefore, the staff had to compile the names and addresses for 606 schools of nursing that had at least a baccalaureate degree program. Two major assumptions underlay the selection process. The first assumption was that the school of nursing's administrator (dean or chair) needed to nominate and write a letter of support for the candidate. Administrative support was viewed as a necessary precondition for a faculty member to accomplish the intended goals of the Nurse Scholars Program. A second assumption was that geographic representation of scholars needed to be ensured. To accomplish this, the United States was divided into nine regions according to procedures used by the American Organization of Nurse Executives (AONE). The regions are divided according to the dis-

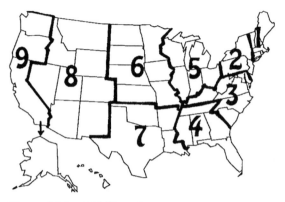

Figure 24.1 AONE regions.

tribution of hospitals across the United States. Figure 24.1 depicts the nine AONE geographic regions.

The most difficult task of the selection process was development of criteria to assess nominees. The selection criteria were developed in collaboration with the Health-Quest/HBO Nursing Advisory Panel. The panel consisted of nationally known nursing management experts who function as deans of schools of nursing, vice presidents of nursing, and others. The panel received the description and goals of the Nurse Scholars Program and an initial draft of selection criteria. In a brainstorming session, selection criteria were proposed. For example, one panel member aptly described a Nurse Scholar as being "hungry"—a self-motivated knowledge-seeker who would use the program as a catalyst. Given this qualitative descriptor, the panel was asked to develop a list of operational definitions for these characteristics and to suggest data collection methods. Upon completion of the brainstorming session, the coordinators established the selection criteria, associated point values for each criteria, developed operational definitions, and designed data collection methods.

The primary data collection method was submission of an application that included completion of a questionnaire, submission of a concept paper, inclusion of support letter from the dean as well as any additional supporting materials. The questionnaire solicited the basic information about each school of nursing and its faculty nominee. The questionnaire was modeled after information collected for standard external reports such as the NLN accreditation report. The faculty nominee or a staff member could complete the questionnaire.

The questionnaire also collected information about student and faculty demographics. The purpose of this section was to describe the sample of nominees and their corresponding schools of nursing. Number of students by degree programs (baccalaureate and graduate) or special program type (RN completion, RN to Master's or MS/MBA programs) were solicited. In addition, schools with graduate programs were asked to specify the major areas of specialization. The number of full- and part-time as well as clinical associate faculty by baccalaureate and graduate divisions was solicited in this section.

The clinical affiliation section solicited information about the top three clinical sites for nursing students. The Nurse Scholars Program also solicited information about the existence of clinical information systems at these clinical sites. Since one of the primary goals of the Nurse Scholars Program is the dissemination of knowledge about clinical information systems, the availability of clinical information systems was an important criterion in the selection process.

The concept paper was designed so faculty nominees could demonstrate their current knowledge of informatics, their current activities in informatics, and the goals they would like to accomplish in the Nurse Scholars Program. To ascertain knowledge of informatics, each nominee had to define the term nursing informatics and how this concept was addressed in nursing education.

The nominee also was asked to explicate how their school of nursing addressed informatics in the curriculum. The final questions requested faculty nominees to generate goals they would like to accomplish as a result of the Nurse Scholars Program. Faculty nominees also had to justify a sufficient foundation to reach the intended goals.

The final component of the application, submission of a support letter from the school of nursing administrator was required for each faculty nominee. If a support letter was not included, the nominee's application was incomplete and not evaluated. Faculty nominees also were encouraged to submit any additional materials to strengthen their application. Support materials included: additional support letters from faculty or clinical affiliates, course materials, curriculum plans, continuing education workshop materials, and publications.

Selection of the Scholars was conceptualized as a two-stage process guided by the principle that the Nurse Scholars Program should serve as a catalyst for faculty currently teaching computer applications courses in the nursing curriculum (Skiba, Ronald, & Simpson, 1991). All applicants were to be reviewed by an evaluation panel that included representatives from Health-Quest/HBO, educational coordinators, and selected nursing advisors. In the first stage of the review, the evaluation panel assessed each application and rated the nominee on three criteria—school characteristics, goals and background, and informatics curriculum. These three criteria were deemed as requisite characteristics by the Health-Quest/HBO Nursing Advisory Panel, who established the selection criteria. The HealthQuest/HBO Nursing Advisory Panel agreed that a nominee must achieve a minimum score of 45 points on these three criteria to proceed to the second stage review.

The first criterion examined school characteristics such as type of degree program, number of students by degree, availability of innovative programs (e.g., weekend programs, MS/MBA options), and specialization areas offered for master's level programs. A total of 30 points was available for this criterion. In general, applicants over the past two years have managed to receive a substantial number of points in this category.

The second criterion examined the nominee's proposed goals to be accomplished as a result of their participation in Nurse Scholars Program. These goals were assessed within the context of the overall goals of the Nurse Scholars Program—the dissemination of knowledge about the life cycle of a clinical information system. Secondary goals included the opportunity for faculty currently working in this area to experience nursing practice in an automated environment and to provide a catalyst for future curriculum development in informatics. Remember HealthQuest/HBO's mission is to ensure that nurses are knowledgeable consumers of information systems. Thus, goals such as "to gain knowledge about computers" or "to develop computer assisted instructional software" were not considered a "good fit" with the intent of the Scholars Program. The evaluation panel also examined the foundation for these goals. For example, a goal of being a systems designer at the end of the program for a person with limited computer experience was not realistic nor did it correspond to the overall goals of the Nurse Scholars Program. A total of 20 points was assigned to this criterion.

The third criterion analyzed the current state of informatics in the nursing curriculum of the nominee's school of nursing. Once again, it is important to note that the Nurse Scholars Program serves as a catalyst and not an agent to institute change in a curriculum. To investigate this criterion, the evaluation panel determined if a computer or informatics course(s) was offered or if computer or informatics content was integrated throughout the curriculum. The course was further evaluated for its status as elective or required course and degree level. If the content was integrated in the curriculum, how was integration defined or conceptualized? If courses or integration were present, was the nominee involved in the informatics curriculum? In general, many schools of nursing did not offer any computer-related courses and of those schools that did, most were elective courses. Relatively few schools integrated content into the curriculum and only a few had general literacy courses required by the university or college. An important consideration with this criterion was the nominee's definition of informatics and how that definition corresponded to the informatics curriculum. Definitions for informatics were either taken from the literature (Grobe, 1988; Ball & Hannah, 1988; Graves & Corcoran, 1989) or the nominee's own derivation. The relationship between the definition and the curriculum was minimal. One trend noted by the panel was the misunderstanding of the term informatics and lack of sophistication regarding informatics. For example, many applicants stated informatics was integrated throughout the curriculum based on computer-assisted instructional software being available for students. A total of 15 points was assigned to this criterion and, in general, most nominees received minimal or no points in this area.

The evaluation panel was instructed to review all nominees on these three criteria and to subtotal these points. If a nominee did not receive at least 45 points, the nominee was not eligible for the second stage review. Thus, a significant portion of the nominee pool was eliminated and only the finalists were reviewed in the second stage. In this stage, applications were reviewed on four criteria—clinical affiliations, support, faculty credentials, and discretionary bonus points.

Clinical affiliations were examined by the evaluation panel for characteristics such as size, type of facility, and availability of a clinical information system. This final characteristic, clinical information system availability, was an important consideration in this assessment phase. For example, if a faculty member or a school had access to an information system in the clinical arena, the Scholars Program might not be as beneficial. Then again, if there was no access to a clinical information system, exposure to the Nurse Scholars Program might be beneficial to the faculty member and eventually to the students at that school. Although this was an important consideration, clinical information system availability was not viewed as an isolated factor but interpreted within the context of the entire application. A total of 15 points was assigned to this criterion.

Support from the dean and additional support materials were also reviewed in this stage. Administrators' letters were examined for their administrative commitment to informatics, their interpretation of the Nurse Scholars Program goals, and their ability to highlight or promote their nominee. The administrator's letter of support was a necessary precondition. Without the support of the administrator, it might be difficult for a nominee to accomplish his or her intended goals. In addition, other support materials were reviewed. The majority of the materials complemented and strengthened the application. A total of 5 points was allotted to this criterion and, in general, there were two distinct distributions of scores—administrators either indicated strong support or a lack of support for the nominee or the Nurse Scholars Program.

Faculty credentials were reviewed by examination of items such as teaching experience, experience teaching computer-related courses, educational preparation, professional involvement in computer-related organizations (e.g., being a member of the NLN Council of Nursing Informatics or American Nurses Association's (ANA)'s Council on Informatics), professional activities (e.g., paper presentations, workshops, involvement on selection committees), and a historical perspective of the nominee's involvement in the profession of nursing. These factors helped the evaluation panel identify "hungry" faculty members who were self-motivated knowledge-seekers to use the program as a catalyst. A total of five points was assigned to this criterion.

The final criterion was the availability of ten discretionary bonus points. Although the evaluators strived for objectivity in the selection process, it was acknowledged that some subjectivity would be a factor and that some skills or talents might be difficult to quantify. The evaluation panel generally used these additional points with discretion and were not overly generous.

The Nurse Scholars Program selection process and criteria were favorably implemented for the 1990 and 1991 cohorts. The evaluation panel has been satisfied with this process and have made only minor adjustments to the criteria. Based on this selection process, nine nurse scholars were selected for each cohort year. The nurse scholars and their schools of nursing for both 1990 and 1991 are listed in Table 24.1 according to AONE region.

EVALUATION

From the conception of the Nurse Scholars Program, program evaluation was considered a necessary and integral component. The primary function of the evaluation component was to provide feedback to various constituent groups and to provide information for continuous improvement of the Nurse Scholars Program. Constituent groups

Table 24.1 HBO/Healthquest Nurse Scholars

Region	1990	1991
1	Margaret Chalmers, EdD, RN Western Connecticut State University	Carolyn A. Lawless, DEd, RN University of Massachusetts at Worcester
2	Ramona Nelson, PhD, RN University of Pittsburgh	Joan O'Leary, EdD, RN Villanova University
3	Nancy Whitman, PhD, RN University of Virginia	Betty J. Paulanka, EdD, RN University of Delaware
4	Nancy M. Longcrier, PhD, RN Clemson University	Carol Patricia Riley, DNS, RN, CS University of Alabama at Capstone
5	Richard Redman, PhD, RN University of Michigan	Carol L. Rossel, EdD, RN Lewis University
6	Marjorie Smith, PhD, RN Winona State University	Bunny J. Pozehl, PhD, RN University of Nebraska
7	Marilyn Murphy, PhD, RN University of Texas Health Sciences Center	A. Susan Nelson, PhD, RN Corpus Christi State University
8	Nancy Kline Leidy, PhD, RN University of Arizona	Barbara McNeill, PhD, RN Lewis-Clark State College
9	Suzanne Henry, DNS, RN University of California at San Francisco	Mary McFarland, EdD, RN Oregon Health Sciences University

who needed feedback included program co-ordinators, the faculty, the scholars, the applicant pool, and the marketing representatives and executive management team of both HealthQuest and HBO companies. The panel provided evaluation summaries in various formats: presentations; internal (e.g., executive management team, Nursing Advisory Panel), and external (e.g., professional nursing organization meetings, informatics-related organizations) reports; executive summaries; press releases; and publications.

The first evaluation component was a postassessment of the Nurse Scholars Program. This postassessment included an evaluation of course objectives, course content, and overall feedback about structure and implementation of the program. Scholars were asked to indicate the extent to which program objectives were met at the end of their four-day experience (i.e., not met, partially met, met). Course content was assessed on three dimensions: relationship to program objectives (i.e., not related, partially related, related, extremely related); depth of the content (i.e., no new knowledge, not new but different perspective, some new knowledge, new knowledge); and overall contribution to the program (i.e., poor to excellent). Overall feedback solicited open-ended responses to a variety of questions related to the structure and implementation of the program. Areas in this section included expectations, new ideas, most and least helpful experiences, "Journey to the Curriculum" discussions, and the hands-on computer experiences with both the minicomputer and mainframe systems.

Another component of the postassessment contained a goal attainment evaluation technique. Each scholar was asked to review their goals as described in their application and determine if there remained goals they wanted to accomplish. Scholars were given an option to generate new projected goals.

For each goal, the scholar explicated the intermediate steps to accomplish this goal and the corresponding timeline for each step. In addition, each goal had to be weighted and the weights had to total 100 percent. The weight was to indicate the importance of a particular goal. Scholars were told that these goals would appear on the follow-up assessment and for their assessment of their progress in the attaining of the projected goals.

A follow-up assessment also was designed to be implemented by two mechanisms. The first mechanism was a structured interview in which scholars were asked a variety of questions about how the Nurse Scholars Program impacted their courses and curriculum and professional activities. Impact on professional activities was divided into several categories such as scholarly publications, research activities, and professional and community presentations and consultations. The interview would be conducted approximately six months after the program. The one-year follow-up was a mailed questionnaire that contained structured questions to measure the dissemination of knowledge to students and nursing colleagues, diffusion of ideas through professional activities, and the attainment of projected goals.

The results of the program evaluation are impressive. Post-assessments are extremely positive and speak to the excellent contribution of this program to the faculty member's own development in the area of informatics. It was difficult to ascertain any negative feedback. There were suggestions for improvement in the organization of class days and the inclusion of more informal discussion time about curriculum issues. The follow-up results for the first group are equally impressive. Highlights of the first cohort's accomplishments include course revisions, postdoctoral programs in informatics, elections to professional organizations related to informatics, and the design of faculty development series by three scholars. The majority of the projected goals were also accomplished by the scholars.

SUMMARY

The HealthQuest/HBO and Company Nurse Scholars Program represents a successful collaboration between industry and academia. This successful venture has generated 18 nurse scholars who have disseminated their knowledge to numerous students and nursing colleagues across the United States. Given the impressive program results, HealthQuest/HBO & Company have renewed their sponsorship. The authors commend HealthQuest/HBO & Company for their continued support to nursing education and informatics.

REFERENCES

Ball, M. J., & Hannah, K. J. (1988). What is informatics and what does it mean for nursing? In M. J. Ball, K. J. Hannah, U. G. Gerdin-Jelger, & H. E. Peterson (Eds.), *Nursing informatics: Where caring and technology meet* (pp. 81–87). New York: Springer-Verlag.

Graves, J., & Corcoran, S. (1989). The study of nursing informatics. *Image, 21*(4), 227–231.

Grobe, S. J. (1988). Nursing informatics competencies for nurse educators and researchers. In H. E. Peterson & U. G. Gerdin-Jelger (Eds.), *Preparing nurses for using information systems: Recommended informatics competencies* (pp. 25–40). New York: National League for Nursing.

Simpson, R. L. (1991). The joint commission did what you wouldn't. *Nursing Management*, January, 26–27.

Skiba, D., Ronald, J., & Simpson, R. (1991). Educating health care professionals in informatics: The scholars program. In E. Hovenga, K. Hannah, K. McCormick & J. Ronald (Eds.), *Proceedings of the Fourth International Conference on Nursing Use of Computers and Information Science.* Nursing Informatics '91. Berlin, Germany: Springer-Verlag.

Zielstorff, R., McHugh, M., & Clinton, J. (1988). *Computer Design Criteria*. Kansas City, MO: American Nurses Association.

Section Six
Development of Computer Applications

This section focuses on computer applications created by authors using both generic and specialized software.

The only interactive video computer application in this text is written by Hassett. She explains the difference between traditional specification computer design and rapid prototyping approach (fast scaled down approach). Production problems and their resolution by the project team are also included. The outcomes of the project and their implications for nursing education are outlined.

The use of expert systems in nursing education is in the beginning stage. Thompson explicates the design of his expert system and its use in teaching nursing students how to formulate nursing diagnoses.

Database applications are described in the next five chapters of this section. The design of an academic database from a generic relational database is shared by Cohen and Lerner including data elements, computer screens, and sample student reports. The use of an application database for record keeping in continuing education is provided by Lauzon-Vallone. The author explains how a database facilitated data manipulation from educational programs and demonstrated employee contributions to organizational goals.

The next three chapters describe the use of the same generic relational database with nurses and nursing students. The work presented is based on one faculty group effort to introduce databases to nurses. Thede uses a scenario to explain the creation and use of databases. She also includes a glossary of terms for the novice. This chapter is an excellent resource for getting started with database software. The next two chapters focus on use of a database as a learning tool with graduate nursing students. These authors developed databases of nursing diagnoses for two nursing specialties—adult nursing and parent-child nursing—thereby adding to the knowledge base of nursing.

This section concludes with two unique computer applications. Merritt demonstrates how a scanner can be used with research instruments to facilitate data entry; and a custom program which measures diagnostic reasoning associated with simulations is described by Arnold. These applications are illustrated through diagrams and computer screens.

25

Rapid Prototyping: A Methodology for Developing Computer-Based Video Instruction Programs*

Mary R. Hassett

INTRODUCTION

Development of computer-based video instruction (CBVI) programs is time consuming (Redland & Kilmon, 1985) and resource intensive. This chapter provides a methodology to improve the development process for CBVI programs: rapid prototyping. Objectives for the reader are to: (1) compare and contrast the specification approach with rapid prototyping methodology for CBVI program development; and (2) describe uses of rapid prototyping for CBVI program development.

Rapid prototyping is defined as the crea-

tion of an early version of the final program, that is, reduced in size and complexity, but functional (Hassett, 1990b). Concepts from the field of software engineering were borrowed and adapted for the rapid prototyped development of the CBVI project presented in this chapter as a model. Prototyping, one of three approaches the software designer may take at the beginning of a project, is discussed. Prototyping tools and the hardware and software constraints associated with rapid prototyping are recognized. The CBVI project prototype evolved into the final product that was beta-tested and used with baccalaureate nursing students. The model project presented includes: background of the CBVI program, hardware and software, the project team, specifications approach, and implementation of rapid prototyping. Examples of design choices and computer screens from the project are used, and the resolution of problems encountered are discussed. Evaluation with reference to students is shared, and a summary provided, with implications for nursing education.

---

* The author gratefully acknowledges: (a) The University of Texas: Dr. George Culp (Project QUEST), Dr. Susan J. Grobe, Supervising Professor, and Dr. Wilhelmina Savenye (now at Arizona State University); (b) C. Michael Hassett, systems analyst; and (c) IBM: Bill Rowell & Jim Slemenda (MultiMedia HelpLine).

THREE METHODOLOGIES FOR DEVELOPING CBVI PROGRAMS

The three approaches (methodologies) were identified by Boehm, Gray and Seewaldt (1984) in an experiment for developing small-size application software. The approaches are build-and-fix, specification, and prototyping. Seven software teams developed versions of the same application software project. Four teams used the specification approach and three other teams used the prototyping approach to develop an interactive version of a particular model for software cost estimation. Build-and-fix was not used in the experiment. The main results of the experiment were: (1) prototyping required about 40 percent less code and 45 percent less effort, with roughly equivalent performance; (2) prototyped software rated somewhat lower on functionality and robustness, but higher on ease of use and learning; and (3) specification software had more coherent design and was easier to integrate.

Brief definitions of requirements and specifications are offered because these teams are important for two of the three approaches. Requirements describe what the software will do (similar to goals). Examples of requirements are: provide a report of learner pretest scores; or provide videodisc segments that support the CBVI content objectives. One needs to begin with good requirements; prototyping can expose the need for additional ones and sometimes requirements change. Specifications are those items that one can define for the software and then test with a pass or not pass (similar to objectives). An example of one specification is: for each learner, pretest questions are listed on a grade report as correct or incorrect, along with a total score. A flowchart may be used as a tool to help define specifications.

Build-and-fix

The build-and-fix approach is constructing the full system using minimal or no specifications. The software is reworked (fixed) as necessary until users are satisfied. Build-and-fix does not work effectively on most projects of a reasonable size (Boehm et al., 1984).

Specification

The specification approach (design-it-first) is the traditional one used to create programs. It entails four steps:

1. developing requirements for the software,
2. developing design specifications to implement the requirements,
3. developing the code to implement the design, and
4. reworking the software as necessary (Boehm et al., 1984).

This approach works well when the program is well understood from the outset. Such is not usually the case with CBVI projects.

Prototyping

The prototyping approach is building scaled down (prototype) versions of parts of the software. It entails three steps:

1. exercising the prototype parts to determine the best way to implement the software,
2. developing the code to implement the design, and
3. reworking the software as necessary (Boehm et al., 1984).

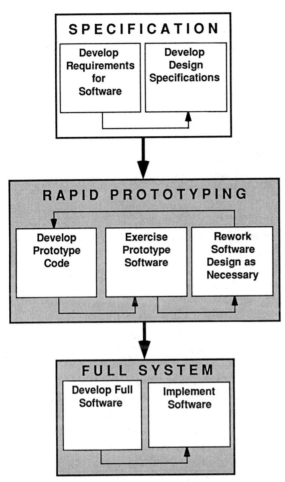

Figure 25.1 Use of methodology for Hassett computer-based video instruction project. (Source: Copyright © 1991 by Mary R. Hassett Consulting. Used by permission.)

Figure 25.1 illustrates the model CBVI project's move from specification to rapid prototyping methodology, about which more will be discussed later.

Fisher (1987) states that prototyping provides users and developers with an effective means to communicate ideas and requirements before a significant amount of effort has been expended. The prototyping approach to software development is particularly useful and cost-effective for CBVI program development. Examples of improved development include:

1. provision of early feedback as to the design, content and look and feel of the program;
2. identification of unneeded or missing parts in the program; and
3. minimizing the deadline effect at the end of the program (Boehm et al.).

Rapid prototyping is a design methodology (fast prototyping), previously defined as the creation of an early, functioning version of the final program. Key parts of the system must be represented. Available software development tools must allow the rapid building and modification of the prototype; rapid prototyping also requires availability of tools that offer modularity and plasticity (Tripp & Bichelmeyer, 1990). Modularity means segments of the instructional unit can be added, removed or modified without causing problems with other segments or the unit as a whole. Plasticity means aspects of the instructional unit can be changed with only minor penalties. According to Miller and Irving (1989) standards to scrutinize for rapid prototyping include: color of background and text, screen design, use of function keys, branching designs, degree of user control and interactivity, type of feedback, and record-keeping ability.

Tripp and Bichelmeyer (1990) provide an example of rapid prototyping: development of a computer-based tutor for foreign students. A rapid prototyped tutorial was built, containing only the major elements presented schematically. The prototype was produced in a matter of hours. Testing with potential users began immediately. This process answered many questions, and the full version of the tutorial was built. This example illustrates the essentials of rapid prototyping: (1) a scaled-down version was quickly built; (2) the available software allowed rapid prototyping with modifications; and (3) the slow traditional approach was replaced by efficient hands-on design. Important to the process was getting the users (students) as active participants in the design.

Prototyping Tools. There are several general classes of prototyping tools including: executable specification language processors, program design languages, and fourth generation languages (4GLs). Languages identified as 4GLs are software systems of integrated tools designed to assist analysts and end users in developing interactive online information systems. A typical implementation consists of: query language, report generator, screen formatter, and high level procedural language. These components may be used to develop prototypes by rapidly building models of data entry screens, reports, and specialized processes (Fisher, 1987). Prototyping tools are also available from the field of software engineering, to support complex software systems (such as an authoring language). One of these tools is the computer-aided prototyping system (CAPS) (Luqi, 1989). No specific prototyping tools were found for CBVI. Nevertheless, most authoring languages can be used for prototyping.

Ideally, a CBVI prototyping tool would include the following: text editor, graphic illustrator, sound editor, video editor, authoring language, and an extensive library of clip art and symbols with a manager. These tools are presently available but not in an integrated form. Operating systems such as Microsoft Windows, and IBM's OS/2 with Presentation Manager will provide such integration. Asymetrix's ToolBook 1.5 recently provided another layer toward integration. ToolBook is a software construction set for

Windows; rapid prototyping is one application (Asymetrix Corporation, 1991). IBM's Storyboard Live! documentation does not specify rapid prototyping as an application, but supports CBVI (International Business Machines Corporation, 1990, October).

Hardware Constraints of CBVI Rapid Prototyping. One constraint that is unique to CBVI is the laser videodisc standard. Repurposing can be used, that is, edited portions of preceding videotape mastered to videodisc, or a videodisc not specifically mastered for the CBVI program. Important reasons for repurposing include: (1) expensive videodisc production signifies that many cannot afford it, and (2) cost-effectiveness of repurposing affords a low-risk means of becoming familiar with the technology (Locatis, 1989).

Traditionally, before a CBVI project is developed beyond the logical design stage, the video must be shot and stored on videotape, edited, and then transferred to a laser videodisc. This leaves little flexibility for revision of the video portion of the design. There are some "work-arounds" to this constraint. For example, dummy screens can show what the video will do when it becomes available. The ultimate solution will be realized through forthcoming technologies such as hardware and software-based compression/decompression algorithms and rewritable magneto-optic disc storage (Newsline: Intel's DVI advances toward desktop mainstream, 1990; Newsline: VideoLogic plans powerful video compression system, 1990; Pioneer buys DVA, develops rewritable videodisc system with KDD, 1989; Technology collision: The Demo Center, 1991). Such technologies will allow video to be edited in real time and stored on hard disc or optical storage media. Hardware such as NEC's PC-VCR (Model PV-S98A) offers yet another alternative: desktop video multimedia. The PC-VCR is a computer-controlled S-VHS/

VHS video cassette recorder with serial cable; one may record, assemble, and edit video and sound (Newsline: NEC unveils PC-VCR for tape-based multimedia, 1990). PC-VCRs provide laserdisc-like frame accuracy and random-access capability, using previously recorded videotape (Knutsen, 1991, May). This capability could eliminate the need for videodisc mastering for some applications or at least delay the point at which a videodisc must be mastered.

BACKGROUND OF PROJECT

The rapid prototyping methodology was employed for a nursing CBVI project entitled *Spiritual Assessment of Christian Clients* (Hassett, 1989a). The project software was beta-tested and then used in a pilot study followed by a research study with baccalaureate nursing students (Hassett, 1989b, 1991). Initially, a specification approach was taken. Rapid prototyping was added later because without it the project would not have been completed within the two-month time frame required for implementation of the full system. The project's rapid prototype evolved into the final system (Connell & Shafer, 1989) as shown in Figure 25.1. Examples from this project will be used to demonstrate rapid prototyping methodology.

PROJECT HARDWARE AND SOFTWARE

A feasibility study compared hardware and software available for CBVI (Hassett, 1990a). An electronic spreadsheet made comparisons, primarily by cost, function, and availability. Companies and vendors were contacted, brochures examined, users inter-viewed, and computer-based environments tested.

Hardware

Hardware comparisons included old and new IBM personal computers (i.e., the IBM-XT and new PS/2 models) and the Apple Macintosh. Upgrading the writer's IBM XT would have required the purchase of expensive add-ons for a computer that already had been phased out by IBM. The Macintosh system would have required a second display for video, separate from the built-in Macintosh text–graphics display. The writer chose an IBM PS/2 Model 70 microcomputer with an InfoWindow touch screen/speech chip color display. IBM's technical support was an important factor in the decision. The PS/2 Model 70 has Micro Channel architecture, a 60 MB hard disk, and 2 MB of memory. The completed hardware environment included the following: an IBM PS/2 Model 70 micro-computer and mouse; an InfoWindow display; a Pioneer LD-V6200A LaserDisc player; and a Hewlett-Packard LaserJet Series II printer.

Software

Software comparisons included CBVI authoring systems (e.g., IBM's InfoWindow Presentation System (IWPS) vs. Allen Communication's Quest Authoring System) and graphics packages. IWPS Level 51A was chosen for authoring because of compatibility with the IBM InfoWindow touch sensitive display. At the time of the feasibility study, the traditional approach was the only one planned. Therefore, IWPS was not examined for rapid prototyping capability. (When the project team added rapid prototyping, it was fortunate that

IWPS was compatible with this methodology.) Since this was the writer's first CBVI project, IBM's MultiMedia HelpLine support was necessary for effective rapid prototyping. This support was excellent.

IBM's Storyboard Plus was chosen for graphics after testing PC Paint 3.1 and finding its graphics would not import into the IWPS graphics library. (Earlier versions imported, but this version did not, due to upgrade file format revisions.) MicroPro's WordStar word processor, already owned by the writer, was used to input text screens. They were captured as graphic screens with IBM Storyboard's PictureTaker function and imported individually into the IWPS graphics library. PictureTaker saved the writer many hours; without it, most text screens would have been manually re-input into graphics mode. The completed software environment included the following: IBM DOS 4.01, IBM IWPS Level 51A authoring system, IBM Storyboard Plus 2.0 graphics package, and MicroPro WordStar 5.5 word processor.

PROJECT TEAM

At the completion of step 2 of the specifications approach (design development), step 3 (code development) was initiated. When moving from abstract design specifications to detailed code development, the project immediately got bogged down. There was a serious gap in the literature about how one actually goes about building a CBVI program. Requirements had been added to automate three paper and pencil research tools, drastically changing the specifications. The flowchart did not include these tools and there were no algorithms for test item scoring and other elements. The writer was the developer and primary user; learners, the secondary users, were brought in later. The writer was also: (1) content expert, (2) instructional designer, (3) hardware and software evaluator, (4) author, (5) graphics artist, (6) videodisc production manager, and (7) programmer. A systems analyst was added to make up a two-person team; this addition immediately speeded up progress on the project. With the help of a systems analyst, problems were quickly solved by using rapid prototyping methodology.

PROJECT SPECIFICATION APPROACH

Requirements

The project requirements (what the software will do) were determined prior to acquisition of the IWPS authoring system. Figure 25.1 illustrated the requirements as a part of the specification methodology. The CBVI project requirements displayed in Figure 25.2 included the four main parts the project covered: (1) demographic data collection, (2) data collection on baseline knowledge of content prior to the CBVI program, (3) the CBVI program on spiritual care that collected data on learner control choices and tested for knowledge gained, and (4) data collection on learner attitudes toward the CBVI program. The time frame for project completion (full system) was two months.

Specifications

The project specifications (how the software will accomplish defined, testable aspects) are displayed in Figure 25.3. Figure 25.1 illustrated the development of design specifications as a part of the specification methodology. The specifications followed the development of requirements. The IWPS documentation listed authoring prerequisites (International Business Machines Corporation, 1986). These also use the spec-

1. Collect demographic data via subject information form (SIF):
   a. Convert SIF paper and pencil form to computer-based
   b. Run computer-based SIF (5 minutes) and collect learner demographics
   c. Provide a list of learner demographics
2. Collect data on baseline knowledge of content prior to CBVI program via screening pretest (SP):
   a. Convert 19-item SP paper-and-pencil form to computer-based
   b. Run computer-based SP (20 minutes) and collect learner score
   c. Provide learner item scores and total score
3. Build CBVI program on spiritual care that collects data on learner control choices and tests for knowledge gained:
   a. Run CBVI on spiritual care (30 minutes); incorporate learner control branching decision points; use videodisc stills at learner control branchings to facilitate decisions
   b. Collect data on each learner control choice
   c. Collect 5-item embedded content questions (ECQ) data and provide learner with item score and total score feedback
4. Collect data on learner attitudes toward the CBVI program via Adjective Rating Scale (ARS):
   a. Convert 24-item ARS paper and pencil format to computer format
   b. Run computer-based ARS (15 minutes) and collect learner scores (factor and total)
   c. Provide learner ARS ite scores, factor scores and total score
Constraint: Two month time frame for completion of full system.

Figure 25.2 Project requirements: Computer-based video instruction (representative examples).

1. Subject information form (SIF): computer-based; all SIF graphics; runs; displays statistical report for each learner, capable of downloading to diskette, that includes student ID#, age, gender, ACT score, SAT score, and semester in nursing program
2. Screening pretest (SP): computer-based; all SP graphics; runs; displays statistical report for each learner, capable of downloading to diskette, that includes answers for each of 19 questions and total SP score
3. CBVI program on spiritual care, with embedded content questions (ECQ): flowchart; hierarchy chart; screen layouts; videodisc script; videodisc map; all CBVI graphics; detailed outline for IWPS authoring; generate IWPS code; Run CBVI program; displays statistical report for each learner, capable of downloading to diskette, that includes: (a) learner control choices for each branch and totals; and (b) answers for each of 5 questions and total score
4. Adjective Rating Scale (ARS) attitude survey: computer-based; all ARS graphics; runs; scoring criteria for factors and total; displays statistical report for each learner, capable of downloading to diskette, that includes responses for each of 24 items, for each of 5 factors and total score

Figure 25.3 Project design specifications: Computer-based video instruction (representative examples).

ification approach and were added to the project specifications. Preparation for specifications included a detailed flowchart, a hierarchy chart, and scripts with videodisc mapping for planned computer usage. An example of videodisc mapping for specifications is taken from the "Mr. Baker" segment[1]

of the project videodisc. In this segment Mr. Baker says, "I was always a drunk. I worked. I had to. But sometimes I wonder . . . I have two daughters; they used to go to church with their mother and I'd stay at home to drink. That's all." The videodisc frame numbers for this segment were written down (23692–24219) and used in the CBVI program.

The detailed flowchart was completed prior to identifying specifications for the

---

[1] Videodisc map segment used by permission of Nurses Christian Fellowship; video segment produced from original script by J. A. Shelly.

main parts of the project. A detailed outline was then attempted (actually pseudocode with script) prior to developing the code (specifications Step 3). After outlining one event for the CBVI program, it was determined that an outline would take far too long. The requirements and specifications were known, but the program design to be used with the IWPS authoring system was still unknown. If an entire comprehensive outline were done as specified, one would still have only a paper model. The writer wanted a special look and feel to the software; how could this be accomplished? And how could the project be completed on time?

Examples

During the process of moving from the project specifications to the program design, the team encountered numerous difficult choices. The following are a few design examples:

1. Color schemes to be used for graphics. A unique look and feel was wanted. The team needed to see a number of color combinations in each section of the software before choosing the final schemes.

2. Transitions between screens. The team needed to experiment with a number of types of screen changes (e.g., dissolves, explosions) before determining final approaches.

3. Use of sound. Other CBVI programs reviewed had some sounds that were annoying, for example, double beeps as feedback for each touch response. The team wanted to try a sampling of sound throughout the presentation before making decisions.

4. Performing calculations. The IWPS documentation recommended performing all required calculations within an event (thus minimizing delays). The

team wanted to branch to outside events for each scored item, to eliminate redundant code.

PROJECT RAPID PROTOTYPING AND POSSIBLE SCREENS

After making design choices, the project team quickly set about creating a rapid prototype (early, functioning version) of the full system software. Figure 25.1 illustrated how the specification methodology merged into rapid prototyping methodology and how the rapid prototype merged into the full system software. Essential elements for each of the four main parts of the software were determined prior to developing the prototype code. Possible screens were considered and tested. Then, prototype versions of these elements were built and the parts exercised and tested. Reworking of the software design was not necessary. Students field tested the prototype. After the prototype was tested, the full system was built with minimal reworking of the project software.

Table 25.1 shows the number of events used for each of the four main parts of the project. The team used 14 events for the rapid prototype, out of a succeeding total of 97 events for the full system; that is, only 14 percent of all the events used were required for the rapid prototype. Sample screens[2] from the four main parts illustrate the results of the project's rapid prototyping. Figure 25.4 is an ACT screen from the subject information form (SIF) tool, using screen

---

[2] Program screens used with permission as follows: Center for Instructional Development, Syracuse University, ARS (paper-and-pencil ver.) item 1; Mary R. Hassett Consulting, ARS (computer-based ver.) item 1, SIF item 1 & SP item 1; Nurses Christian Fellowship, CBVI assessment data (screen 76).

Table 25.1   Rapid Prototype Events: Computer-Based Video Instruction Program

Main Part Represented	No. of Events Used
1. Subject Information Form (SIF)	3
2. Screening Pretest (SP)	3
3. CBVI program introduction w/graphics, text & video	1
4. Adjective Rating Scale (ARS) w/5 factors	7
Total	14

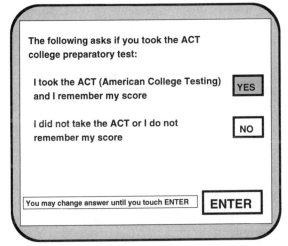

Figure 25.4 Subject information form (SIF): American College Testing sample item. (Note: Copyright © 1989–1991 by Mary R. Hassett Consulting. Used by permission.)

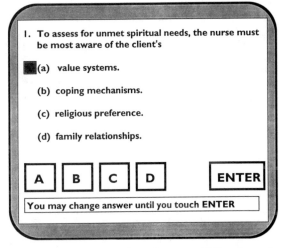

Figure 25.5 Screening Pretest (SP): Sample item. (Source: Copyright © 1989–1991 by Mary R. Hassett Consulting. Used by permission.)

buttons (*yes, no, enter*) that change color after selected; an indicator switch is set after *enter* is selected by the learner (branches to the ACT score event if *yes*). Figure 25.5 is item 1 from the screening pretest (SP) tool; this screen uses feedback for learner's input (for a, b, c, or d); the speech chip states the letter touched ("a" in this case) and a colored square appears to left of answer; the *enter* button changes color after it is touched (If *enter* is touched before an answer is input, the speech chip suggests, "Touch letter a b c or d at the bottom,"); an indicator switch is set after that question is answered by the learner; data handling of correct response results in +1 to SP total score event. Figure

25.6 is a screen from the CBVI program that introduces assessment data content before a video segment is shown that illustrates the text (the interactive videodisc is activated after the learner touches *continue*). Figure 25.7 is item 1 from the Adjective Rating Scale tool, computer-based from paper and pencil; if *enter* is touched before an answer is input, the speech chip suggests, "Touch answer box one two three or four"; this screen uses feedback for the learner's input (1, 2, 3, or 4), the button changes color after an answer has been touched ("2" in this case); the *enter* button changes color after touched and the speech chip issues a "tock" sound; an indicator switch is set after answered by the

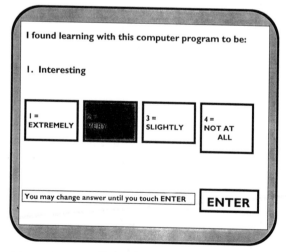

> **In gathering assessment data, the nurse observes the affect (facial expression) and attitude of the client, and the client's behavior. The next video segment shows what the nurse observes about Mr. Mason's affect, attitude and behavior, prior to an interaction.**
>
> **CONTINUE**

Figure 25.6 Computer-based video instruction program: Assessment data. (Source: Copyright © 1989–1991 by Nurses Christian Fellowship. Used by permission.)

> **I found learning with this computer program to be:**
>
> **I. Interesting**
>
> | 1 = EXTREMELY | 2 = VERY | 3 = SLIGHTLY | 4 = NOT AT ALL |
>
> You may change answer until you touch ENTER   **ENTER**

Figure 25.7 Kelly's adjective rating scale (ARS): Sample item. Note: Adapted by permission of the Center for Instructional Development, Syracuse University.

learner; data handling of response: loop to ARS total score event.

IMPLEMENTATION: PROBLEMS ENCOUNTERED AND RESOLUTION

Rapid prototyping represents a fundamental shift in methodology. The responsibility for defining requirements changes from talking about building the software to actually building the system project. Success with this methodology, therefore, required a shift to a bias for action (Boar, 1985). One does not just document, but demonstrates; one moves from the static to a dynamic; and instead of linear action, one moves to iterative actions. The team used a combination of specification and rapid prototyping that was effective. Nevertheless, specifications used valuable time and the team will not use a combination for the next CBVI project. Instead, a rapid prototyping approach will be taken from the outset because it is efficient and effective.

A sample videodisc was mastered before the rapid prototyping began, from repurposed videotapes (Heather, Wiebe, Shelly, & Hassett, 1981). Videotape segments were edited in one week. A sample videodisc was mastered from the edited videotape master and arrived within two days. Miller and Irving (1989) document that a rapid prototype module should be ready in about four weeks, yet the team completed the rapid prototyping module in two weeks, probably because the project was a small (60-minute) program. (Including time for team adjustment to all-new hardware and software, the process would have taken five weeks.) If one is familiar with hardware and software, two or three weeks would be necessary for rapid prototyping a one-hour CBVI program. The following are examples of problem resolutions:

1. A unique look and feel for graphics was achieved with a few complementary pastel colors and patterns.

2. Transitions between screens included simple dissolves and curtains, with occasional explosion effects.

3. A few well-chosen sounds were used. For example, the author-defined on-screen keyboard had a tick sound as feedback for each touch of an on-screen "key."

4. Performing calculations with branches to outside events for each scored item worked well.

As stated earlier, designing and programming CBVI programs is time consuming (Redland & Kilmon, 1985). Development of the full CBVI project took the writer approximately one year. Rapid prototyping reduced the time needed to author, and the rapid prototype became a part of the final software. The time needed for just the programming portion of the full project (rapid prototyping included) was 11 weeks for the writer and approximately one week for the systems analyst. The full system project was completed five weeks after the rapid prototyped version was finished and included evaluation of the full system by a panel of content experts. No changes were deemed necessary by the panel of judges.

EVALUATION WITH REFERENCE TO STUDENTS

Students field tested the prototype and, as active participants in the design, they helped in reworking the prototyped software. The CBVI project's full software was pilot tested with excellent results (n = 10); few changes were necessary (Hassett, 1989b). The full software met the requirements and specifications and was used successfully, on time,

in a study with baccalaureate nursing students (n = 32) (Hassett, 1991). The exploratory descriptive study examined whether differences existed among nursing student subjects of sensing (S) and intuitive (N) psychological type who used a CBVI program with learner control options. Hassett's CBVI Model was used (Hassett, 1991), based on Gagne's conditions of learning and Jung's psychological type operationalized by the Myers-Briggs Type Indicator (MBTI) Gagne's constructs about the ways in which people receive and then use information to achieve learning objectives and his constructs about attitude toward learning were used (Gagne, 1985). Jung's constructs describe basic personality differences, such as how people prefer to use their minds in perceiving the world. The two ways of perceiving are sensing (S, directly aware through the five senses) or intuition (N, indirectly aware by way of the unconscious). The MBTI was used to determine S or N (Myers & McCaulley, 1985).

A nonprobability convenience sample of volunteer generic baccalaureate students was recruited (47% were S and 53% N). Chi-square for differences between subjects' psychological type and learner control choices made in the CBVI program (i.e., to SEE MORE information, or REPEAT selected program segments) yielded no significant differences. Both psychological types showed positive attitudes toward CBVI (Hassett, 1991). A study limitation was too few SEE MORE options (allowing learners to see more information about the content just covered) related to the repurposing of an existing videotape to videodisc for the CBVI program. Recommendations included: continued testing of Hassett's CBVI Model, additional SEE MORE options in the CBVI program, and mastering videodiscs from videotapes designed specifically for CBVI (Hassett, 1991). The pilot study and the study yielded similar results. Students in the pilot study and the study reported the program was easy to use, fun, and the look and feel of the program was pleasing. Branchings worked well, and students were not frustrated with timing sequences. The full project software (described by Bolwell, 1991) was robust in that aborts or crashes did not occur and reasonableness tests worked.

Modularity and plasticity in the IWPS authoring system were important; because of these attributes, changes were made within a matter of hours. Segments of the instructional unit were added, removed, or modified without causing problems. Aspects of the instructional unit were changed with no penalties. Standards worked well because they were scrutinized during rapid prototyping: color of background and text, screen design, use of function keys, branching designs, degree of user control and interactivity, type of feedback, and record-keeping ability.

SUMMARY WITH IMPLICATIONS FOR NURSING EDUCATION

The model project presented in this chapter included: background of the computer-based video instruction (CBVI) program, hardware and software, the project team, specifications approach, and implementation of rapid prototyping. Examples of design choices and computer screens from the project were used, and the resolution of problems were discussed. Evaluation with reference to students was shared: field testing of the rapid prototype and the positive attitudes of nursing students toward CBVI found in a pilot study and a study.

The major implication of rapid prototyping for nursing education is the potential for improvement of the CBVI development process. The addition of rapid prototyping

methodology to the specification approach markedly improved the CBVI project. Rapid prototyping worked well and greatly reduced the time needed to finish the CBVI project. Rapid prototyping allowed the team to build a small, functional program with a minimal amount of effort. Having a physical working model gave encouragement to the team, and brought the project to life! Modifications were easy to make because needed features were added early, without having to go through the full program later, and each new understanding was implemented immediately.

Rapid prototyping provides nursing education with a formal methodology to facilitate and improve the development of computer-based video instruction (CBVI) programs. Rapid prototyping requires minimal resources (e.g., time, money, and video). It saves time on programming revisions, and provides an accurate picture, in miniature, of the CBVI program. Needed changes are identified early in the development process, thus saving money and video resources. One can capture and then master to videodisc only what is needed. Advantages of beginning with a specification approach include a formal structure for the full system. Nevertheless, rapid prototyping alone may be all that is needed for some CBVI projects.

REFERENCES

Asymetrix Corporation. (1991). *ToolBook ideas: An author's introduction to programming in ToolBook*. Bellevue, WA: Author.

Boar, B. H. (1985). *Application prototyping: A project management perspective*. New York: American Management Association.

Boehm, B. W., Gray, T. E., & Seewaldt, T. (1984). Prototyping versus specifying: A multiproject experiment. *IEEE Transac-*

tions on Software Engineering, SE10 (8), 290–302.

Bolwell, C. (1991). *Directory of educational software for nursing* (4th ed.). Athens, OH: Fuld Institute for Technology in Nursing Education.

Connell, J. L., & Shafer, L. B. (1989). *Structured rapid prototyping: An evolutionary approach to software development.* Englewood Cliffs, NJ: Yourdon.

Fisher, G. E. (1987). *Application software prototyping and fourth generation languages* (NBS Special Publication No. 500-148). Washington, DC: U.S. Government Printing Office.

Gagne, R. M. (1985). *The conditions of learning and theory of instruction* (4th ed.). NY: Holt, Rinehart & Winston.

Hassett, M. R. (Producer & Author). (1989a). *Spiritual assessment of Christian clients* [Unpublished Level III interactive videodisc and IBM InfoWindow® computer program]. Hays, KS: Mary R. Hassett Consulting.

Hassett, M. R. (1989b). Differences in attitude toward computer-based video instruction and learner control choices made by baccalaureate nursing students of sensing and intuitive psychological type (preliminary data). In Proceedings of the 31st Conference of the Association for the Development of Computer-Based Instructional Systems: Creativity through analogy (pp. 112–119). Bellingham, WA: Western Washington University, Association for the Development of Computer-Based Instructional Systems.

Hassett, M. R. (1990a). Computer-based video instruction in nursing: One nurse's experience as author. *The Kansas Nurse, 65* (9), 3–4.

Hassett, M. R. (1990b). Rapid prototyping: A methodology for developing computer-based video instruction programs [Abstract]. In *Eighth Annual Computer Conference Abstracts, Nursing Informatics: Current Trends and Future Directions* (p. 1). Newark: Rutgers, The State University, College of Nursing.

Hassett, M. R. (1991). Differences in attitude toward computer-based video instruction and learner control choices made by baccalaureate nursing students of sensing and intuitive psychological type. (Doctoral dissertation, The University of Texas at Austin, 1990). *Dissertation Abstracts International, 51* (9), 4277-B.

Heather, J. (Exec. producer), Wiebe, C. (Producer-Director), Shelly, J. A. (Script Writer), & Hassett, M. R. (Actress & Script Consultant). (1981). *Spiritual needs assessment practicum and nursing process practica.* [Videotape set 1-5.] Madison, WI: Nurses Christian Fellowship.

International Business Machines Corporation. (1986). *InfoWindow presentation system: Editor.* Atlanta, GA: Author.

International Business Machines Corporation. (1990). *Storyboard Live! User guide.* Boca Raton, FL: Author.

Kelly, E. F., Pascarella, E. T., Terenzini, P., & Chapman, D. (1976). *The development and use of the Adjective rating scale: A measure of attitude toward courses and programs.* Paper presented at the annual convention of the American Educational Research Association, San Francisco, CA.

Knutsen, E. (1991, May). *VCR videos for "controlled" use* [with demonstration of MPG & IBM LinkWay computer program]. Paper presented at the seminar Multi-Media Review III, International Business Machines Corporation, Kansas City, MO.

Locatis, C. N. (1989, Jan.). *Videodisc repurposing* (Lister Hill monograph; LHNCBC 89-2). Bethesda, MD: National Library of Medicine.

Luqi, A. (1989, May). Software evolution through rapid prototyping. *Computer, 22* (5), 13–25.

Miller, A. W., & Irving, J. W. (1989). Rapid prototyping: Solving the "mystery" of IVD. In *Proceedings of the 31st Conference of the Association for the Development of Computer-Based Instructional Systems: Creativity through analogy* (pp. 200–201). Bellingham, WA: Western Washington University, Association for the Development of Computer-Based Instructional Systems.

Myers, I. B., & McCaulley, M. (1985). *Manual: The Myers-Briggs type indicator* (2nd ed.). Palo Alto, CA: Consulting Psychologists.

Newsline: Intel's DVI advances toward desktop mainstream. (1990). *The Videodisc Monitor, 8* (12), 4.

Newsline: NEC unveils PC-VCR for tape-based multimedia. (1990). *The Videodisc Monitor, 8* (10), 8.

Newsline: VideoLogic plans powerful video compression system. (1990). *The Videodisc Monitor, 8* (11), 3.

Pioneer buys DVA, develops rewritable videodisc system with KDD. (1989). *The Videodisc Monitor, 7* (11), 1, 3.

Redland, A. R., & Kilmon, C. (1985). Interactive video: Rationale and practicalities of one experience. In *Proceedings of the First Annual Nursing Conference on Computer-assisted Interactive Video Instruction.* Sacramento: California State University, Sacramento, Division of Nursing.

Technology collision: The Demo Center. (1991). *Multimedia & Videodisc Monitor, 9* (7–8), 24–25.

Tripp, S. D., & Bichelmeyer, B. (1990). Rapid prototyping: An alternative instructional design strategy. *Educational Technology Research and Development, 38* (1), 31–44.

26

NursEXPERT: A Nursing Diagnosis Assessment Expert System

Brent W. Thompson

INTRODUCTION

"No computer will ever take the place of the nurse!"

This comment has been spoken by nurses since computer applications first made their appearance in nursing practice. Add the prospect of artificial intelligence and expert systems and the emotional level of the discussion only increases. It is thought that the art of nursing is too complex to be reduced to a computer program. It does not seem possible that the cognitive skills that have evolved over millennia, the accumulated professional knowledge of the past 100 years, and the interpersonal skills acquired over one's own lifetime could be entered into a computer as series of 1s and 0s. Does this mean that if a computer cannot duplicate the cognitive processes of a human nurse then no attempt should be made to explore how these cognitive processes work? This chapter will examine how nursing decisions and diagnoses are made, discuss the need for computerized nursing diagnosis decision support, describe a nursing diagnosis assessment expert system under development, and consider the future of artificial intelligence in nursing education and nursing practice.

MAKING NURSING DECISIONS

Research into clinical decision making has grown tremendously in the past 30 years. The first problem-solving tool of nursing practice was the nursing process, which is an application of the scientific method. The nursing process alone was not sufficient to define nursing practice (Henderson, 1982). In the 1970s the development of nursing diagnosis assessment gave standardized labels to groups of signs and symptoms of interest to nurses (Ziegler, Vaughn-Wrobel, & Eielen, 1986). Nursing diagnoses refined the definition of nursing practice but did not simplify the practice of nursing. A nurse making a nursing diagnosis assessment must sort through the tremendous amount of available data to determine the relevant data, then must decide what those data mean. How does a nurse learn to make these decisions?

Identification of the decision-making process by expert nurses is the focus of current research in clinical decision making. Benner (1984) has described the process of growth from novice to expert. As nurses progress to stages of advanced beginner, competence, proficiency, and expert they are increasingly able to identify the relevant aspects of the whole client situation. Expert nurses can then unconsciously apply a deep understanding of the situation to implement appropriate actions. Becoming an expert nurse is a lengthy process that begins in nursing school and continues throughout a nurse's practice. Learning how to recognize the significant elements in a given nursing situation is not usually taught directly. It is considered an intuitive process that can only be learned through experience (Benner, 1984; Benner & Tanner, 1987).

Computers are good repositories of information that novice nurses can use to draw on the expertise of experienced nurses. Expert systems are one way to provide decision-making assistance or decision support. Decision support is the use of a computer to assist nurses to make decisions that are better than those they would make if they were unaided (Brennan, 1990).

Expert systems are a branch of artificial intelligence that also includes robotics and natural language processing (Stallings, Hutchinson, & Sawyer, 1988). Expert systems have been designed for mainframes and personal computers in many domains of knowledge, including nursing. Any expert system consists of four parts: (1) a natural language, or interface with the user, (2) a knowledge base (or the rules from which decisions can be made), (3) a database of facts specific to the domain of the problem, and (4) an inference "engine" to solve problems by linking the knowledge base rules with the database facts (Hart, 1986; Brennan, 1990). Expert systems, unlike traditional computer programs, are easily open to alteration as knowledge changes. Advantages of using expert systems as decision-making assistants include (1) comprehensiveness (they consider all options), (2) consistency (they have no bias nor will they jump to conclusions), and (3) they are always available (Hart, 1986).

Making Nursing Diagnosis Decisions

Many authors have documented the need for decision-making assistance with expert systems for nursing diagnoses (Chang, Roth, Gonzales, Caswell, & DiStefano, 1988; Bloom, Leitner, & Solano, 1987; Laborde, 1985; Evans, 1984). A key feature of all expert systems is the ability to transfer the knowledge of an expert to a novice (Hart, 1986). The novice nurse, or student nurse, often has difficulty in applying the data collected about a client when formulating nursing diagnoses. Most students use one of the many books on nursing diagnosis to make their diagnoses. These books usually provide a list of diagnoses in alphabetical order or in unprioritized accordance with the Taxonomy I diagnosis classifications of the North American Nursing Diagnosis Association (1990). Students then use a brute force method of comparing every diagnosis with the data they have collected about the client. The brute force method consists in first considering definitions of "A" diagnoses (starting with Activity Intolerance), then going alphabetically down the diagnosis list to "Z" (actually "V" for Violence Potential). This method of assessment is typical for novices acquiring almost any skill (Benner & Tanner, 1987). Those with experience have learned to combine, or "chunk," related problems unconsciously.

This unconscious aspect of diagnosis also

means the nursing instructor often has difficulty explaining to the student how a nursing diagnosis is determined. To teach the process of forming a diagnosis, it is sometimes necessary to model the process for the student. It can be difficult to explain to a novice a process that has become automatic for the teacher.

There is a need for more research on the cognitive processes of diagnosis (Tanner, Padrick, Westfall, & Putzier, 1987). The cognitive processes of nursing diagnosis are largely unexplored. Additionally, both nursing students and instructors would benefit from computerized nursing diagnosis assistance for teaching, learning, and research. Nursing can use diagnosis expert systems in research of nursing diagnosis as both process and product (Abraham, 1990). Process questions explore how nurses make diagnoses. The product under question is each diagnosis, its validity, and its definition. This research confirms or contests the definitions of every nursing diagnosis (Abraham, 1990). The adequacy of diagnostic language and classifications also need to be constantly examined and tested (Pinkley, 1991). A decision support tool in the domain of nursing diagnosis assessment can contribute to this research as a mode of clinical testing.

NURSEXPERT

In 1987 work began on an expert system to teach nursing diagnosis assessment to undergraduate students. NursEXPERT is a nursing diagnosis knowledge-based expert system under development at the University of Delaware. Project goals include:

1. Input is quick and requires little or no use of the keyboard.
2. The database and knowledge base are easily modified.

3. Incorporation of all accepted NANDA nursing diagnoses.
4. Output is quick and easy to read.
5. Users receive a list of existing and potential nursing diagnoses for their actual clients.

These goals were chosen because of the need to examine diagnostic cognitive processes in the clinical area on actual clients. Previous research on diagnostic reasoning has been done with simulated clients and without the use of decision-support software (Tanner et al., 1987). It was also desirable to create a program that was easy to use, provided information in a timely manner, and was easy to modify.

NursEXPERT uses a hypertext program, HyperCard™ (version 1.2 or greater) running on an Apple Macintosh™ (with $\geq$1 MB RAM, System 6.0.5 or greater). This program's graphic ability and ease of distribution made it ideal for this project. HyperCard is included with all Macintosh computers, thus distribution of the NursEXPERT file, or "stack," can be made without copyright infringement. Expert systems that use commercial shells require the purchase of the shell or permission to distribute a "read-only" program from the shell manufacturer. Another advantage is that NursEXPERT can also be translated into a hypertext file for the IBM-PC™ program, Toolbook™.

The graphics ability of HyperCard allows the user to enter data with just clicks of a mouse. A single screen display can ask many questions of a student and the student can respond quickly by moving the cursor to one of the screen buttons and clicking. NursEXPERT was designed as a program that could be used quickly by students with limited knowledge of computers. The only skill required is the ability to turn on the computer and use the mouse.

The NursEXPERT nursing diagnosis database is from NANDA's *Taxonomy I—Revised*

1. Oxygenation	10. Activity	18. Emotional integrity
2. Circulation	11. Cognition	19. Knowledge
3. Elimination	12. Family function	20. Self-care
4. Nutrition	13. Meaningfulness	21. Rest
5. Physical regulation	14. Sexuality	22. Recreation
6. Physical integrity	15. Spirituality	23. Growth
7. Comfort	16. Socialization	24. Activity of daily living
8. Communication	17. Self image	25. Participation
9. Perception		

Figure 26.1 Prioritized nursing diagnosis categories used by NursEXPERT.

1990 by the North American Nursing Diagnosis Association (1990). This taxonomy provides the definitions and defining characteristics of all accepted diagnoses. NursEXPERT uses the defining characteristics of each diagnosis as the data for confirming or contesting the existence of a diagnosis for a client. The use of NANDA diagnoses and their definitions standardizes the database, eases updates as new diagnoses and definitions evolve, and facilitates research of the process and product of diagnosis.

The NursEXPERT knowledge base has two components: the diagnosis classifications and their organizational structure. First is the taxonomy that classifies diagnoses into related groups. For example, the NANDA Taxonomy I groups the diagnoses of altered airway clearance, altered breathing patterns, and impaired gas exchange as part of the human response pattern Exchanging. Exchanging is the name for the group of all physiologically based diagnoses. The three diagnoses are also part of a subgroup within Exchanging (grouped as 1.5.1) but are unnamed in Taxonomy I. NursEXPERT names the Exchanging subgroup 1.5.1 as the classification Oxygenation. Figure 26.1 shows the 25 NursEXPERT classifications.

The second component of the NursEXPERT knowledge base organizes the classifications according to Maslow's Hierarchy of Needs (see Figure 26.1). This approach of prioritizing diagnoses from the physiological to the self-actualization needs was first pro-

posed by Halloran (1983). Maslow's Hierarchy of Needs provides a logical order for the expert system to validate the existence of diagnoses in clients. NursEXPERT uses these classifications as a heuristic to organize the pathway of questioning. Instead of asking questions about all 108 nursing diagnoses, NursEXPERT asks broad questions to confirm or contest diagnoses in each classification. This speeds the input process and more closely approximates the diagnostic reasoning process of experienced nurses (Benner & Tanner, 1987).

Figure 26.2 shows the pathway of questioning for the classifications of Oxygenation, Circulation, and Elimination. An

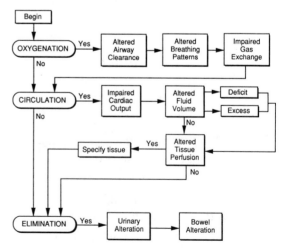

Figure 26.2 Sample pathway of questioning used by NursEXPERT.

advantage of the classification system is the ability of the student to avoid unnecessary and time consuming questioning about nursing diagnoses that are not present. It also allows the student to see if sufficient data was collected to make a decision.

Using NursEXPERT

Nursing students in a microcomputer laboratory are the initial users of NursEXPERT. Students collect data on their clients and return to the laboratory for assistance in determining the existing nursing diagnoses of their clients. The program tests hypotheses about the existence of nursing diagnoses by asking broad questions about a client's condition. If the user responds "yes" then more detailed questions about the possible diagnoses of that classification are asked. The expert system uses deductive inference, moving from the global to the specific, and efficiently sifting the available data.

An example of how NursEXPERT functions follows. After a welcome screen is displayed the user can go to a help screen (see Figure 26.3) or start the program. The user may quit, start over, or print a list of diagnoses at any time by clicking on the buttons that are always available at the bottom of the screen. The first question screen determines if any diagnoses under the Oxygenation classification exist for the client (see Figure 26.4). The top of the screen always displays the classifications or the diagnosis under question. If the user responds "No" to the Oxygenation question, the program skips to the next classification—Circulation. If the answer is Yes, it then asks more detailed questions about the possibility of ineffective airway clearance (Figure 26.5), altered breathing patterns, and impaired gas ex-

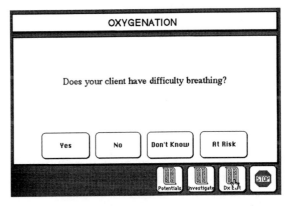

Figure 26.4 NursEXPERT's question to determine if any oxygenation category diagnoses exist for the client.

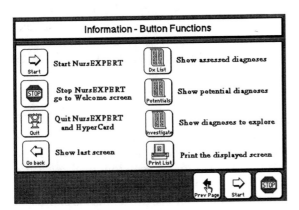

Figure 26.3 Example of a NursEXPERT help screen showing how each button functions.

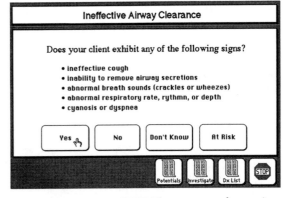

Figure 26.5 NursEXPERT's screen to determine if the nursing diagnosis Ineffective Airway Clearance exists for the client.

change. NursEXPERT compiles and prints out three lists: confirmed diagnoses, potential or at-risk diagnoses, and diagnoses that need further data collection to confirm, called Investigate.

Current State of Development

NursEXPERT is being tested with nursing students at the University of Delaware. Students collect data on their clients in the clinical area and then use NursEXPERT to assist them in creating a list of prioritized diagnoses for their client. Diagnoses that need more data are explored the following clinical day. Ideally this program should be used on a portable or laptop computer to allow use directly in the clinical area.

NursEXPERT has spawned many research questions. Comparison of diagnosis lists made by students using decision assistance and those not using it is the first investigation. Future research will examine the validity of the classification priority system and the use of NANDA diagnosis defining characteristics as the database.

The user interface is also being tested. Interface design follows the guidelines for HyperCard stack design by Apple Computer, Inc. (1989). These guidelines give suggestions for screen design, button function, and user control of the stack. The graphics capability of the program allows an interface that requires only mouse clicks or single keyboard strokes to answer. Such input methods speed use and should be less intimidating for the novice computer user. As students use and evaluate the program, new features can be added or modified.

THE FUTURE OF NURSEXPERT

Expert systems will not replace nurses, nor should they. NursEXPERT is a sim-

plistic starting point for more research into the quantification and examination of nursing diagnosis decision making. The analysis of apparently intuitive decisions can contribute to the describable practice base of nursing (Field, 1987). Expert systems are open to change. The expert system knowledge bases and databases will expand as nursing knowledge expands. This program will contribute to research regarding the process of nursing diagnosis and nursing diagnoses themselves.

The future of expert systems in nursing is very promising and exciting. NursEXPERT is a start in providing computer-aided assistance to assessment, the first step of the nursing process. Expert systems for nursing practice are still in their infancy. The potential uses of expert systems will increase as computer storage space and computing speed increase. The next step will be to extend the use of diagnostic expert systems to the next steps of planning, intervention, and evaluation.

Another potential use of expert systems is their integration into hospital information systems. As nurses care for their clients, they would answer questions about the client posed by the system, make decisions with the system's assistance, and input the results of nursing actions. Such a system would have a two-fold use as both nursing documentation for an individual client record and as a database for nursing practice research.

Decision-making assistance will not take nurses away from the bedside. Expert systems will help keep nurses at the bedside collecting data, making assessments and goals, implementing interventions, and evaluating outcomes. Judgments on the suggestions given by an expert system will still require nursing expertise. Computerized decision assistance will help us ask the right questions and make decisions in "consultation" with hundreds of experts. The question is not *should* nurses use expert systems in our practice, but rather, *when* will nurses use expert systems in our practice?

REFERENCES

Abraham, I. L. (1990). Issues in the application of artificially intelligent decision support technology to nursing diagnosis. In J. G. Ozbolt, D. Vandewal, & K. J. Hannah (Eds.), *Decision support systems in nursing* (pp. 91–96). St. Louis: C. B. Mosby.

Apple Computer, Inc. (1989). *HyperCard stack design guidelines.* New York: Addison–Wesley.

Benner, P. (1984). *From novice to expert: Excellence and power in clinical nursing practice.* Menlo Park, CA: Addison–Wesley.

Benner, P., & Tanner, C. A. (1987). Clinical judgment: How expert nurses use intuition. American Journal of Nursing, *87*, 23–31.

Brennan, P. F. (1990). Decision support systems in nursing: An overview. In J. G. Ozbolt, D. Vandewal, & K. J. Hannah (Eds.), *Decision support systems in nursing* (pp. 3–14). St. Louis: C. V. Mosby.

Bloom, K. C., Leitner, J. E., & Solano, J. L. (1987). Development of an expert system prototype to generate nursing care plans based on nursing diagnoses. *Computers in Nursing, 5,* 140–145.

Chang, B. L., Roth, K., Gonzales, E., Caswell, D., & DiStefano, J. (1988). CANDI: A knowledge based system for nursing diagnosis. *Computers in Nursing, 6,* 13–21.

Evans, S. (1984). A computer-based nursing diagnosis consultant. In G. S. Cohen (Ed.), *Proceedings of the Eighth Annual Symposium on Computer Applications in Medical Care.* New York: IEEE Computer Society.

Field, P. A. (1987). The impact of nursing theory on the clinical decision-making process. *Journal of Advanced Nursing, 12,* 563–571.

Halloran, E. (1983). RN staffing: More care-less cost. *Nursing Management, 14* (9), 18–22.

Hart, A. (1986). *Knowledge acquisition for expert systems.* New York: McGraw–Hill.

Henderson, V. (1982). The nursing process—is the title right? *Journal of Advanced Nursing, 7,* 103–106.

Laborde, J. M. (1985). Expert systems for nursing? *Computers in Nursing, 2,* 130–135.

North American Nursing Diagnosis Association. (1990). *Taxonomy I—Revised 1990.* St. Louis: North American Nursing Diagnosis Association.

Pinkley, C. L. (1991). Exploring NANDA's definition of nursing diagnosis: Linking diagnostic judgments with the selection of outcomes and interventions. *Nursing Diagnosis,* Jan./March, *2* (1), 26–32.

Stallings, W. D., Hutchinson, S. E., & Sawyer, S. C. (1988). *Computers: The user's perspective.* St. Louis: Times Mirror/Mosby.

Tanner, C. A., Padrick, K. P., Westfall, U. E., & Putzier, D. J. (1987). Diagnostic reasoning strategies of nurses and nursing students. *Nursing Research, 36,* 358–362.

Ziegler, S. M., Vaughn-Wrobel, B. C., & Eielen, J. A. (1986). *Nursing process, nursing diagnosis, nursing knowledge: Avenues to autonomy.* New York: Appleton-Century-Crofts.

27

Creation and Utilization of a Database for Student Advisement

Barbara Cohen
Helen Lerner
Marcia Brown

INTRODUCTION AND BACKGROUND

A student database was created for the Division of Nursing, Lehman College to provide comprehensive and accessible information about each nursing student for academic advisement. Providing academic counseling is essential in working with students from economically and academically disadvantaged backgrounds. The nursing students at Lehman College are similar to students enrolled in most public urban universities today. That is, they consist primarily of minority students who are older, working, and responsible for child care while attending college. Many students lack adequate backgrounds in science and mathematics and given their personal responsibilities may encounter difficulties that prevent successful completion of the nursing program. Providing students with academic advisement may mean the difference between their success or failure.

Academic advising requires that faculty have easy and quick access to students' records. Although in most educational institutions this information is available from the office of the registrar, attaining the needed data may prove frustrating due to the time and effort required. Even when faculty have access to a terminal permitting entry into students' records, information that can be accessed may be limited. Obtaining students' entire transcripts is time consuming. This paper addresses how a comprehensive database was established and how this information was utilized. The steps involved included: (1) identifying purposes of the database and equipment needed; (2) design of the database; (3) trial and modifications of design; and (4) implementation and uses.

IDENTIFYING PURPOSES OF THE DATABASE AND EQUIPMENT NEEDED

The primary goal for creating this database was to provide faculty with com-

Acknowledgment: Preparation of this article was supported in part by a grant from the Department of Health and Human Servvices, Health Resources and Services Administration, Division of Nursing D19 NU 22164 to Dr. Rosanne Wille.

prehensive information for student advisement. The literature on student attrition and predictors of academic success was reviewed prior to developing the database. Also the writers further identified data necessary for faculty to have available. Data included scores obtained on the assessment tests in writing, mathematics, and reading; grades in college core courses (courses providing the foundation for study in sciences and liberal arts); academic grades in courses prerequisite to the nursing program; grades attained in nursing courses; transfer status; and selected attributes of students (Allen, Higgs, & Holloway, 1988; Safian-Rush & Belock, 1988; Mckinney, Small, O'Dell, & Coonrod, 1988; Felts, 1986). Student characteristics included: age; country of birth; primary language; gender; ethnicity; marital status; number of children under 21 years of age; responsibility for child care; employment status; RN status; and general health status. Academic variables were obtained from the office of the registrar while demographic information was solicited directly from students through a short questionnaire.

Several printed reports that would assist faculty in giving appropriate academic advisement were identified. These reports included individual students' records and a list of students who had a grade point average (GPA) of 2.0 or less in nursing courses. It was also decided that a report that listed all students who were at risk of academic failure was needed.

Software and Hardware

The database was created using the program dBASE III PLUS (Ashton Tate 1985, 1986). Although there are other commercial databases available, e.g., Paradox (Borland), Alpha3 (Alpha Software Inc.), our decision to purchase dBASE III PLUS was a pragmatic one. The authors opted to use the database that was used on campus since support ser-

vices were available. Computer support personnel highly recommended dBASE III PLUS as a software program that would serve our purposes. The hardware used was an IBM PS 2 Model 50 with 640K. Students' records are stored on hard and floppy disks. In preparation for using the database for advisement purposes, the authors examined the relationships among students' academic and demographic variables to predict academic failure. To accomplish this the software program SPSS/PC+ V.3 (SPSS Inc. 1988) was used. Data from dBASE III PLUS can be imported to SPSS PC+ V.3.

DATABASE DESIGN

Creating a database calls for the entry of fields. It further requires naming each field and identifying the type of field. A field refers to each item of information within a specific record. For our purposes a field is each item of information we wanted to record about each student (e.g., name, ethnicity, course grades). The naming of fields entails creating a truncated name for each variable entered in the database. Examples of truncated names are DOB and ROCC that refer to date of birth and responsibility for child care respectively. The rationale for using a shortened name was that a field name cannot be more than 11 characters (numbers or letters). An eight-character length is the standard for a DOS system.

When shortening field names it is important to use names that will mean something to the individuals entering and retrieving data. A code of fields and their explanations was established and maintained.

The type of field refers to whether data are entered as character, date, logical field, numeric, or a memo. A character refers to alphanumeric entries such as letters, numbers, and punctuation marks. Entry in the format of a date is the recording of a specific month, day, and year. A logical field refers to a true or false response or a yes or no response. The term numeric field refers to numbers that are to be calculated. A memo permits room for anecdotal material, or additional information one wants to document.

The number of fields depends on the number of variables one wishes to document. This software allows for 128 fields. This particular database design consisted of 98 fields.

One also needs to anticipate how many spaces are needed for the information to be entered. For example a true (T) or false (F) response only requires one space; an address may require 25 spaces. This needs to be anticipated at the beginning of establishing the database. Examples of fields, type of fields, and width (number of characters) are illustrated in Table 27.1.

As in the development of other software programs, creating a database requires the expertise and labor of more than one individual. The two faculty members involved specified what they deemed necessary to know about students and what relationships should be analyzed. They obtained institutional review board consent, designed a short student questionnaire, identified variables to include, and utilized the statistical program. The computer consultant established the criteria for the fields, entered the data, and created additional programs (e.g., computing GPAs and customizing the database for the division of nursing). The student database is menu driven. Easy entry to the database was created by the computer consultant. Faculty did not have to learn dBASE commands to use the program.

Data entry is an arduous job in that it is time consuming and must be accurate and consistent. Approximately three and one-half to four weeks were needed for establishing the original database. This included entering data for about 400 students. Subsequent information, such as additional course

Table 27.1 Structure of the Database

Field	Field Name	Type	Width	Explanation
1	FIRSTNAME	CHARACTER	15	
2	MI	CHARACTER	1	
3	LASTNAME	CHARACTER	17	
4	ADDRESS	CHARACTER	25	
5	CITY	CHARACTER	15	
6	STATE	CHARACTER	2	
7	ZIPCODE	CHARACTER	7	
8	TELEPHONE	CHARACTER	13	
9	SOCSEC	CHARACTER	11	
10	DOB	DATE	8	date of birth
11	COB	CHARACTER	10	country of birth
12	PRIMLANG	CHARACTER	10	primary language
13	GENDER	CHARACTER	1	
14	ETHNICITY	CHARACTER	10	
15	MARRIED	LOGICAL	1	
21	ROCC	LOGICAL	1	(responsible for child care)
26	HEPW	NUMERIC	2	(hours employed per week)
29	FINAID	LOGICAL	1	(financial aid)
50	NUR 250	CHARACTER	9	(one of the nursing courses)

grades and new students, took approximately one week. This update is completed every semester.

TRIAL AND MODIFICATIONS OF DESIGN

There were two areas in which modifications were made. Changes were needed because it was not anticipated that analyses of relationships among student variables would be conducted. As mentioned before, a statistical program was used for this purpose. To use SPSS/PC+ V.3 some field names had to be shortened and numerical values assigned to demographic data. For example, logical fields using responses of either yes or no were changed to numbers 1 or 2 respectively. The demographic variables of sex, country of birth, and ethnicity were also given numeric values. An example is Black was changed to 1, Caucasian changed to 2, and so forth.

The second area involving changes was the decision to calculate students' GPAs. The computer consultant wrote a program to compute the grade point averages. This permitted faculty to refer to a student's overall GPA in addition to reviewing performance in individual courses. Letter grades were converted to the their numeric equivalents.

FINAL IMPLEMENTATION AND OUTCOMES

Full implementation of the database occurred in the semester following completion of data entry. The authors gave faculty individual instructions in using the database. Once faculty entered the code to access the student database, the menu illustrated in Figure 27.1 would appear.

Faculty have the option to input data by pressing the numbers 1–3 or obtain output of data by using the numbers 4–8. Once the original database is created, faculty have the

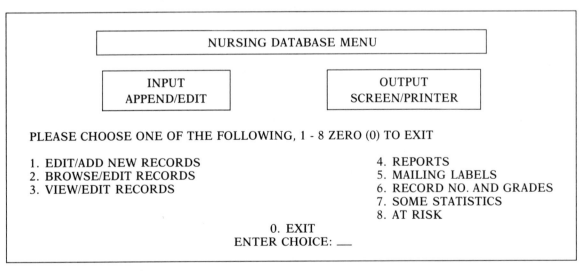

Figure 27.1 Customized menu.

option to input additional data. The distinctions between 1, 2, and 3 shown in the customized screen in Figure 27.1 are: (1) edit/add new records refers to accessing existing individual students' records or adding new records; (2) browse/edit option provides a listing of all student records; (3) view/edit uses the dBASE screen format.

The types of output available include printing: (4) a report of an individual student; (5) mailing labels; (6) records without students' names or other identifiers other than the record number; (7) summary reports on descriptive data; (8) a list of students identified at risk of academic failure.

A sample of one student's report as it appears on the computer screen is illustrated in Figures 27.2 and 27.3. On this screen one notes that the student, Sarah Green, lives in the Bronx, NY and was born in Jamaica in 1960. Ms. Green transferred to Lehman College in 1986 and entered the nursing program one year later. Her demographic data discloses that she is Black, female, single, and is responsible for the care of her own child. Ms. Green works 30 hours per week as a licensed practical nurse and is receiving no financial aid. Her grade point average in prerequisite nursing courses was 3.0 while her nursing grade point average is 2.32. Course grades attained at Lehman are as shown.

Although in dBASE III PLUS faculty can request a printout of a report by pressing the number 4, another database software program, Alpha 3 (Alpha Software Corporation), was frequently used to print a report similar to Lehman College's transcripts. Alpha 3 is used independently of dBASE III PLUS but is capable of reading dBASE III files. This program prints a report in less time and in a format we prefer compared to the reports printed using dBASE III PLUS. dBASE III is column oriented—it prints the report horizontally. Alpha 3 can print a report in rows or in columns. Each piece of information is shown on a separate line.

Name: Sarah Green
ADDRESS: 1516 Morris Avenue
Bronx, NY 10056
TELEPHONE: (212) 833-8500

ID NUMBER: 055-31-9187
COUNTRY OF BIRTH: Jamaica
PRIMARY LANGUAGE: English

TRANSFER STUDENT?: T (*SEE NEXT PAGE FOR STUDENTS GPA ***)
YEAR ENTERED LEHMAN: 09/30/86 ENTERED NURSING: 09/30/87
GRADUATED: / /

DATE OF BIRTH: 11/09/60 GENDER: F ETHNICITY: Black
MARITAL STATUS: M: F S: T D: F SEPARATED: F
                        WIDOWED: F
NUMBER OF CHILDREN IN HOUSEHOLD UNDER 21: 1
RESPONSIBLE FOR OWN CHILD CARE?: T
GENERAL HEALTH STATUS: Good

HOURS EMPLOYED PER WEEK: 30 HEALTH FIELD?: T
IF YES IN WHAT CAPACITY: LPN
FINANCIAL AID?: F IF YES, TYPE: (see below)
REGISTERED NURSE?: F COUNTRY: PROGRAM

Figure 27.2 Sample student report: demographic data.

HAS THE STUDENT BEEN IDENTIFIED AS BEING AT RISK OF ACADEMIC FAILURE: F
IF YES, WHAT SEMESTER: / /

** GRADE POINT AVERAGE + GRADES **
GRADE POINT AVERAGE (TRANSFER CREDITS ARE NOT INCLUDED)
PGPI 3.00 (PREREQUISITE)   NURGPI 2.32 (NUR ONLY)
OGPI 2.35 (OVERALL)
 BIO 181
 BIO 182
 CHEM 114
 CHEM 115
 CHEM 120   B
 NUR 250   B+
 NUR 251   A−   ETC. ALL COURSES LISTED

COLLEGE ENTRY EXAM:
WRITING 8
READING 30
ARITHMETIC 18
ALGEBRA 13

Figure 27.3 Sample student report: grades and GPA.

The database has facilitated the advisement process in the division of nursing. As previously stated information obtained (academic and demographic) was entered into a database. Using this information, the relationships among students' demographics, grades in basic assessment tests, grades in courses prerequisite to the nursing program, and grades in nursing courses were analyzed. Each of the three assessment tests had significant relationships with academic performance in nursing courses. The strongest relationships between basic skills assessment tests and grades in nursing courses were students' reading scores. The best indicator for predicting student performance in a specific nursing course was performance in previous nursing courses (Cohen & Lerner, 1990). Subsequent data analyses verified that students who previously earned a C− did not do well in subsequent nursing courses and were in jeopardy of attaining a GPA of less than 2.0 in their major. A 2.0 is required in the major to graduate from the college.

Factors associated with placing a student at risk for academic failure were shared with faculty. Students at risk of academic failure are contacted. When a student is scheduled to meet with a faculty advisor the adviser now has all the student's latest grades at hand. Advisors working with students identify why students are having difficulty. That is, are they having trouble with child care, time management, test taking, other areas? The faculty advisors and students discuss interventions that are feasible and beneficial (e.g., number of credits that can be managed, courses the student is ready for, or referrals to other resources on campus).

A direct outcome of student advisement with the database is that faculty in the division of nursing have changed their grading policies. A grade of C, instead of C−, will be the required passing grade for any nursing course. The rationale for this was provided by computing correlations among grades in courses prerequisite to the nursing program and grades attained in all nursing courses.

Additional benefits from using the database have been the ability to generate mailing labels and create summary reports requested by organizations such as the National League for Nursing and the American Association of Colleges of Nursing.

CONCLUDING REMARKS AND RECOMMENDATIONS

Creation and use of the database have met the creators' expectations and those of faculty and administrators. Based on the success of using dBASE III PLUS in the undergraduate nursing program, a database was established for the graduate program. The same format is used with the necessary adjustments reflecting the requirements of the graduate curriculum. At this point it is difficult to document that establishment of the database has resulted in increased student retention, although it is suggested. The database has been extremely valuable in facilitating student advisement. The writers are satisfied with dBASE III PLUS as a data management system and Alpha 3 for printing reports. Other than anticipating and ad-

dressing the modifications that needed to be made to use SPSS/PC+ V.3 with dBASE III PLUS prior to entering data, the same procedure would be used again.

REFERENCES

Allen, C. B., Higgs, Z. R., & Holloway, J. A. (1988). Identifying students at risk of academic difficulty. *Journal of Professional Nursing, 4*, 113–118.

Cohen, B., & Lerner, H. (1990). Database utilization: Identifying students at risk of poor academic performance. *Dean's Notes, 11* (4), 1–2.

Felts, J. (1986). Performance predictors for nursing courses and National Council Licensing Examination NCLEX-RN. *Journal of Nursing Education, 25*, 372–377.

McKinney, J., Small, S., O'Dell, N., & Coonrod, B. A. (1988). Identification of predictors of success for the NCLEX and students at risk for NCLEX failure in a baccalaureate nursing program. *Journal of Professional Nursing, 4*, 55–59.

Safian-Rush, D., & Belok, S. (1988). Ethnicity academic skills and nursing student achievement. *Journal of Nursing Education, 27*, 71–77.

28

Computerized Continuing Education Record Keeping: A Marketing Tool for Nurse Educators

Claire Lauzon-Vallone

INTRODUCTION

Marketing requires offering useful services to consumers. Computerized data provides a basis from which information for quantitative analysis is derived; information assembled by compiling, manipulating, and massaging data provides a qualitative basis for decision making (Sanders, 1983). Computer derived reports from basic continuing education data provide quantitative and qualitative information for different nurse consumers. Application of basic continuing education data in report form provides validation of an educator's service to the organization.

A review of the literature from 1980 to 1989 revealed few articles on the use of continuing education documentation for marketing that service. Only one article (Bell, 1986) identified needs for data management and development in three focus areas: financial data, participant records, and mailing lists.

Educational inquiries need to be more ac-curate and efficient if we are to serve our consumers. Computerized answers or reports support the need for efficient and effective methods of collecting and reporting information (Robinette & Selensky-Weitzel, 1989).

Integrated database systems provide ideas on how to store, access, and manipulate the information (Armstrong, 1987). A database management system (DBMS) facilitates coding of data specifically for the purpose of manipulation and retrieval; all elements to be stored in the system must be defined and characterized (Zielstorff, 1980). In a database program, course coding, attendee demographics, class characterization, and evaluation classification are sorted and analyzed according to the consumer's need.

Consumers of a staff education department are defined as external and internal users within the nursing division. External consumers are nursing personnel in administration, management, and staff who require reports to support aspects of employee staffing and performance. Internal consumers are nursing educators who utilize data to project future projects based upon past educational productivity and attendance.

Each nurse consumer has different education information management needs. An educator can sort and analyze variables of an educational offering and match it to the consumer's need. A standardized, high frequency, or customized report satisfies requests in a timely and efficient manner. Variable-specified reports support consumer goals and create an interdependence for this type of documentation.

SOFTWARE CHOICE: ED-U-KEEP II

Current information management software are varied in what they can offer the nurse educator who wishes to maintain computerized records. The inability to define certain fields can be a deterrent to purchasing a program. Some information management systems only allow a percentage of personnel data to be devoted to education. The purchase cost of information database software ranges from slightly under $800 to over $3,000 (Hales, 1989). Utilizing a current database program to create your own information management system will deliver a highly specialized product, but one which could take years to implement (Robinette & Selensky-Weitzel, 1989).

This article will demonstrate the advantages of a marketing tool for the nurse educator using a computerized record keeping application called ED-U-KEEP II. The cost of the program is under $1,000.

The software requires 640K of RAM and can be run as a single or multiuser system on a personal computer. If the educational record volume is large, then the preferred method is to install it onto a mainframe. ED-U-KEEP II is written in programming language called Dataflex. The Dataflex language system supports different computer systems, such as VAX and UNIX-based machines. Entering data according to some standard coding scheme can contribute to an economical and efficient system (Sanders, 1983).

ED-U-KEEP II, a database software, makes use of several master files. The master files use a coding system, established by the user, to retrieve information associated with that code. Data is entered into fixed education fields that are defined by the user. Information which is used repetitively is entered only once into a master file. It is then entered automatically by the computer as needed by the user (Taylor, 1988). The information associated with the code is sorted and re-indexed into specific files for fast and easy recall for viewing or printing.

All menus and functions are called from a central menu. Within ED-U-KEEP II there are several submenus to guide you through the software program.

One of the strengths of the software is that it allows the user to establish codes or guidelines for certain fields in the master files, which assists the user in identifying departments requesting, conducting, or attending an educational program (Taylor, 1988). Figure 28.1 shows the main selection menu. A subscreen of this menu, entitled the Master File Menu, connects the user with the template files that serve as the foundation of the database. Standards or definitions of codes help the user form a baseline of how information is entered. Successful sorting and reporting on department education goals depend upon compliance of entry standards. It is recommended that code selection and legends be consistent to support retrieval of the data in the way you need it.

Once definition and coding of the fields in the master files system are established, equivalent fields in each of the master files will serve as the foundation for superimposing information into many destinations in

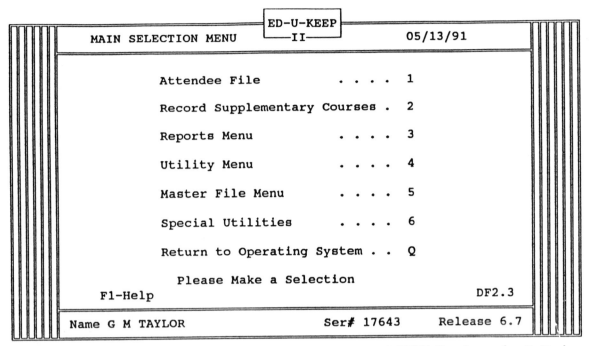

Figure 28.1 Main selection menu. (Source: Opening screen ED-U-KEEP II software by G. Taylor. Copyright © 1988 by JMT Enterprises. Reprinted by permission.)

the educational record. These equivalent fields of the master file system decrease the need for the user to double-enter information already existing in the database. In each of the master files, a designated unique field helps the user retrieve data quickly to assign new or changed information applicable to that educational event or participant.

In the master files, participants are recalled by a unique identification number. This unique number must be one that the employee will easily remember when asked to register at an educational event. Courses have a similar unique field that differentiates one educational activity from another. Simple entry of that key number recalls demographic information of the participant or course to complete the educational record. Identification codes eliminate duplication of data due to a double check by the computer for an equal past entry.

Each of the master files incorporate necessary details of an educational endeavor. Each event requires facts about course programming, attendance, evaluation, and any credentials that are extended to the participants of that program. The master files— course, department, employee, location, licensing requirement and evaluation—provide the foundation support for data retrieval through a merging of master file information for reports.

The employee master file has fields related to employee demographics. The employee identification number serves as the unique field in simplifying registration problems due to illegible signatures or nicknames. An accreditation field links the employee to a hospital licensing requirement such as CPR. This field loops to the course master file accreditation field which automatically updates the employee master file when an

```
                              ┌──ED-U-KEEP──┐
┌─────────────────────────────┤             ├─────────────────────────────┐
│      COURSE MASTER FORM      └────II───────┘   ADD/MODIFY COURSES   Page One │
│ ┌──────────────────────────────────────────────────────────────────────┐ │
│ │ Course No: _____        Name: _____ │ │
│ │                                                                      │ │
│ │ Course Date: _____  Time: __:__ __  Scheduled Hours: _____  CEU: _____ │ │
│ │ Location: _____       Course Fee: _____    │ │
│ │                                                                      │ │
│ │ Course Type: _ (0-9)   Course Classification: _____  Accreditation: _ │ │
│ │ Audience: _____  Department Given  For: _____  Inhouse: _ │ │
│ │                                                                      │ │
│ │ Instructor: _____ _ _____  On Staff: _  Evaluation: _ │ │
│ │ Secondary Instructor: _____  Coordinator: _____     │ │
│ │                                                                      │ │
│ │ Comments: _____ │ │
│ │                                                                      │ │
│ │     COURSE NUMBER - MUST BE UNIQUE                                    │ │
│ │                                                                    _  │ │
│ └──────────────────────────────────────────────────────────────────────┘ │
│ ┌──────────────────────────────────────────────┬───────────────────────┐ │
│ │ Evaluated: _  Costs: _____  Attendees: ____ │  Total Courses: 0     │ │
│ └──────────────────────────────────────────────┴───────────────────────┘ │
└────────────────────────────────────────────────────────────────────────────┘
    F1 - Help      F7 - Location List     F8 - Costs Page      Esc - Quit
```

Figure 28.2 Course master form. (Source: "Professional record keeping system: User guide and technical reference manual" by G. Taylor. Copyright © 1988 by JMT Enterprises. Reprinted by permission.)

employee attends this required cyclical course. Thereby compliance of licensing requirement is noted for that individual.

Figure 28.2 shows the course master form. The unique course code was defined by the writers' institution as three characters followed by numerics. The characters identify a course by the department requesting the educational offering or as an abbreviation of a course title. The course master file contains data that is entered only once and then is applied to the attendance master file without double entry. Classes in the course master file are assigned a number from one through eight in a field entitled "course type." A listing of these course types may be found in Table 28.1. This field helps all our nurse consumers identify class content focus. A subscreen of the course master form enables the user to record any costs incurred for that program.

The attendance master file computes and enters participants in a program faster and with more accuracy than a manual method. Entering the course code immediately brings up a brief course description to apply to attendee data. This method shortens the time it takes to apply consistent roster data to each participant. Data entered by the unique attendee I.D. numbers brings the participant name and demographics from the employee master file on the screen. Inaccuracy of matching participant and course is alleviated and the speed of crediting educational records is increased.

There are many system checks and adjustments available to the user while working within the attendance master file. Double entry of a participant for the same class is rejected as an error because the computer associates the unique identification number with the course code. Educational hours and

Table 28.1 Course Type Legends for the Course Master Form

Legend	Course Type
CE internal educational program	1
CEC internal educational program	2
CE external educational program	3
CEC external educational program	4
CE, trauma focus; internal educational program	5
CEC, trauma focus; internal educational program	6
CE, trauma focus; external educational program	7
CEC, trauma focus; external educational program	8

```
                                    ┌──ED-U-KEEP──┐
  COURSE EVALUATION SUMMARY         └────II────┘      add/modify evaluations

  Total Eval's:    0 Course No: _____   Name: _____
  Course Date: _____   Time: __:__ __       Scheduled Hours: _____
  Total Attendees: _____   Instructor: _____

 OBJECTIVES   TOPIC        SPEAKER        MATERIAL    TEACHING     PRESENTATION
   MET        HELPFUL      PRESENTATION   QUALITY     METHOD       LENGTH

 E   S   U    E   S   U    E   S   U    E   S   U    E   S   U    E   S   U

 _   _   _    _   _   _    _   _   _    _   _   _    _   _   _    _   _   _

              Total E (Excellent)      _____
              Total S (Satisfactory)   _____
              Total U (Unsatisfactory) _____
                       Overall Score  _____     Rating _____
      General Comments: _____

  F1 - Help    _____   Esc - Quit
```

Figure 28.3 Evaluation master file. (Source: Screen 7 ED-U-KEEP II. Copyright © 1988 by JMT Enterprises. Reprinted by permission.)

continuing education credit may be adjusted on the screen manually if only a portion of the educational program was attended by a participant. A current list of attendees for the class may be called up at any time by pressing a function key.

Two other master files aid the user in coordinating data on speakers or course evaluations. The instructor master file contains fields resembling a speaker's biographical data form. A speaker entered into a course master file will be bumped to the instructor master file to establish their credentials screen for future use in brochure or advertising. Figure 28.3 depicts the evaluation master file which allows the user to enter feedback data to the class by calling up the course code number. Descriptors from the course appear on the screen and the user proceeds to log in the course ratings as they relate to topic, objectives, speaker, material, teaching method, and presentation.

REPORTS

Evidence of contributions to organizational goals conveys a message of educational support to nursing administration. Reports outlining numbers of classes, participants, and average participants per educational offering demonstrate an education department's productivity. Information on course demographics, speaker qualifications, costs, audience type, and evaluation addresses the scope of coordination required to run a continuing education program. Data compiled on course title, type, classification,

continuing education credits, and participant demographics represent the overall impact on an organization's goals. Course, attendee, class costs, or speaker reports summarize information to benefit the organization.

Once data is entered into the respective master files, the user can request the reports menu for standard high frequency reports. The software program has a custom report generator for specialized report requests from nurse consumers. Ten user-select criteria, from the master files, can be sorted and compared in the custom report option.

Several standard reports taken from data in the course and attendance master files validate attendance, time, and cost of an educational offering. Figure 28.4 depicts the course summary report which highlights attendance and budgetary considerations for a program. It also reports average attendance

JMT HEALTHCARE ASSOCIATES
COURSE SUMMARY REPORT

Date: 03/14/88   Page: 1

Course Number	Course Name		Course Date	Hours	CEU	Fee	Class
A02	CRITICAL CARE 101-A		01/01/80	2.50	1.00	0.00	CLAS3

Attendee Name		Dept		Hours	CEU	Id Number	Fee Paid	Date Paid	Balance Due
HALLEY	MATTHEW	H	FIVE	2.50	1.00	107	0.00	01/01/80	0.00
HALLEY	CRISTY	A	FIVE	2.50	1.00	108	0.00	01/01/80	0.00
HICKMAN	CLYDE	H	FIVE	2.50	1.00	86	0.00	01/01/80	0.00
HOFFMAN	ELISE		FIVE	1.50	1.00	90	0.00	01/01/80	0.00
DEBRANIN	DAVID	M MD	FIVE	2.50	1.00	93	0.00	01/01/80	0.00

Summary for Course:
A02   CRITICAL CARE 101-A

Attendees	Credit Hours	Credit CEU	Contact Hours	Fees Collected	Fees Due
5	11.50	5.00	57.50	0.00	0.00

Figure 28.4 Course summary report. (Source: "Professional record keeping system: User guide and technical reference manual" by G. Taylor. Copyright © 1988 by JMT Enterprises. Reprinted by permission.)

and projects potential gross profits. Reports on courses that show a profit and good attendance market a successful educational contribution to the hospital or community.

A major challenge in reporting which content met licensing stipulations, continuing education credit, or trauma center continuing educational hours, was solved by using the category field in the course master file. Table 28.1 represents the code system we established. The continuing medical education (CME) report displays categories along with class title, educational, and contact hours. The CME also summarizes and totals each category at the end of the report. Progress updates on attainment of the required eight hours per nurse per year of trauma continuing education was made efficient by the computerized totalling of an individual's category hours. This field helps all our nurse consumers identify class content focus.

Data captured in the employee, course and attendance master files can reveal in report form employee or course demographic comparisons with attendance. This information can measure education participation by separate or all nursing departments, note areas of productivity for nursing education, and improve staff compliance with licensing requirements. Staff compliance with licensing requirements was improved by identifying by department and individual, those persons who do not meet current licensing requirements by their expired course date. The required classification report prints department summaries and individual reminder letters that request the employee to comply with hospital policy.

In evaluating a course, the strength of strategic educational planning comes from reporting participant survey results. Data entered into the evaluation master file was adapted for expanded use by our educational department. The five standard evaluation questions did not provide enough answers for course planning. Redesign of the screen

meant added cost and time. A method of coding comments made by attendees enabled retrieval of a requested code and course title easy. This report serves as the internal control mechanism for speakers and course content.

NURSE CONSUMERS

Head Nurses

Computer applications that cumulatively record each employee's "job growth" activities can be used in the employee job evaluation system (Dixon, Gouyd, & Varricchio, 1980). Reports on compliance with Joint Commission on Accreditation of Healthcare Organizations (JCAHO) guidelines, attainment of current continuing education requirements, fulfillment of professional development, and maintenance of yearly certification are goals of any nursing department. A department, individual, or licensing requirement summary report informs the department head of educational progress for his or her staff.

Administrators

A ready source of quantitative data is available for compilation of reports for administration. Cross referencing with qualitative class or program information can give the "whole picture" (Dixon, Gouyd, & Varicchio, 1980). A nursing administrator uses data to compare educational hours versus clinical time at the bedside to define what is needed in Full-Time Equivalents (FTEs) and budget to support the required education for a nursing unit. Retrospective comparison of educational hours and patient care coverage can justify more FTEs if the coverage was below what was required. A department summary report, shown in Fig-

Department Summary Report

Date 05/13/91   For 01/01/80 thru 12/31/99   Page: 1

Department 5001

No.	Course Name	Employee Id.	Last Name	Crs's	-----Credit----- Hours	CEU
1	CPR					
		1001	CODY		0.50	0.50
Total for 1001			CODY	1	0.50	0.50
1	CPR					
		1235	STROUD		0.50	0.50
Total for 1235			STROUD	1	0.50	0.50
1	CPR					
		5538	TAYLOR		0.50	0.50
Total for 5538			TAYLOR	1	0.50	0.50
1	CPR					
		66372	TIMMONS		0.50	0.50
Total for 66372			TIMMONS	1	0.50	0.50
Totals for Department 5001				4	2.00	2.00

Figure 28.5 Department summary report. (Source: "Professional record keeping system: User guide and technical reference manual" by G. Taylor. Copyright © 1988 by JMT Enterprises. Reprinted by permission.)

ure 28.5, specifies educational hours per nurse per unit and assists the administrator in building a case for budgeted FTEs.

Directors of Education, Educators

Directors of education and educators need reports representing instructor time, scope of continuing education coordination, program completion, program evaluation, and current consumer needs in order to remain a viable asset to the organization. Documentation of educational activities in a meaningful, accessible format is a challenge for the nurse educator (Robinette & Selensky-

Weitzel, 1989). A created or purchased database system assists the educator in producing the report style which communicates the essential data. Information management and rapid coordination of data in nursing education turn liabilities into assets.

Evaluation data serves as an internal control mechanism for examining feedback on speaker qualifications, applicability to nursing practice, and general course comments. It validates instructor competency through data from learner evaluation and data comparisons. Feedback from programs guides the educator in strategic planning of future nursing education offerings. An evaluation report provides the necessary feedback for program evaluation.

JMT HEALTHCARE ASSOCIATES
INDIVIDUAL SUMMARY REPORT

Date: 03/14/88   Page: 1

ALLEN H HONEYWELL ID: 101   Department: FIVE

COURSE NO	DATE	COURSE NAME	HOURS	CEU
AB01	02/04/81	TUMOR CONFERENCE	2.50	1.00
AB102	03/04/83	TUMOR CONFERENCE	2.00	0.00
ZZ501	10/10/87	NEW EMPLOYEE ORIENTATION #1	0.50	0.00

Summary for   ALLEN H HONEYWELL   Id: 101

3 Total Course(s) ————————— 5.00 Total Hour(s) ————————— 1.00 Total CEU(s)

Figure 28.6 Individual summary report. (Source: "Professional record keeping system: User guide and technical reference manual" by G. Taylor. Copyright © 1988 by JMT Enterprises. Reprinted by permission.)

Documentation from the database files promotes revenue producing capacities of nursing education. Brochures created from speaker bibliographies advertise prospective conferences. Self-produced mailing lists from attendee files saves time and money. A database report can also sort and print those employees from a particular department or course in which follow-up attendance is essential.

Staff

Nursing staff need a cumulative record to use in demonstrating their pursuit of job improvement (Dixon, Gouyd, & Varricchio, 1980). Many states require mandatory continuing education for maintaining yearly licensure. Reports specifying licensure requirements or cumulative educational hours can be distributed at the request of the staff nurse. The individual summary report, shown in Figure 28.6, can assist the staff nurse in quickly assessing where he or she stands in the attainment of educational goals within the organization's career ladder system.

IMPLICATIONS FOR STAFF DEVELOPMENT

Certain challenges face the nurse educator in order to produce this marketing tool. Establishing resources enhances the educator's ability to produce the reports essential for marketing contribution and productivity. A manual that serves as a resource for guidelines on software operation and code definitions aids in recalling established standards. A course code log-in book tracks code assignment. Networking with data processing personnel, computer support groups, and other users of this software provides an objective viewpoint on problem-solving database applications. Utilizing available clerical staff or work study students for data entry frees the educator to pursue potential marketing avenues with this tool.

CONCLUSION

Reports from computerized continuing education records serve as a marketing tool by linking a consumer need with an educational service. Easy entry, manipulation and retrieval of data into tangible reports can validate your productivity and contribution to the organization. The benefit will be increased consumer awareness and confirmation of the existence of that service.

REFERENCES

Armstrong, M. (1987). *Contemporary strategies for continuing education in nursing.* Rockville, MA: Aspen Publishers.

Bell, E. (1986). Putting the PC to work in continuing education. *Computers in Nursing, 4* (3), 119–122.

Dixon, J., Gouyd, N., & Varricchio, D. T. (1980). A computerized education training record. In R. D. Zielstorff (Ed.), *Computers in Nursing* (pp. 59–62). Wakefield, MA: Nursing Resources.

Hales, G. D. (1989). Software Exchange. *Computers in Nursing, 7* (2), 38–40.

Robinette, J., & Selensky-Weitzel, P. (1989). Design and development of a computerized education and records system. *The Journal of Continuing Education in Nursing, 20* (4), 174–181.

Sanders, D. (1983). *Computers Today.* New York: McGraw-Hill.

Taylor, G. (1988). Professional record keeping system: User guide and technical reference manual. *ED-U-KEEP II Manual.* Webster, TX: JMT Enterprises.

Zielstorff, R. D. (Ed.). (1980). *Computers in Nursing.* Wakefield, MA: Nursing Resources.

29

Databases: An Untapped Potential

Linda Q. Thede

PROLOGUE

Vicky is the assistant unit manager on 2 East. She has just received the lab report of a wound culture for Mr. Peterson, a postsurgical patient on her unit. He has a Staph infection, the unit's second one in less than a week. After gaining the cooperation of the staff 18 months ago, this unit has been relatively free of most postsurgical infections, a fact of which the whole unit is proud. Somewhat disquieted, Vicky makes a note to tell the unit manager and to discuss with the staff the importance of good aseptic techniques. Then she calls Sarah, the infection control nurse, to ask if Staph infections are occurring in other places in the hospital.

"I'm not certain," replies Sarah. "I get so many of these reports that it's hard to keep track. We'll know for sure in a few months when the computer printout comes out."

Vicky groans. "I wonder how many more we will have before then. Isn't there some way you can go through your records and get this information now?"

"Sorry, Vicky, but these days with the workload I have I am lucky to even get all these recorded. There is no way I can manually go through all these reports."

Vicky hangs up the phone and says aloud, "We spend hours collecting these data and there is no way to use them!"

"What did you say?" comes a reply from Joan, her counterpart on 3 West who had just entered the office.

"I said that as nurses we are prolific data gatherers, but the information just falls into a black hole. By the time we can have it in a usable format, it's too late to do anything."

"What caused this sudden realization?" replies Joan.

"I just recorded another Staph infection, our second in a week."

"That's interesting, I just got our second yesterday, too. I wonder, do you suppose there is something we can do about this?"

"Like what?"

"Don't you have a personal computer on this unit? All the units are supposed to have one."

"Well, yes, but the unit manager uses it for budgeting and staffing."

"Vicky, have you ever heard of a *database*?"[1]

"Sure, but that's something the management information systems people are responsible for with their big computer."

"Not necessarily. Chris, the assistant unit manager on 4 West was telling me about a workshop she attended last week. She said that by using a commercial software database, anyone can design and use a database to keep track of information. Chris seemed quite enthusiastic about it."

"But who has the software?"

"We do! I remember being told that a database program had been installed on each of the computers."

"But I don't know that much about computers. How can I do this?"

"Not 'I'," replies Joan, " 'We!' Let me call Chris and see if she would be interested in helping us."

At lunch Chris informs the group that despite her enthusiasm, she too is a little intimidated by starting in on a database project. Somewhat tentatively, she says, "The workshop leader, Susan, did offer to assist anyone who was interested in starting to use a database."

"Do you think Susan would work with absolute neophytes?" asks Vicky.

"Chris, you said that Susan is used to working with people at all levels of computer knowledge," states Joan.

With renewed confidence Chris says, "I did, didn't I. Let's at least try; let me call her and arrange for us to meet."

With more than a little trepidation, they all agree. "I only hope that I haven't gotten in over my head," Vicky says. They all agree,

but believe that the possible benefits are worth the risk.

FLAT DATABASES

Several days later, Vicky, Joan, and Chris find themselves answering Susan's questions at their first meeting. Susan wants to know what kind of information they wish to get from the database. "What data you collect and how you structure the database depends on the kind of information you want to get from it," explains Susan. "Too many people decide first what information they wish to collect, then later try to figure out how to make these data solve their problems. There is no substitute for a well-written plan detailing exactly what information you want a database to give you before you ever sit down to create a computer database."

"Before we go on," Vicky says, "Could you please explain to me what a database is and how it can answer our questions."

"Of course," replies Susan. "We'll look at it in relation to your situation. But first, let's talk about databases in general. Tell me, do you have an address book in your pocketbook?"

"Well, yes," replies Vicky. "Why?"

"Because an address book is a database, as is a phone book and the Physician's Desk Reference. These, however, are paper databases. In a paper database you can gain information easily only if you know the piece of information used to index the data. For example, in a phone book, you can only easily find a number if you know the name. But, if I gave you a number, and asked you to find the name to whom it belonged, you would have a very tedious and long job.

"If the phone book were computerized, you could find the name to whom a number belonged in one of two ways. Search for it, or

---

[1] Words that are italicized are in the Glossary at the end of this chapter.

temporarily reorganize the records so they are ordered, or indexed, by number. Many people are familiar with the searching capabilities of databases because they have performed a library search using one of the computerized indexes. Reorganizing, or sorting records, however, is not so familiar.

"Sorting records, based on one piece of information, not only enables you to find a specific piece of information, but to gain a picture of the data as a whole and produce reports with current information. This, I believe, is what you wish to do with the information you have about postsurgical infections. To give you an idea of how to go about this, let's analyze your problem, create a small subset of information, enter it into the computer, and produce some *reports* using this information.

"What I have heard you say is that you wish to see if there is a pattern for postsurgical infections on your respective units. Let's say that you believe that to gain this knowledge you would need to record the patient's name, unit, pathogen causing the infection, type of surgery, and physician."

They all agree that this would be helpful. Susan helps them create a small database to do this. She explains that the program they are using calls this collection of data a *table*. To create this table, they make a place for each category of information they have decided to collect: patient's name, the unit she or he is on, the name of the pathogen responsible for the infection, the surgery, and the name of the surgeon. These are illustrated in the headings in Figure 29.1.

Susan explains that Name, Unit, Pathogen, Surgery, and Surgeon are each *field names* and that each column is called a *field*. They then make up some information and enter it into the database. Susan adds that in doing this they are creating a *record* for each patient. For example, the record for Georgette Brandt contains her name, unit, the pathogen responsible for her infection, the surgery, and surgeon. They enter 10 records, *indexing* them by name, creating a

Name	Unit	Pathogen	Surgery	Surgeon
Brandt, Georgette	4 West	Strep	Tonsillectomy	Black
Danforth, Barbara	2 East	Staph	Herniorrhaphy	Smith
Hearn, Jack	4 West	Strep	Appendectomy	Black
Jensen, George	3 West	Staph	Open reduction, lt femur	Smith
Jones, Carolyn	3 West	Staph	Hysterectomy	Smith
Johnson, Charles	3 West	E coli	Cholecystectomy	Black
Munson, Florence	4 West	E coli	Herniorrhaphy	Greene
Neilson, John	2 East	E coli	Herniorrhaphy	Greene
Olson, Susan	3 West	Strep	Tubal ligation	Jones
Peterson, Ken	2 East	Staph	Cholecystectomy	Smith

Figure 29.1 Records of patients with infections sorted by name.

Name	Unit	Pathogen	Surgery	Surgeon
Danforth, Barbara	2 East	Staph	Herniorrhaphy	Smith
Neilson, John	2 East	E coli	Herniorrhaphy	Greene
Peterson, Ken	2 East	Staph	Cholecystectomy	Smith
Jensen, George	3 West	Staph	Open reduction, lt femur	Smith
Jones, Carolyn	3 West	Staph	Hysterectomy	Smith
Johnson, Charles	3 West	E coli	Cholecystectomy	Black
Olson, Susan	3 West	Strep	Tubal ligation	Jones
Brandt, Georgette	4 West	Strep	Tonsillectomy	Black
Hearn, Jack	4 West	Strep	Appendectomy	Black
Munson, Florence	4 West	E coli	Herniorrhaphy	Greene

Figure 29.2 Records re-sorted with primary sort unit and secondary sort name.

table which, in database language, is the complete collection of all the records. The results can be seen in Figure 29.1.

"Now the fun begins," says Susan. "Let's re-sort these records using the unit field as a *primary sort*. This means that we will tell the computer to reorder the records so that all those with the same entry in the unit field are together. To make it more interesting, we will use name as a *secondary sort* which will order the records so that the names on each unit are alphabetized."

After sorting the records with the designated primary and secondary sort, Susan says, "Notice that all the records for patients on Unit 2 East are grouped together, and that within that unit, the records are ordered by name." (See Figure 29.2.)

"From this information we can produce a report that counts the number of infections on each unit and even produce a graph of the information," Susan tells them. Because all the information that this report would use is generated from this table only, we say that this is a flat table and that we are using a *flat*

database. A little later we will experiment with creating reports with information from more than one table. When more than one table is used to produce information, the tables are relational and one uses a *relational database*.[2]

"You can also tell the computer to do what is called a *crosstab*. In simplified format, this means taking some of the *field entries*, that is, the information in each field, and making them field names, then counting the number of times they occur and where. It is sort of a rotation of a table. The rotation enables you to count the number of times each pathogen occurred on each unit." Using the table in Figure 29.2 Susan creates the crosstab seen in Figure 29.3.

---

[2] Generic database software is sold as a flat or relational database. All relational database software can be used as a flat database, but flat database software cannot be used as a relational database.

Unit	E coli	Staph	Strep
2 East	1	2	0
3 West	1	2	1
4 West	1	0	3

Figure 29.3 Crosstab of pathogens/unit.

"This information could also be put into a bar or line graph," says Susan.

"That would be very helpful," says Joan, "but to get back to the basic table (Figure 29.1), quite often a culture report shows that more than one organism is involved in an infection. When that happens what would we do?"

"Just put in another pathogen in the pathogen field," replies Chris.

Problems with Flat Databases

"That would cause two problems," interjects Susan. "First, the field is not long enough to hold that information, but even more important, this entry would look different to the computer and would therefore prevent sorting by pathogen. If after making this entry, you used the pathogen field to sort the records, the entry in the pathogen field in Florence Munson's record would be regarded as a separate entity because it did not match either E coli or Strep. When you counted the number of infections per pathogen you would get a total for 'E coli, Strep,' but nothing in this entry would be included in either the E coli or Strep count.

"That is one problem with computers: entries must be absolutely identical to be grouped together. The addition of a comma, or a letter capitalized in one entry and not another, produce two entirely different computer entries, although they may look similar to a human. You are lucky, the database

program you are using will allow you to control what is entered into a field so that different users will use the same data entry format. These techniques also save keystrokes in data entry, so they are appreciated by data enterers as well as the individuals analyzing the database."

"Can you think of another solution?" asks Susan.

"Create a record in which all the information is the same except for the pathogen?" inquires Vicky.

"That is one solution, but it creates its own set of problems," replies Susan. "Let's suppose that Florence Munson's culture has shown that Strep as well as E coli are responsible for her infection." She duplicates the information for all the fields in Florence Munson's record except the Pathogen field, putting Strep in that field. "Now, what will happen if we try to count the number of infections per unit?" asks Susan.

"4 West will have four instead of the three seen in Figure 29.1," replies Vicky.

"I know," says Chris, "We'll create another field for pathogen so we will have pathogen 1 and pathogen 2."

"Which pathogen field will you sort on if you wish to reorder the records by pathogen?" returns Susan. "And, how will you handle it if a patient has more than two pathogens responsible for an infection?"

"I see your point. Is this the time when you need the relational database you told us about earlier?" responds Chris.

RELATIONAL DATABASES

"Yes! I realize that relational database sounds somewhat complicated, but it really is not. It just means that we tap more than one table to get the information needed in a report. In essence it involves conceptualizing the data in a multidimensional format.

"As you can see, working with only one table becomes cumbersome when you are working with categories of information that refuse to be organized one per record, such as the pathogens. To solve this, we create two tables. One contains all the information except the field with more than one entry per main record, the other contains this 'problem' field, and another field that is also found in the first table. This common field will have identical information in both tables and is called the *relational field*.

"Let's see how the information in which you are interested would be structured to allow you to record more than one pathogen per patient, but still preserve the ability to accurately count and sort. First we would create a *master table* containing identifying information about a patient in which each field is mutually exclusive and for which there is only one piece of data per record in that category. Then we would create another table, sometimes called a *detail table*, that has a field for the pathogen and a field that is also in the master table."

Implementing this, Susan creates a master table with fields for: name, unit, surgery, and surgeon, and a detail table containing the fields, name and pathogen. The name field is the relational field, that is, it occurs in both tables. (See Figures 29.4 and 29.5.)

"You can now sort or count pathogens in the pathogen table and information in any of the fields in the patient table," Susan tells them.

"But now," queries Joan, "How can we tell which surgeon was associated with which pathogen, let alone on which unit which pathogens were a problem?"

"By relating the tables," Susan explains. "What you do is to take specified fields from each table, and using a relational field as the criteria for matching, create another temporary table that answers your question. I'll demonstrate by helping you create a temporary table that shows who was the surgeon associated with each pathogen.

"To answer this question you need two fields, the surgeon and pathogen field. To make this easier to follow, let's also say we

Name	Unit	Surgery	Surgeon
Brandt, Georgette	4 West	Tonsillectomy	Black
Danforth, Barbara	2 East	Herniorrhaphy	Smith
Hearn, Jack	4 West	Appendectomy	Black
Jensen, George	3 West	Open reduction, lt femur	Smith
Jones, Carolyn	3 West	Hysterectomy	Smith
Johnson, Charles	3 West	Cholecystectomy	Black
Munson, Florence	4 West	Herniorrhaphy	Greene
Neilson, John	2 East	Herniorrhaphy	Greene
Olson, Susan	3 West	Tubal ligation	Jones
Peterson, Ken	2 East	Cholecystectomy	Smith

Figure 29.4 Patients with infections—master table.

Name	Pathogen
Brandt, Georgette	Strep
Danforth, Barbara	Staph
Hearn, Jack	Strep
Jensen, George	Staph
Jones, Carolyn	Staph
Johnson, Charles	E coli
Munson, Florence	E coli
Munson, Florence	Strep
Neilson, John	E coli
Olson, Susan	Strep
Peterson, Ken	Staph

Figure 29.5 Pathogens—detail table.

Name	Surgeon	Pathogen
Johnson, Charles	Black	E coli
Brandt, Georgette	Black	Strep
Hearn, Jack	Black	Strep
Munson, Florence	Greene	E coli
Neilson, John	Greene	E coli
Munson, Florence	Greene	Strep
Olson, Susan	Jones	Strep
Danforth, Barbara	Smith	Staph
Jensen, George	Smith	Staph
Jones, Carolyn	Smith	Staph
Peterson, Ken	Smith	Staph

Figure 29.6 Results of relating client master table and pathogen detail table and sorting by surgeon.

wish to see the name associated with these two fields, although the results would be the same whether you included the name or not. To achieve the desired results, you give instructions to the computer to use the information in the master table to create a new table with fields for name and surgeon. For each name in the new table, the computer receives instructions to look in the pathogen table and take the entry in the pathogen field of the record with the same name and place it in the new table's pathogen field with the record that contains that name.

"If this seems hard to follow, go to Figure 29.4, the master table, and note each surgeon and the name of the patient in the same record. Then look at the pathogen table in Figure 29.5 and select the appropriate pathogen for that patient. Check your results with Figure 29.6. Note that if there are two pathogen entries for one name, such as with Florence Munson, this will produce two records for that name. This table, however, is temporary and is created only to answer the ques-

tion of which surgeon cared for which patient with what infection. Because the basic tables are left undisturbed by this manipulation, they can still be used to answer other questions.

"Because we are interested in each physician, let's also sort this table using physician as the primary sort and the pathogen as the secondary sort." This creates the table in Figure 29.6.

"Look at Dr. Smith," cries Vicky. "Can you imagine how long it would take us to figure this out, if we ever did, using the information we get now?"

EPILOGUE

When Vicky, Joan, and Chris start work on their database they will probably discover some other facts. For example, the relational field needs to be something that can belong to only one record in the master table. Names are easily duplicated, thus they would probably use patient number as the relational field. Additionally, they may discover that more than one physician cares for a patient which may lead them to create a separate table for physicians. Or, if they wish to track the nurses who care for a patient, they may need a nurse table.

In this manner, what seems like a simple database can easily become more complicated. It is expected that when this group first starts creating databases, they will resist the temptation to record every possible piece of data. To gain comfort with database techniques, it will be best if they concentrate on the most important question and collect only the data needed to answer it. They can always expand and collect more data later.

Susan should also suggest that when they start manipulating data to answer questions, they experiment with a small subset of the data to which answers can be easily seen without computer manipulation. An example is the samples used in the demonstration. This allows the creators to check their results to learn if the procedures they are using to obtain answers are accurate. It takes a while to become comfortable with a database package and to learn to "think as the software thinks."

Beginning to use a new tool is always a little frightening. There are, however, many resources. Books about the specific database software, in addition to the program's manuals, are very helpful. Someone who is already using the program is another excellent source of help. User groups, or associations of people who use or who are learning to use a program, exist for this purpose. To find one in your area call a store that sells the product you use, or contact the company that produced your database. User groups consist of people at all levels of experience who share one thing in common: a desire to learn and teach about the program. Attending one

meeting usually yields some phone numbers, often of people who can help you when you have a question.

One reason why databases are not used more is that being able to manipulate data is not a tool with which we are familiar. Our present standard for record keeping is paper records. They contain much data, but finding it, let alone using it for a report, is time consuming. Even if one is able to produce one timely report from paper records, the ability to produce reports that manipulate the data in different ways is too costly to consider. As such, we have not developed the concepts necessary to use data manipulation as a way of gaining information.

Whether you are a practicing nurse, researcher, or educator, once you learn to "think data base," the situations that lend themselves to this tool become numerous. Keeping track of when employees are due for CPR or other annual considerations is one. Using an electronic database, it would be possible to print a list of employees each month (or more frequently) who need CPR recertification. Recording grades with a database not only provides computation for final grades, but conversion into a letter grade. The same information can then be used to print an overall list of grades, another list specific to each instructor, and a report for each student giving him or her the grades they received for each entity that was graded, and information on how the grade was computed.

With still another focus, at Kent State University School of Nursing, several years ago the author and some colleagues started a database for graduate students centered around nursing diagnoses. Like all beginners, this group made many mistakes, but slowly this project has evolved into a useful tool. The biggest mistake was thinking paper record instead of electronic database. This caused the collection of too much data, most of which was not in a format that lent itself to analysis. Additionally, at the beginning a flat database was used, creating extra records that made some analyses difficult.

This problem has been alleviated by the group's change to Paradox (Borland International Inc.), a relational database. The original table was broken down into five tables, all related by a nurse and client number. Moreover, various techniques are used to ensure that entries that mean the same are entered identically. Even during its evolution, students were able to analyze some items which helped them to see data as a whole in relationship to individual patients. Now, however, special commands are preprogrammed to allow the students to obtain specific information from the database. The results of these efforts to date are seen in chapters 30 and 31.

If nursing is to be an important entity in contemporary day health care in which outcome is used for evaluation, it is imperative that we become proficient with databases. Databases will be used, if not by us then by others who will decide what our priorities are. Despite the appearance of objectivity, every database is imbued with a subjective premise.

Roszak (1986) reports on an experiment done in early 1985 in which a financial columnist created a hypothetical middle-class family with a given set of financial resources, needs, plans, and preferences and submitted them to four different financial plan database services. "The result was four strikingly different sets of recommendations, covering such options as investments, savings, liquidity, insurance, and retirements. Why? Because the advice of each plan was programmed with different assumptions, a fact which none of the services mentioned" (Roszak, 1986, p. 118).

In the example Susan used, it is easy to come to the conclusion that Dr. Smith is responsible for the outbreak of Staph infections. This database manipulation was based on the assumption that relating a surgeon with a pathogen would provide answers as to which surgeons were responsible for which infections. A prudent institution would of course check Dr. Smith to see if he was a Staph carrier; but suppose this check were negative? Other questions must be asked. Even if Dr. Smith is a Staph carrier, it would be wise to look further; these patients may have something else in common. This something could explain why Dr. Smith is a carrier.

Databases are excellent tools, but caution is advised in assuming that what they tell us is carved in stone, or that their answers explain everything. Databases, like all computer programs, only generate reports based on the directions given by the database creator for manipulating the data they have; computers cannot think. Nor are they capable of interjecting common sense into their answers. It is up to the users to supply these other ingredients.

What assumptions will be encompassed in the databases that are used to make nursing care decisions? If nurses do not have a working knowledge of databases, how they work, and how they are designed, the assumptions will not have a nursing focus. The choice is still ours to make, but time is running out.

GLOSSARY

Crosstab—a result of manipulating data in a rotational manner, that allows field entries to become field names for the purpose of specifying how many of each occurs in a specific instance.

Database—a collection of well-defined, mutually exclusive data elements.

Detail table—a table of "details," or information that does not fit the structure of the main table. It is related to the main table by an identical field.

Field entries—the data placed into a field.

Field names—the name given to a column of data, or a field, in a database.

Field—a mutually exclusive data element in a database.

Flat database—a database in which all the information pertaining to one record, or case, is in one table.

Indexing—sorting or rearranging of records in a database. Often a database has one field that is its fixed index, or its default sort. Any records entered into the table will be placed in the table in an order determined by the index field.

Master table—the main table in a relational database. Detail tables are "related" to it by a common field.

Primary sort—the field which will be used first in determining the order records will be arranged. After being ordered based on this field, further sorts of groups of records with identical entries in the primary sort field can be performed.

Record—a row in a database table. The collection of data belonging to one case.

Relational database—a database that allows information from many tables to be used in creating knowledge. The prerequisite is that each table have at least one field that is identical.

Relational field—the field that is identical in two or more tables in a relational database.

Report—an up-to-date summary of what is in the database. Report templates can be created, then used periodically with a table. The report uses the current table for its information, thus the same report template will produce different results when information in the table is updated.

Secondary sort—a field used for arranging the records within each group generated by a primary sort. If the secondary sort yields groups of identical entries, tertiary or more sorts are possible with some commercial databases.

Table—a collection of data synonymous with a file of data in database format.

REFERENCES

Roszak, R. (1986). *The Cult of Information.* New York: Pantheon.

30

Creation and Use of a Nursing Diagnosis Database Related to Nursing of Adults

Margaret O'Bryan Doheny
Diane M. Eddy
Sharon Oetker Black
Mary A. Wyper
Harriet V. Coeling
Beatrice B. Turkoski

The purpose of this chapter is to describe the creation and use of a nursing diagnosis database that was designed to increase graduate students' nursing process and computer literacy skills. The faculty anticipated that this project could facilitate the following learner outcomes: (1) understanding of the importance of valid defining characteristics for nursing diagnoses, (2) understanding of the link between identified etiologies for nursing diagnoses and selection of nursing interventions, (3) knowledge and understanding of a repertoire of independent nursing interventions, (4) beginning skill in use of computers for data management, and (5) appreciation of the role of computers in nursing education. An overview of computer use in nursing education will be presented followed by a description of the database project and its outcomes.

USE OF COMPUTERS IN NURSING EDUCATION

Reports in the nursing literature indicate that computers are used extensively in both practice (Bailey, 1988; Chang, Roth, Gonzalez, Caswell, & DiStefano, 1988; Halloran, 1988; Saba, 1989; Saba & McCormick, 1986; Simmons & Ryan, 1984; Werley, Devine, & Zorn, 1988) and research (Cox, Harsanyi, & Dean, 1987; Polit & Hungler, 1991). Few references, however, support various instructional uses of computers in nursing education. Computer use in nursing education has historically centered around computer aided instruction (CAI). This instructional mode was defined by Norman (1982) as a way of teaching and learning by computer that can be adapted to individual needs. Bolwell (1988) stated that the advantages of CAI were related to the computer's ability to provide students with interactivity, rapid calculation, animation, and sound. This approach can be cost effective when the computer and software are used frequently.

Although the primary use of computers in nursing education has been for CAI, other aspects of computer technology that have been used in nursing practice and research could be used in nursing education as well. According to Cox, Harsanyi, and Dean (1987), cognitive and affective domains in nursing education can be measured through computer-based discovery, dialogue, and simulation gaming strategies. These authors also suggested the use of databases in nursing education. They viewed the future of computer technology in nursing education from a very broad perspective and predicted uses that include information management, theory development, instruction, research, evaluation, and administration. A nursing education study regarding the use of nursing diagnosis in graduate nursing education was reported by Van Steeg (1988). This project used Gordon's work on nursing diagnosis as a system for documenting the encounters of second-year masters' students and their clients. The researchers in this project suggested the computerization of student and client encounters for research in nursing practice.

A computer program for graduate students was developed by Hirsch, Chang, and Gilbert (1989) at the University of California at Los Angeles. This project was named CARIN (Computer-Associated Research in Nursing) and occurred in two phases based on the North American Nursing Diagnosis Association's (NANDA) Taxonomy I. The first phase consisted of an automated guide for screening, interviewing, and physical assessment. The second phase centered on the identification of abnormal signs and symptoms that might contribute to a nursing diagnosis. One benefit of this program was assistance with organization of data to improve the diagnostic phase of the nursing process.

Another use of data bases in nursing education was described by Shellenberger (1991). Shellenberger used a database to record skills students completed as well as to maintain records on the types of patients cared for by students. She found that the use of a database was a quick and efficient method to assist with student assignments and evaluations.

In reviewing computer and nursing literature, it can be seen that nursing faculty are beginning to use computers in new and creative ways that promise great potential for the future. One area that is still seriously underaddressed, however, is the inclusion of computer education in the nursing curriculum, despite general agreement that it should be included. Nursing educators must recognize their responsibility for preparing students for a world in which those without computer skills will be educationally disadvantaged. The use of computers in nursing must focus not only on the technology but also on the nature of information, its access, and its use in decision making (Heller, Romano, Damrosch, & McCarthy, 1988). Computers are transforming the way individuals, groups, and organizations think and interact with one another (Jenkins, 1988).

PROJECT

Overview

This project grew out of the perceived need to assist students to become familiar with databases as a means for generating information. Over a two and one-half year period, 77 graduate students enrolled in the Nursing of the Adult program were involved in this project. The Nursing of the Adult major consists of three sequential clinical courses. The first course focuses on health appraisals of individuals in ambulatory care areas using Gordon's functional health patterns to organize assessment data (Gordon, 1987). The second course focuses on development of nursing diagnoses and related interventions for clients in acute care settings. The third course focuses on clients in rehabilitation or long-term care settings and on evaluation of nursing care delivery. Since students in both the second and third courses were caring for several clients and were developing nursing diagnoses and related interventions, the faculty decided that a database program built on nursing diagnoses would be most useful and therefore included students from the second and third courses. Each record in the database was developed from information from clients for whom students provided care. Initially a flat database program (Reflex)® was used, but due to the complex nature of the data manipulation, the program was changed to a relational database (Paradox).®

PROCEDURE

Prior to involving the students in this project, faculty working with graduate Nursing of the Adult students met with another faculty member who had an extensive computer background to develop the structure for the database and data-entry worksheets. Four major worksheets were developed for data entry. One worksheet was for general client information such as demographic data and medical diagnoses (see Figure 30.1). Two other worksheets were used for nursing diagnoses. One was for nursing diagnoses already included in the database and the second one for nursing diagnoses formulated by the student. This particular worksheet was also used when the student wished to add new etiologies to a previously identified diagnosis. A fourth worksheet was used if the student needed to edit previously entered data. The structure of the worksheets was identical to the data-entry prompts that appeared on the computer screen.

Figure 30.2 depicts the worksheet used for existing nursing diagnoses. This worksheet included fields for the name of the diagnosis, defining characteristics, etiologies with sup-

---

Data Entry for Client table with form F1: Record 1 of 1   Data Entry

  Type requested information, press enter for next field.

Last four numbers of your SS# _____   Client # _____
                                                   (a 2 digit number you assign)

Date you saw client _____ Client's age _____ Client's sex _____

For fields in blue, tap F1 to see acceptable, move cursor to your choice and tap F2.

Marital status _____ Culture _____ Place of visit _____

When choose next entry, read specifics column for help with specifics field.

Type of visit _____ Specifics _____

Comment:

  Tap F4 to enter Medical Diagnoses, enter after each one.

Medical Diagnosis

Tap F4 and Page Down to enter another client.   F2 Quit.

Figure 30.1 Worksheet for general client information.

Data Entry for Nxdx table with form F1: Record 1 of 1 _____ Data Entry _____

Last four numbers of your SS# _____ Client # _____ (Be sure it is identical with one entered in client record)

Date _____ Nursing Diagnosis _____

Tap F4 to enter defining characteristics, enter after each entry.

Defining Characteristic

Tap F4 to enter etiology and interventions, enter after each entry.

Etiology
Short Term Goal:
Intervention:
Bibliography:
Evaluation Date   Outcome
Comment

If another etiology, tap PgDn, else F4 & PgDn for next nxdx. F2 to Quit.

Figure 30.2 Worksheet for existing nursing diagnosis.

porting data, goals, nursing interventions, and evaluation of goal achievement. Faculty and students alike found this extra step of completing the worksheets helpful in preparing the data for computer entry. It was easier for the students to think through the process ahead of time on the worksheet rather than to organize their thoughts during data entry. When possible, the worksheets were reviewed by a faculty member to ensure accuracy and consistency among ideas.

After selecting a client to include in the database and completing the worksheets, students used an IBM compatible computer equipped with a hard drive and the Paradox database program to enter the data. Students were encouraged to select nursing diagnoses that had been a priority for that client, and most did so. However, because the selection of diagnoses for entry into the database was arbitrary, the diagnoses entered cannot be considered representative of any patient population. Some students selected nursing diagnoses that were of special interest to themselves, but were not necessarily priorities for their patients.

Findings

At this time the project is ongoing with the intent of developing a more comprehensive database. Even though students selected nursing diagnoses of their own preference, some nursing diagnoses were selected more frequently than others. The most frequently occurring nursing diagnoses were ineffective individual coping, fear, knowledge deficit, powerlessness, and constipation. Figure 30.3 depicts the various nursing diagnoses en-

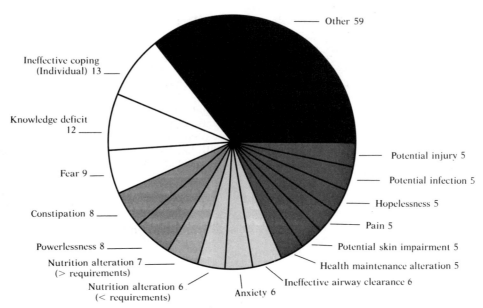

Figure 30.3 Nursing diagnoses entered in database.

tered in the database. Of the identified diagnoses (n = 168), about one-half were physiological in nature and the other half were psychosocial in nature.

The information contained in the data base can be manipulated in various ways to generate new knowledge. Through this manipulation some interesting findings are beginning to emerge. By sorting records in different ways, we have been able to create various reports. Reports which combine nursing diagnoses with defining characteristics for that diagnosis are useful to validate or refute the defining characteristics identified by NANDA and also to provide evidence for new defining characteristics. Reports which combine the nursing diagnosis field with the etiology fields for that diagnosis have supported the need to identify etiologies whenever possible as one diagnosis can be associated with a variety of etiologies. Such reports have also identified the need to explicate etiologies that are amenable to nursing intervention. Reports that combine etiologies, short-term goals,

and nursing interventions allow examination of the logic behind these links between nursing diagnoses and various aspects of the nursing process. Reports for two frequently occurring nursing diagnoses, ineffective individual coping and pain, are illustrated in Tables 30.1 and 30.2. These tables include nursing diagnosis, etiologies, and interventions.

Outcomes

This computer project increased the nursing process and computer skills of the participating graduate students as evidenced by their comments and completed assignments. Students also recognized the value of sharing their observations and plans with others so as to build the body of nursing knowledge.

Nursing Process Skills. Saba (1989) suggested that areas related to nursing diagnosis requiring future research include developing defining characteristics for each

Table 30.1 Composite for Nursing Diagnosis: Ineffective Individual Coping

Etiologies	Interventions
Problem solving skills deficit	— Instruct client on problem solving techniques followed by discussion or demonstration. — Use counseling skills to identify effective coping skills.
Negative beliefs about self	— Encourage patient to verbalize feelings about self. — Encourage use of positive self affirmations.
Inadequate support systems	— Provide frequent contact with client. Encourage communication with family and associates to help patient identify potential sources of support.
Presence of multiple stressors	— Help patient to identify stressors that can be eliminated. — Encourage use of relaxation techniques during the day to decrease stress. Review discharge plans to identify further stressors. — Assist patient to use cognitive restructuring.

Table 30.2 Composite for Nursing Diagnosis: Pain

Etiologies	Interventions
Powerlessness	— Have patient become more active with pain management by using an analog scale to document when pain medication is given and the results.
Absence of distraction activities	— Provide client with diversional activities.
Lack of knowledge of pain management techniques	— Teach relaxation techniques in a quiet restful environment. — Have client give return demonstration of techniques.
Inability to modify activity secondary to chronic physical disability	— Teach techniques of work simplification.

nursing diagnosis, establishing valid nursing-care planning measures, clarifying the relationship between medical diagnoses and nursing diagnoses, and identifying cost-of-care measures for each nursing diagnosis. The use of this database program in nursing education has begun to address Saba's first three recommendations by increasing graduate students' insights and skills in these areas.

Students, using the NANDA diagnoses, developed an appreciation for the need to validate the current nursing diagnoses. They indicated they could now understand how comparing defining characteristics listed by a variety of nurses for a specific problem statement could assist in identifying the most important characteristics for currently existing nursing diagnoses. They were excited by the cumulative data which began to suggest new defining characteristics as well as new nursing diagnoses. Nevertheless, they also began to realize how difficult and time-consuming it is to build a solid database. This realization developed an increased appreciation for researchers who laboriously gather the data that will ultimately serve to increase our nursing knowledge. This experience also enabled the students to appreciate the need for a unified nursing language system. Although the human mind can translate "nausea and vomiting," and "N & V" to mean the same thing, the computer cannot. Problems in searching and sorting arose from these deviations.

Use of this program helped students to become more skilled in establishing etiologies. When sorts were performed on a certain nursing diagnosis, the reports showed students what other etiologies had been used with this diagnosis. The program provided the ability to search data entries in a variety of ways and to look for patterns or themes such as those that emerged after combining etiologies with interventions or combining nursing diagnoses with the client's medical diagnosis.

This experience also enabled students to become more consistent and logical in their thinking by increasing their ability to make logical connections between the problem statement, etiology, and selected interventions. The worksheet used for data entry helped students to organize data in a concise and logical manner. Reviewing the information they had entered into the database helped students to evaluate and critique the logic and consistency of the data in relation to the entire nursing process. Bulechek and McCloskey's (1985) definition of nursing interventions, as autonomous actions executed to benefit the client in a predicted way related to the nursing diagnosis, also facilitated this logical thinking by students.

As students become more skilled with manipulation of the information contained in the database, they can use the information provided by their peers as a basis for their own nursing care. Searching the database for a particular nursing diagnosis (problem and etiology) will allow students to identify interventions that other students have used and, ideally, the outcomes of those interventions. Such information may also provide

the stimulus for nursing research projects related to evaluating the effectiveness of specific interventions. This type of activity can help bridge the gap between research, education, and practice.

Information concerning evaluation of patient outcomes is sparse to date. Patients were often discharged from acute care settings before such data became available. Evaluation data may be more easily obtainable in long-term care facilities or in ambulatory care settings where clients are seen over time. These settings may also be more conducive to nursing diagnoses and interventions focusing on wellness than those identified thus far in acute care settings.

Computer Skills. This experience helped the students to increase their confidence in data entry abilities. At the end of the year they indicated an increased inclination to use computers in the future, however, they also indicated that learning to use the program was frustrating. As might be expected, students having little or no computer background were often the most frustrated. Student recommendations to decrease this frustration included: (1) more instruction in basic computer operation prior to instruction related to the database program, (2) increased availability of a computer resource person during data entry, and (3) more opportunities to learn and practice data manipulation.

Format Modification. Modifications in the procedure are currently being implemented. They include: (1) converting from a flat (Reflex) to a relational (Paradox) database to improve the efficiency and accuracy of data entry and knowledge generation, (2) developing selection menus for each field to ensure consistency of terms, (3) developing a field where students can enter suggested readings about a particular intervention, thus increasing the resource value of the data base, (4) modifying the evaluation fields to describe the actual outcomes in more detail, and (5) setting up menus to allow students greater opportunity for program application and data manipulation.

SUMMARY

Findings from this project show that computers have vast possibilities for future use in nursing education. The use of computers in nursing education is just beginning and can open new avenues for teaching strategies that facilitate knowledge acquisition and critical thinking skills among diverse student populations. With a database program such as the one presented here, current nursing diagnoses can be further validated, new nursing diagnoses can be developed, and nursing interventions for particular etiologies can be identified and evaluated. The role of the nurse educator is to be aware of the capabilities of computers and to use them more fully and creatively to develop new teaching strategies. Nurses need to be familiar with data entry process as well as organizing and manipulating data so that outcomes of the data manipulation yields knowledge. Additionally, as nurses become familiar with database capabilities, they develop ways of thinking about information that allow a given data set to generate more knowledge than was previously thought to be easily accessible.

REFERENCES

Bailey, D. (1988). Computer applications in nursing: A prototypical model for planning nursing care. *Computers in Nursing, 6* (5), 199–203.

Bolwell, C. (1988). Evaluating computer assisted instruction. *Nursing and Health Care, 9* (9), 511–515.

Bulechek, G., & McCloskey, J. (1985). *Nursing interventions: Treatments for nursing diagnoses.* Philadelphia: W. B. Saunders.

Chang, B. L., Roth, K., Gonzales, E., Caswell, D., & DiStefano, J. (1988). CANDI: A knowledge-based system for nursing diagnosis. *Computers in Nursing, 6* (1), 13–21.

Cox, H., Harsanyi, B., & Dean, L. (1987). *Computers in Nursing.* Norwalk: Appleton & Lange.

Gordon, M. (1987). Nursing diagnosis: Process and application (2nd ed.). New York: McGraw-Hill.

Halloran, E. J. (1988). Computerized nursing assessments. *Nursing and Health Care, 9* (9), 497–499.

Heller, B. R., Romano, C. A., Damrosch, S. P., & McCarthy, M. R. (1988). The need for an educational program in nursing informatics. In M. J. Ball, K. J. Hannah, U. Gerdin Jelger, & H. Peterson (Eds.), *Nursing Informatics* (pp. 331–343). New York: Springer-Verlag.

Hirsch, M., Chang, B. L., & Gilbert, S. (1989). A computer program to support patient assessment and clinical decision making in nursing education. *Computers in Nursing, 7* (4), 157–160.

Jenkins, T. (1988). New roles for nursing professionals. In M. J. Ball, K. J. Hannah, U. Gerdin Jelger, & H. Peterson (Eds.), *Nursing Informatics* (pp. 88–95). New York: Springer-Verlag.

Norman, S. (1982). Computer assisted learning: Its potential in nurse education. *Nursing Times, 78* (35), 1467–1468.

Peterson, M., & Hannah, K. (1988). Nursing management information systems. In M. J. Ball, K. J. Hannah, U. Gerdin Jelger, & H. Peterson (Eds.), *Nursing Informatics* (pp. 190–205). New York: Springer-Verlag.

Polit, D., & Hungler, B. (1991). *Nursing Research* (4th ed.). Philadelphia: J. B. Lippincott.

Saba, V. (1989). Nursing diagnoses in computerized classification systems. In R. Carroll-Johnson (Ed.), *Classification of nursing diagnoses: Proceedings of the eighth conference* (pp. 84–88). Philadelphia: Lippincott.

Saba, V., & McCormick, K. (1986). *Essentials of computers for nurses*. Philadelphia: J. B. Lippincott.

Shellenberger, T. (1991). Use of a database for clinical assignments and student evaluations. *Nurse Educator, 16* (2), 39–41.

Simmons, S., & Ryan, L. (1984). The implementation of nursing diagnosis using a computerized information system. In M. J.

Kim, G. K. McFarland, & A. M. McLane, (Eds.), *Classification of nursing diagnoses: Proceedings of the fifth national conference* (pp. 276–286). St. Louis: Mosby.

Van Steeg, D. (1988). Computer use and nursing research. *Western Journal of Nursing Research, 10* (4), 506–509.

Werley, H., Devine, E., & Zorn, C. (1988). Nursing needs its own minimum data set. *American Journal of Nursing, 88* (12), 1651–1653.

31

A Computerized Database
for Parent–Child Nursing

Greer Glazer

This chapter focuses on the history of the development of a computerized database for the Parent–Child Nursing master's program at Kent State University. The database will be presented and is then followed by a discussion of findings from three years of student experience with the database.

REVIEW OF LITERATURE

Nursing diagnoses can make a significant contribution to nursing practice by defining and organizing knowledge as a prerequisite for practice and by providing a means for communicating this knowledge in a systematic way (Tanner & Hughes, 1984). The nursing diagnosis model enables the nurse to gain cognitive control over the unmanageable diversity of nursing practice (Gordon, 1985). Nevertheless, Aspinal (1976) and Anderson and Briggs (1988) found that nursing diagnosis is a weak part of the nursing process. Allen (1989) delineated six problems public health nurses had using nursing diagnoses in their practice. Nursing diagnoses do

not: (1) deal with families and communities, (2) describe wellness/well care, (3) describe prevention, (4) describe health promotion, and (5) describe health behaviors. In addition, there is a preponderance of a negative/deficit orientation instead of a positive/wellness orientation. The Missouri Department of Health, Bureau of Community Health Nursing addressed the problem of focus on illness and disease by using North American Nursing Diagnosis Association (NANDA) approved diagnosis categories but changing modifiers such as "inadequate" and "ineffective" to "adequate" and "effective" where appropriate (Allen, 1989). Despite present difficulties with using nursing diagnoses in nursing practice, the author believes they are the best classification system that exists today.

USE OF THE DATABASE AT KENT STATE UNIVERSITY

There were five purposes of using a computerized database with graduate nursing students. They were to: (1) increase computer skills, (2) provide more effective nursing assessment, diagnosis, intervention, and evaluation, and therefore, better client care, (3) increase analytic skills, (4) increase students' ability to link practice and research, and (5) provide student nurses with an opportunity to look at all nurse and client data and therefore see a global picture rather than learning only from their own clients.

Specifically, in their three specialty courses, students begin with development of computer skills because most students do not have prior experience with computers. Students then quickly move on to a working knowledge of databases, how to use a specific database program (Paradox), and most importantly, how to analyze the database for predominant nursing diagnoses, client strengths and weaknesses, effective nursing interventions, and researchable questions. In the 1990–1991 academic year professors have emphasized further development and refinement of wellness-oriented nursing diagnoses.

Four groups of students have worked with the database. Group I consisted of 14 parent–child nursing (PCN) students working in acute-care settings with 88 cases; Group II included 13 PCN students working in ambulatory-care settings accounting for 135 cases; Group III consisted of 11 PCN students working in ambulatory care settings with 54 cases; and Group IV consisted of 10 students working in ambulatory- and acute-care settings accounting for 276 cases in fall, 1990 and 54 cases in spring, 1991. Forty-eight students worked with a total of 607 cases which provided the database.

DESCRIPTION OF THE DATABASE

The database of PCN client information was created as a substitute for paper and pencil health records using nursing diagnosis as a framework. The original database had two problems that have been described by Pryor, Califf, Harrell, Hlatky, Lee, Mark, & Rosati (1985). There was too much data to be collected and entered, and the original function of the database subsequently changed. The amount of data has been reduced to two screens that are readily filled out in no more than 15 minutes per client. The process of data entry is facilitated by having students work in pairs; one student reads the data and the other enters the data. Whereas students originally had the opportunity to enter any amount of data, there are now limits placed on the number of characters per field. Moreover, look-up tables have been developed so that students are able to see the choices they have for data entry in a specific field. For instance, a student wishing to fill out the field for nursing diagnosis may look up what other wellness-oriented nursing diagnoses have been developed by students as well as the NANDA-approved nursing diagnoses. In addition, the function of the database was altered. Whereas students perform complete health assessments on the clients, only pertinent data are recorded. A field was added related to success or lack of success of the nursing intervention with the hope of someday using this data to obtain direct reimbursement for nursing services.

The first screen contains the following data: last four numbers of student's social security number; client number; date the client was seen; client's age, sex, marital status, and race or ethnicity; place of visit; type of visit; and medical diagnosis. Figure 31.1 depicts the information completed by student 1960 on the first screen.

The second screen that students observe includes the following data: the last four numbers of their social security number; client number; date; nursing diagnoses (a star denotes a student-developed wellness diag-

Editing Client Table with Form F1: Record 27 of 154   Edit M

Type requested information, press enter for next field.

Last four numbers of your SS# 1960 Client # 01 (a 2 digit number you assign)

Date you saw client 10/18/90   Client's age 9 months   Client's sex M

For fields in blue, tap F1 to see acceptable, move cursor to your choice and tap F2.

Marital status S   Race Caucasian   Place of visit Home

When choose next entry, read specifics column for help with specifics field.

Type of visit WCC   Specifics

Comment:

Tap F4 to enter Medical Diagnoses, Enter after each one.

Medical Diagnoses: Tap enter after each
Otitis media

Tap F4 and Page Down to enter another client

F2 Quit.

Figure 31.1 PCN database: first screen.

nosis); defining characteristics; etiology; short-term goal; nursing intervention; evaluation date; outcome; bibliography; and comment. An example of the second screen is presented in Figure 31.2. The space bib (bibliography) is included for students to document references that assisted them in providing nursing care to their clients. The comment field enables the students to add additional pertinent information that is not included in the fixed fields. The use of wellness-oriented nursing diagnoses and client strengths are necessary to describe the client's health status and can facilitate more complete health assessments for the client with emphasis on the positive aspects of health. Life processes were added to the NANDA definition of nursing diagnosis in 1990. As Carson, Craft, McGuire, and Popkess-Vawter (1991) point out, nursing diagnosis is supposed to describe the nature of nursing practice (which includes health promotion, illness prevention, and restoration of health). Therefore, there must be inclusion of wellness-oriented diagnosis. In addition, as Lyons and Hester (1987) argue, clients can

see their own progress and improvement and take an active interest in their own health and self-care. Nurses should be better able to promote client health-seeking behaviors.

STUDENT RESPONSIBILITIES

All PCN students used the database while providing care to PCN clients in their clinical experience. Students were expected to input data into the computer on a weekly or biweekly basis. At the end of the course, students analyzed the database for predominant nursing diagnoses, client strengths and weaknesses, effective nursing interventions, and researchable questions. The final exam included a question on the advantages and disadvantages of using a computerized database. Students beginning the Parent–Child master's program in 1990 were given a pretest at the beginning of the semester and posttest at the end of the semester in which they identified nursing diagnoses related to a case study.

Viewing Nnxdx table with form F1: Record 1 of 1   Main

Last four numbers of your SS# <u>1960</u>   Client # <u>01</u> (Be sure is identical with one entered in client record.)

Date <u>10/11/90</u>   Nursing Diagnosis * <u>Parent/Child relationship intact</u>

Tap F4 to enter defining characteristics, enter after each entry.

Defining Characteristics

Appropriate caretaking behaviors

Attentive to child needs

Presence of attachment behaviors

Tap F4 to enter etiology and interventions, enter after each entry.

Page Down to enter another intervention, Ctrl-D to repeat the etiology

Etiology <u>Relation fostering G&D</u>

Short Term Goal <u>Maintenance of intact parent/child relationship</u>

Intervention <u>Support & reinforcement</u>

Evaluation Date <u>11/11/90</u>   Outcome <u>4</u> (1, 2, 3, 4, or 5)

(1 Not Successful - 5 Very Successful)

Bib:

Comment

If an Escape Only Active when menu is displayed - Press [F10] to display menu

Figure 31.2   PCN database: second screen.

OUTCOMES OF USING THE DATABASE

Group I: Acute-Care Setting

The most frequently reported nursing diagnoses were knowledge deficit, alteration in nutrition, anxiety, sensory deprivation, and ineffective airway clearance. The effective nursing interventions identified included presence, active listening, distraction, guided imagery, diversional play, support, teaching, music therapy, infant stimulation, counseling, and relaxation.

Group II: Ambulatory-Care Setting

The most frequently reported nursing diagnoses from this group were knowledge deficit, alteration in nutrition, pain, good physical health, sound or improved nutritional status, intact parent–child–family relationship, and potential for improved adequate health maintenance.

There were a total of 90 nursing diagnoses with 45 new wellness-oriented nursing diagnoses representing 26 different diagnoses. These diagnoses represented a good beginning but were subsequently refined.

Little data about sexuality-reproductive, value-belief, and self-perception functional health patterns appeared. There were two reasons for this: the client usually only made one visit and there was not enough time to develop a rapport to be able to assess these areas. Students most frequently identified strengths and weaknesses in health perception, health maintenance, and nutritional-metabolic functional health patterns. Out of 45 antepartum and gynecologic patients, only eight had medical diagnoses. The data suggests that these women do not need to routinely see physicians, but could be seen by master's-prepared nurses.

Group III: Ambulatory-Care Setting

The most frequently reported nursing diagnoses were knowledge deficit (60%), and alteration in nutrition. Only seven out of 54 clients had a medical diagnosis that required treatment by a physician.

Students in this group identified five new wellness-oriented nursing diagnoses: (1) family coping—potential for growth, (2) adequate support system, (3) good dental health, (4) adequate knowledge base, and (5) sustained emotional health.

Group IV: Ambulatory-Care Setting and Acute-Care Setting

Great strides have been made in the development and analysis of the database during the 1990–1991 year. The four major goals for this year were creating wellness-oriented nursing diagnoses; developing defining characteristics for wellness-oriented nursing diagnoses; critical analysis of the database to reconceptualize diagnoses, cleanup coding problems, and combine similar diagnoses; begin gathering data to see if students were meeting the five purposes of using a computer database that were originally set up. Namely, were students prepared to identify nursing diagnoses and focus on the whole person including wellness-oriented nursing diagnoses?

In fall, 1990, students practiced in ambulatory-care settings. The most frequently reported nursing diagnoses were adequate prenatal care, growth and development progressing, fatigue, knowledge deficit, anxiety, nutrition alteration, and pain. In spring, 1991, students practiced in a pediatric or maternity acute-care setting with a focus on high risk conditions and illness. As evidenced by the large amount of wellness-oriented nursing diagnoses, students maintained an awareness of health promotion and wellness. The most frequent nursing diagnoses were: health-seeking behaviors, knowledge deficit, parent–child relationship intact, anxiety, effective coping, growth and development progressing, and knowledge reinforcement need.

All of the nursing diagnoses entered into the database for the 1990–1991 academic year were analyzed for frequency and type of diagnosis. As evidenced by the graph in Figure 31.3, the most frequently entered nursing diagnoses were wellness oriented. Sixty-three of the nursing diagnoses were either health-seeking behaviors or growth and development progress. Other nursing diagnoses in order of frequency were: knowledge deficit, parent–child relationship intact, anxiety, knowledge reinforcement need, pain, and effective individual coping. The category "other" contained nursing diagnoses entered less frequently than seven times during the academic year.

Originally, 24 new nursing diagnoses were entered by the students. After analysis of the database, at the end of last semester, new nursing diagnoses were reduced to a list of the 14 that appear in Table 31.1. Of the ten new nursing diagnoses that were eliminated, three were already NANDA-approved nurs-

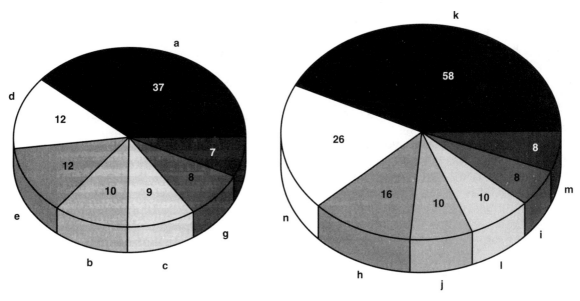

Figure 31.3 Number of nursing diagnoses in database—academic year 1990–91.

a = *Health-seeking behavior
b = *Knowledge reinforcement
c = *Nutritional status sound
d = *Parent–child relationship
    intact
e = *Anxiety
f = Anxiety anticipatory
g = Fatigue

h = Knowledge deficit
i = Nutrition alteration, less
    than
j = Pain, acute
k = other
l = *Coping effective individual
m = *Family relationship intact
n = *Growth & development
    progress

Table 31.1   New Nursing Diagnoses Developed by PCN Students 1990–1991

* Emotional health sustained
* Family processes, intact
* Growth and development, progressing
* Health maintenance, good
* Nutritional status, sound; improved
* Parent–child relationship, intact
* Parenting progressing, well
* Body image disturbance, potential
* Self-esteem disturbance, potential
* Anger
* Coping, effective individual
* Coping, effective family
* Coping, progressing family
* Dental health, good

ing diagnoses. Students combined categories that were coded differently but signified the same thing (e.g., coping effective and coping effect). Seven nursing diagnoses were recategorized to fit into already preexisting nursing diagnoses. Last, categories that fit together were combined. For instance, strong parent–infant attachment and parent–infant relationship intact were combined into parent–child relationship intact. Some of what nursing students listed as new nursing diagnoses were recategorized into defining characteristics for health-seeking behaviors.

Nursing diagnoses were grouped into

broad areas by combining altered, sound, and improved into one category. By doing this, students were able to see pivotal areas where nursing intervention needed to be directed. When nursing diagnoses were grouped into broad areas the most frequent areas were health-seeking behaviors, growth and development, nutrition, anxiety, parent–child relationship, knowledge deficit/reinforcement, fatigue and sleep pattern, and coping. As can be seen from Table 31.2, originally nutrition showed up on the most frequent nursing diagnoses, in terms of nutritional alteration, less than with the frequency of 6, and here became the third most frequent area.

The greatest contribution to date has been development and refinement of the wellness-oriented nursing diagnoses. This is the first year that the students have added to the database by putting in defining characteristics of new nursing diagnoses. Students have identified defining characteristics for health-seeking behaviors, effective coping, intact family relationships, growth and development progressing, good health maintenance, parent–child relationship intact, and progressive or good parenting.

As an example, when adequate prenatal care and adequate well-child care were re-categorized into health-seeking behaviors related to adequate prenatal and well-child care, the following characteristics were developed: individual and family coping effective, growth and development progressing, nutritional status improved, health maintenance good, strong parent–infant attachment, progressive parenting, and seeking knowledge reinforcement. Thirty-three percent of the cases fit into health-seeking behaviors. The following three criteria were added to the NANDA-approved defining characteristics for health seeking behaviors: (1) attends classes to increase knowledge of health promotion behaviors, (2) follows health routines, and (3) receives health care at appropriate times.

One more example of defining characteristics that students developed for wellness-oriented nursing diagnosis will be provided. Growth and development progressing was the second most frequently used nursing diagnosis. Defining characteristics developed by students for growth and development progressing are achieving age-appropriate tasks, adequate physical growth, communication skills typical for age group norms; evidence of cognitive growth mastery for age group norms; health promoting, enriching lifestyle; meeting normal growth parameters per height and weight chart; receiving health care at appropriate times; performing health care abilities typical for age group norms; progression/improvement in skill performance, and social skills typical for age group norms.

Students entering in 1990–1991 had a pre and posttest to assess the impact of using the computerized database. The students were given the same case study the first and last day of class in Parent–Child Nursing I. The case study was based on the neonatal assessment tool developed by Terhaar and Bunton (1989). The case study very briefly involved a mother, who was 22 years old, married for

Table 31.2 Nursing Diagnoses Grouped Into Broad Areas

Health-seeking behaviors (adequate prenatal care)	23
Growth and development*	22
Nutrition*	22
Anxiety	14
Parent–child relationship*	12
Knowledge deficit/reinforcement	12
Fatigue/sleep pattern	10
Coping*	9

* Altered, sound, and improved

two years, and who had preterm labor with premature rupture of membranes. She delivered an infant at 34 weeks, who was transferred to the intensive care unit and received respiratory assistance with oxygen, monitoring, and IV. The case study disclosed that the parents were touching, stroking, and talking to their baby and had recognized family friends for support as well as grandparents and siblings. The findings were remarkable. Prior to being exposed to the PCN program the students were able to label nursing diagnoses quite accurately. Students documented between six and 14 nursing diagnoses for this mother and baby unit. Nevertheless, one-half of the students, five out of ten, had no relationship statement. No student identified a wellness-oriented nursing diagnosis. In addition, students did not identify any nursing diagnosis related to support systems, coping, or spiritual integrity. After exposure to the database for one semester, students identified between five and 27 nursing diagnoses. Six out of seven students included relationship statements in their nursing diagnosis statement. Every student included at least one wellness-oriented nursing diagnosis, with students including between one and ten wellness-oriented nursing diagnoses. In addition, students investigated things they had not considered before—coping, spiritual integrity, and support systems.

The most exciting thing for the author was that students gained a new perspective in looking at clients by focusing on strengths and wellness as well as health problems. For example, one student went from documenting alteration in parenting related to prematurity and infant in ICU to, at the end of the semester, adequate parenting related to positive parent–infant attachment behaviors as evidenced by talking, stroking, and touching. Students were able to identify more advantages of using a computerized database

than the faculty found documented in the literature. These advantages include:

1. synthesizes data faster than by pencil;
2. can perform calculations;
3. can form researchable questions;
4. gives more global picture; enables one to look at multiple forms of data at the same time;
5. able to sort, search, and group data as needed; can sift through data not needed;
6. can make changes as often as needed and rearrange data with minimal work;
7. can focus on data one is interested in at a given time;
8. all data are in one place and not scattered on many pieces of paper;
9. may enable nurses to cost out nursing care;
10. everyone uses the same language, which gives way to a mutual understanding of information;
11. data can be networked and worked on by a number of people at the same time;
12. can provide a printout of desired information any time;
13. decreases the need for writing and record keeping;
14. content can be displayed in a wide variety of formats; can be helpful in presentation of data to prove or disprove a point, argument, or hypothesis;
15. can be maintained over a long period of time to reflect an historical perspective.

Disadvantages, on the other hand, included:

1. frustration when unfamiliar with computer or database;

2. time to learn how to use the computer or database was limited;

3. there were limits on how the data could be entered and students had to keep looking at the manual for help;

4. there was the fear of inadvertently losing data;

5. the ability to retrieve data is dependent upon the data that were entered.

CONCLUSIONS

A lot has been learned since a nursing database was incorporated into the PCN curriculum. Based on four groups of students the following conclusions have been made. Most important, students can be taught to focus on wellness as well as illness. Client strengths and weaknesses can be identified. Wellness-oriented nursing diagnoses can be developed and used. Students can develop defining characteristics for wellness-oriented nursing diagnoses. Effectiveness of nursing interventions can be ascertained. Students' abilities to organize, structure, and analyze data improved. Students improved their abilities to ask reasonable questions based on data. Students understood principles of using a database.

Three major directions for the future have been identified. Students will be encouraged to develop new wellness-oriented nursing diagnoses with defining characteristics. Students will be encouraged to assist the faculty by doing research so that some of the wellness-oriented nursing diagnoses may be submitted to NANDA. The process has begun by providing evidence that the defining characteristics occur in the ambulatory- and acute-care settings in which the students practice. Second, the database will continually be refined by adding, deleting, and combining items. In particular, a field will be added to

include time of nurse client interaction so that cost of nursing care can be ascertained. Last, the database will be analyzed for congruence with the nursing minimum data set.

The possibilities for the future are exciting. Whereas not every student reaction has been positive, their commentary does provide data that confirm that inroads have been made in assisting students to visualize the importance of a computerized nursing database. As one student answered:

Computerized databases have advantages and disadvantages. Disadvantages can be taken care of with proper instruction, guidance, and most of all, time. The advantages can be very beneficial to nursing and the future of nursing research.

REFERENCES

Allen, C. J. (1989). Incorporating a wellness perspective for nursing diagnosis in practice. In R. M. Carroll-Johnson (Ed.), *Proceedings of the 8th Conference of the North American Nursing Diagnosis Association: Classification of nursing diagnoses* (pp. 37–42). Philadelphia: J. B. Lippincott.

Anderson, J. E., & Briggs, L. L. (1988). Nursing diagnosis: A study of quality and supportive evidence. *Image, 20* (3), 141–144.

Aspinal, M. J. (1976). Nursing diagnosis: The weakest link. *Nursing Outlook, 24*, 433–437.

Carson, J., Craft, C., McGuire, A., & Popkess-Vawter, S. (1991). *Nursing diagnosis: A case study approach.* Philadelphia: W. B. Saunders.

Gordon, M. (1985). Nursing diagnosis. In H. Werley & J. Fitzpatrick (Eds.), *Annual review of nursing research* (Vol. 3, pp. 127). New York: Springer.

Lyons, J., & Hester, N. (1987). Research-generated nursing diagnoses for healthy school-age children. *Issues in Comprehensive Pediatric Nursing, 10*, 149–159.

Pryor, D., Califf, R., Harrell, F., Hlatky, M., Lee, K., Mark, D., & Rosati, R. (1985). Clinical data bases: Accomplishments and unrealized potential. *Medical Care, 23* (5). 623–647.

Tanner, C. A., & Hughes, A. M. G. (1984). Nursing diagnosis: Issues in clinical practice research. *Topics in Clinical Nursing, 5* (4), 30–38.

Terhaar, M., & Bunton, S. (1989). Neonatal assessment tool. In C. Guzetta et al (Eds)., *Clinical assessment tools for use with nursing diagnoses* (pp. 328–342). St. Louis: C. V. Mosby.

32

Using a Scanner in Nursing Research

Sharon L. Merritt

Computer technology has simplified many aspects of information processing for nurse faculty. In spite of the emergence of optical scanning equipment, few faculty in higher education seem to be taking full advantage of this technology to enter and manage data.

Faculty often use central facilities to complete test scoring tasks, but are unaware that these facilities can be used for tasks other than grading examinations. Furthermore, desktop scanners that either stand alone or are connected to a personal computer are available for examination scoring and data entry. This capability in a school of nursing can make it possible for faculty to grade tests and compile an item analysis within 30 minutes of exam completion. But equally important, with the right scanning equipment and forms it is possible to create a quantitative database more efficiently than with keyboard data entry. The purpose of this chapter is to acquaint the reader with scanner technology and some software that can be used to enter and process data.

HARDWARE

A scanner is a piece of equipment that uses optical mark reading and a scannable form to record and interpret data. Central scanning devices available in university test centers are often high speed devices that scan forms rapidly and perform a multitude of tasks such as uploading data to a mainframe computer and creating ASCII (American Standard Code for Information Interchange) data files on disk for use on a personal computer as well as test scoring. The major difference between a stand alone, large scanner and a desktop version is the speed with which the former can process data and the complexity of the tasks that it can execute. The focus of this chapter will be on desktop scanning devices that can be located practically anywhere in a school of nursing. The readers are encouraged to inquire about large, central scanning facilities and the capabilities available in their own settings.

A desktop scanner consists of an input

tray, the feed bed or "body" of the device in which the forms are transported and read with a read head, and an output stacker in which forms are collected after they are scanned. Usually, one or both sides of a form can be read as it passes through the feed bed. Options for automatic feeding of forms one at a time and a printer for printing information on the form are often available for specific models of the basic scanner equipment, sometimes at an increased cost. Since feeding forms into the equipment one at a time can be quite tedious, the author recommends that autosheet feed capability be purchased with the basic desktop equipment. If the scanner is to be used for test scoring purposes, a printer is necessary so that the test score can be printed on the answer sheet as it is graded (see Figure 32.1).

The cost for basic equipment (e.g., for the Opscan 5™ from National Computer Systems (NCS)), runs around $5,000 plus freight charges. For local processing, the scanner requires a host personal computer (PC) preferably with a hard drive and at least 256K of RAM internal memory. The PC does not have to be dedicated to scanning tasks since it is needed only when the scanner hardware is being operated. After the sheets have been scanned and a database is developed, a variety of software can be used to complete a particular task.

NCS manufactures the Sentry™ 2050, a specialized scanner that is a stand alone version and can be used to score tests and tabulate surveys. It contains a microcomputer that has been preprogrammed to scan 14 standard NCS forms. The capability of this equipment is limited since some of the usual measurement properties of an achievement test (full descriptive statistics, item difficulty, and others) are not computed with this equipment, nor can it create a database that can be exported for use with other applications programs. Limitations such as these make the applications for which it can be used somewhat limited. Nevertheless, the forms used can be read by any other Opscan™ scanner so this stand alone desktop version can be used to obtain immediate results, and the sheets can be scanned again later for more complete item analysis processing.

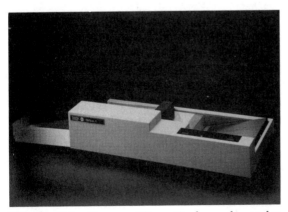

Figure 32.1 Opscan 5™ optical mark reader desktop scanner.

FORMS

Scanning equipment requires the use of specialized forms. The forms contain a timing track at the bottom or guide edge which is made up of small black rectangles (National Computers System, 1989b). Skunk marks located at the top line of the form are used to identify which form is being processed (see Figure 32.2). This edge is called the "leading edge" because it is the first edge of the form that goes into the computer. Various response positions consisting of bubbles or ovals that can be marked by a respondent make up the rest of the form.

A wide variety of forms that can be used for processing data are available from NCS.

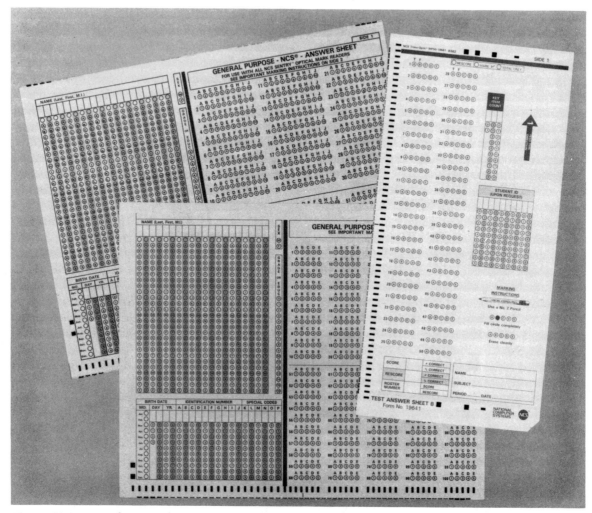

Figure 32.2 Sample general purpose NCS answer sheets.

They include half-sheet and whole-sheet forms that look like the typical answer sheet used by many nursing faculty to collect students' examination responses. These general purpose answer sheets include either five or ten options for responses. Typically, the five-option sheet has room for up to 240 responses. The ten-option sheet has room for 200 responses. In addition, some basic identifying information such as name and stu-

dent ID is collected. People mark their responses on the form by filling in the appropriate bubble with a number 2 pencil. The scanner collects data by projecting light onto these forms and measuring the amount of light that passes through the form at various points.

Besides general purpose answer sheets, forms for collecting attendance, scheduling information, class rosters, and course registration are also available. Others include forms for some of the major standardized tests used in primary and secondary schools. Survey and ballot forms allow the user to overprint appropriate information for collecting responses (e.g., survey questions or nominees for office). Additionally, by working with NCS, completely customized forms containing items specified by the purchaser can also be developed. The cost for standard forms runs about $25.00 plus shipping per box of 500 forms.

SCANNER OPERATION

Operation of a desktop scanner is relatively simple. The operator either feeds forms into the scanner one at a time or stacks them in the hopper where they are automatically picked one at a time from the stack. The operator determines the direction for feeding the forms by where the skunk marks and the timing track are placed. The edge with the skunk marks is fed in first, and the timing track is placed along the guide rail of the input hopper. The NCS scanner has a light on the automatic sheet feeder that lets the operator know when a stack of sheets is appropriately placed for feeding. The light is green when the stack is correctly placed and changes to red if the stack has been placed too far into the hopper. The operator panel on the feed bed assists in selecting and starting the scanning procedure. By pressing a couple of switches on the panel, the operator chooses the scanning and start procedures.

As with any piece of equipment, some maintenance procedures are required to keep the equipment in optimal condition. The read head needs to be cleaned periodically and calibrated to make sure that data are being recorded accurately. If a printer is purchased, the ribbon needs to be changed

periodically and the print head cleaned. The ribbon cartridge design could be improved because it tends to wear out rather quickly compared to the length of time ribbons usually last on computer printers. Troubleshooting and diagnostic procedures are provided with the equipment in order to aid the user in correcting operations if the scanner does not operate properly.

With a PC, the NCS equipment, and appropriate forms, the user can scan forms, use an auxiliary device such as a printer or display terminal in addition to the host PC, and score one examination answer sheet form (see Figure 32.3). The scanned data are transmitted to the host computer in an ASCII file format. In order to use the data, programs must be written for processing them. Fortunately, NCS has two application packages available for use with the scanner that allow the user to process data in usable form.

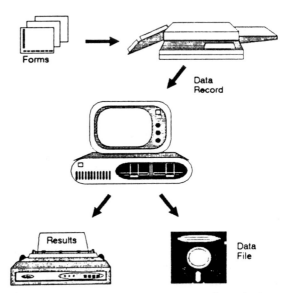

Figure 32.3 Processing, storing, and retrieving scanner data.

SOFTWARE

MicroTEST Score II Plus™ (MTSII)

Many nurse faculty have experienced the frustration of a backlog from central examination scoring facilities, particularly during final examination time. Perhaps even more frustrating is a lack of good central support services. Using an answer key that has the appropriate bubble punched out to hand grade examinations can often seem to be a waste of time, to say nothing of hand calculating examination psychometrics in order to compute final grades because testing services will not provide timely information.

The MTSII software is an easy-to-use, menu-driven software package that allows the user to scan, score examinations based on normative or mastery criteria, and store achievement test results, select reports, and print reports of test results (National Computer Systems, 1989a). Additionally, file utilities (e.g., deleting files and upgrading files) and data importing procedures are available with this software. The software is installed and accessed from the PC to which the scanner is attached. To score examinations, additional forms (i.e., the test header and test identification header) are needed in addition to an answer sheet key and the answer sheets completed by the students. About 20 different answer sheet forms can be scanned in simple or multiple batches; users need to consult the manual before purchasing forms to make sure their choice is compatible with the software. A helpful feature of this program is a screen that provides information relative to each form as it is scanned and interrupts the procedure if a form is rejected (the program automatically error checks each sheet). At the bottom of the screen, information is provided about why the form was rejected and assists the operator in making appropriate corrections. The report selection options include individual test results (for posting the results, this may be printed by identification number only); item analyses that include item discrimination and difficulty and frequency data; and test score distribution information that includes z-score and percentile rank. A report queue of up to 12 reports is generated as the reports are selected and printed in order of selection when the print report menu is chosen.

The manual accompanying the software is easy to read and follow. Based on the author's experience, even a novice computer operator can be taught to successfully use the software in less than one hour. A few nuances associated with use of the software can be annoying. Unless bar code reader capability is purchased with the equipment, students must properly place their identification number on the answer sheet in order for it to be scanned. In the author's experience student mistakes in completing the answer sheets with this information are the most frequent reasons for scanning failure. Another troubling feature is the need to supply report header information as each report is selected following scanning and scoring (e.g. test name, faculty name). Nevertheless, this is a minor inconvenience since after the report header information is supplied during the first report selection procedure, it can be quickly recalled for subsequent reports by pressing the enter key.

ScanTools™ (STS)

Keyboard data entry is tedious work that often requires extensive training of the people who enter the data. Depending upon the number of subjects and variables, it can be a time consuming task that may delay data analysis. Other than mentioning transferring data to scannable answer sheets as an alternative data entry procedure, nursing research texts offer little guidance about these procedures (Cox, Harsanyi, & Dean, 1987;

Polit & Hungler, 1991). The focus of research texts continues to be on transferring data to coding sheets or coding on the questionnaire prior to hand entering data into the computer. With careful planning, both of these steps can be virtually eliminated from the process of computer data entry.

ScanTools™ (STS) is a menu-driven, three-part software package that allows the user to

1. scan data documents and manage files created after scanning (the application base [AB]);
2. create form applications by defining where data are located on a NCS form, and install them on a main menu so they can be used whenever the particular form is scanned (the document system [DS]); and
3. validate and modify (clean) data in a file during scanning or after the file has been created (the editor [SE]) (National Computer Systems, 1988).

The AB part of STS contains main menus for scanning forms and is the module through which the DS and SE are reached. The DS procedure to create form applications is analogous to defining the fields in which data are located in a format statement that is used with a statistical package, but is easier to compile since field option choices are provided in a menu and easily selected with the enter key. The SE module allows the user to identify and correct errors made by the respondent on the answer key (e.g., filling in two response options when instructed to make only one selection). The SE assists in making data organized through scanning complete and error-free.

An ASCII data file is created during scanning and can be used by any other computer program that accepts files in this form. The record length depends on the form that has been used and the number of items used to record data on the form. A record length of as long as 480 columns can be created. Many PC statistical packages accept data in this form and allow a variable record length, that is, as many as 480 columns per record, making direct importing of scanned data relatively easy. Mainframe packages may require that data be presented in an 80-column format so that the user may have to do some editing prior to uploading to a mainframe. Nevertheless, this can be done once for a particular form and saved in the SE so that future uses of the form can be converted to an 80-column format. Data recorded in identification number and special codes fields are scanned into the file as they appear on the form, for example, 1017 as the value of a subject number. Item options recorded on the answer sheet are scanned as a 1, 2, 3, and so on, depending upon the option chosen by the respondent. File utilities in the AB make it possible to change the file to a different format, such as the data interchange format, if this is required by the particular application package being used to analyze data.

Although ScanTools™ is somewhat more complicated to use than MTSII, with a reasonable amount of computer literacy and some time devoted to learning it is not difficult to master. An earlier version of the package contained some form applications making it easier to use immediately. It is the author's opinion that NCS has lessened the "user friendliness" of the package by not providing at least some forms applications with the software.

ScanTools™ Applications. The author has conducted a number of studies dealing with validation of a patient learning style questionnaire. The instruments used with this research have been carefully planned so that data are transferred onto standard NCS answer sheets and entered into the computer using the ScanTools™ software. This same procedure can be used for a wide variety of applications in a school of nursing. For example, many schools perform follow-up surveys of their graduates to collect information about program quality. Designing survey instruments that can be answered directly on answer sheets by the graduates can save considerable time with data coding and entry. In the author's experience patient and subject answer sheet completion has not proven to be successful. Nevertheless, it is easier to train student workers or research assistants to transfer data from questionnaires onto answer sheets than to input data from the keyboard into a computer. Additionally, the answer sheets are a permanent hard copy of the data; they can be rescanned easily if errors occur in data file management once the database has been created. Who has not experienced frantic calls from assistants claiming that "the data are no longer in the file" and, therefore, a significant amount of data need to be reentered by hand.

Descriptive and survey data are most easily adapted for scanned input. Self-report measures of personal characteristics, attitudes, and traits are usually the focus of this type of research. Items measuring these characteristics often present a limited number of options to which the person is asked to respond. Depending upon the number of options provided, the five- or ten-option answer sheet can be used to record characteristics. The identification number and special codes sections of the answer sheet can be used to record information about a limited number of interval level variables such as subject number and age. A sample of scannable coding is provided in Figure 32.4.

DATA SCANNING RECOMMENDATIONS

The author recommends the following steps to make scanning as a way of data entry as easy as possible:

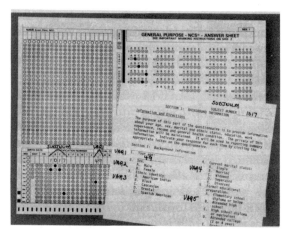

Figure 32.4 *Sample answer sheet coding.*

1. If you have central scanning procedures, check that the office has the capability to scan data and create a usable file. If they have scanning equipment and are not providing this service, lobby for it because full capability of scanning potential should be realized.

2. Select the standard answer sheet that will be used to record data while the questionnaire is being developed.

3. Define where each piece of data will be recorded on the answer sheet form. Modify items and options as necessary to fit the fields provided on the answer sheet assuming this does not compromise studying the particular research questions being addressed.

4. Code a copy of the questionnaire with the names of variables and the fields where the data will be located during scanning.

5. Decide on the statistical package that will be used to analyze data and determine what file form is needed to input data into the package. If possible, choose a package that imports an ASCII file and allows a variable record length to be used in order to avoid having to make file conversions after the data have been scanned.

SUMMARY

Optical scanning technology can speed up many of the daily tasks of data management that take place in a school of nursing. In spite of the fact that desktop scanners are available, few faculty seem to be taking advantage of this technology to locally score examinations and build a database for further analysis. Being able to use these data in a timely manner close to their point of origin could result in smoother operations and greater data accuracy.

REFERENCES

Cox, H. C., Harsanyi, B., & Dean, L. C. (1987). *Computers and nursing: Application to practice, education and research*. Norwalk, CT: Appleton & Lange.

National Computer Systems. (1989a). *Micro-TEST™ Score II Plus User's Guide* [Computer program, Pub. #202 157 327, Revision E.]. Minneapolis: Author.

National Computer Systems. (1989b). *Operator's Guide for the Sentry™ 3000 Scanner* [Computer Program, Pub. #202 151 981, Revision D.]. Minneapolis: Author.

Polit, D. F., & Hungler, B. P. (1991). *Nursing research: Principles and methods* (4th Ed.). Philadelphia: J. B. Lippincott.

National Computer Systems. (1988). *Scan-Tools™ Application Base User's Guide* [Computer program, Pub. #202 158 317, Revision C.]. Minneapolis: Author.

33

A Computerized Diagnostic Reasoning Evaluation System for Nursing Practice and Education

Jean M. Arnold

INTRODUCTION

This chapter describes a computerized diagnostic reasoning evaluation system based on decision theory. The idea for its development emerged from a study of undergraduate and graduate nursing students' responses to written simulations. That research has been described previously (Arnold, 1988). The goal of the study was to develop a generic software program that would score simulations (situations) objectively and consistently.

The writer participated in the first Measurement Conference sponsored by the University of Maryland. Participants were expected to develop a measurement tool for nursing practice and education. The computerized diagnostic reasoning evaluation system known as U-Diagnose® Program (see note p. 320) evolved from this experience and subsequent research by the writer.

REVIEW OF LITERATURE

The review of the literature consisted of an examination of the use of written simula-

tions in nursing. Early descriptions of nurses' reasoning processes focused on the decisions nurses made about observations and data collection. Researchers questioned what determined the clinician's selection of observations and data. Clinicians' choices were referred to as clinical judgments (Verhonick, 1968). According to information processing theory, the human's memory capacity affects its cognitive processing of data. The short-term memory of the human mind causes people to narrow their data choices. A human's experience and education affects the information stored in his or her long-term memory, which in turn affects choices of data and observations (Tanner & McGuire, 1983). The data sorting process is thought to conclude with problem identification.

Nurses and physicians tend to select multiple problems (hypotheses) (Barrows & Tamblyn, 1976). The collection of additional information results in a further narrowing of the hypotheses called diagnoses. Nurses are expected to act upon their diagnoses by formulating a plan of action and then intervene. The nursing process consists of a series of steps including assessment, planning, intervention, and evaluation. The diagnosis process occurs at the end of the assessment stage and provides the basis for the plan of care (Yura & Walsh, 1978). Written care plans include goals to provide direction for their implementation and criteria to evaluate their effectiveness. Rationale may not be written, but are inherent in the nursing process. Nurse educators ask novices to identify verbally, or in writing, their rationale for their action choices. Each component of the written care plan involves decision making. The categorization of data for the assessment and action plans comprises the diagnostic reasoning model used in the software.

COMPUTERIZED DIAGNOSTIC REASONING EVALUATION SYSTEM

The computerized diagnostic reasoning evaluation system (U-Diagnose Program) measures the cognitive processes associated with diagnostic reasoning. In the U-Diagnose Program, assessment consists of problem identification and data collection. Figure 33.1 illustrates the flow of information required for the problem identification stage

of diagnostic reasoning. Planning consists of delineating major diagnoses and selecting related objectives, criteria actions, and rationale. Figure 33.2 illustrates the diagnostic reasoning processes for action plans.

The diagnostic reasoning model inherent in the U-Diagnose Program evolved from the use of six simulations with 141 subjects. A three-member expert panel judged the subjects' answers for the six simulations. The reliability and validity procedures used in this study have been described elsewhere (Arnold, 1988). This research confirmed the diagnostic reasoning protocols and provided a foundation for the scoring system.

Design

The diagnostic reasoning model was transferred to a flow chart which was used as the algorithm for a computer program. The writer collaborated with a systems analyst at Rutgers, The State University of New Jersey in producing the U-Diagnose Program. The development process was tedious and time consuming, requiring more than two years. PASCAL was the programming language choice because it was the only

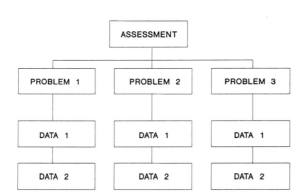

Figure 33.1 U-Diagnose assessment model. (Source: *U-Diagnosis Situation Tests* by J. M. Arnold, 1991. Copyright © 1991, by J. M. Arnold. Used by permission.)

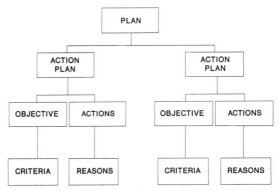

Figure 33.2 U-Diagnose plan model. (Source: *U-Diagnosis Situation Tests* by J. M. Arnold, 1991. Copyright © 1991, by J. M. Arnold. Used by permission.)

structured and compiled language available for the IBM personal computer (PC) at the time of development. The IBM PC was selected because of its availability both in the nursing and computer services divisions at the development site. Initially, the U-Diagnose Program consisted of a scoring system, and users read a written situation and wrote their responses on an answer sheet. Written answers were necessary because, at the time, a low level of computer literacy existed among nursing students and practicing nurses. Other design considerations included the following:

1. All responses would be made as choices from lists.

2. All answers would be numeric data.

3. Assessment component would be comprised of initial problems with supporting data taken directly from the scenario within the situation.

4. Planning component would consist of action plans including major hypotheses with related objectives, criteria, actions, and rationale.

5. No feedback would be provided during the entering of responses.

6. Six diagnostic reasoning protocols would be divided into a two-part answer sheet. Part one would consist of problem identification (assessment) and part two, planning.

7. Scoring system would generate a quantitative score for the assessment and planning sections.

8. Scoring system would yield ratings for assessment, hypothesis, actions, and rationale components.

9. A printout would provide a profile of an individual's diagnostic reasoning processes for a given situation.

10. Computerized diagnostic reasoning evaluation system would be a testing tool and be treated with corresponding security measures.

11. Definitions of terms would be provided to respondent.

12. Each U-Diagnose Situation Test would consist of one situation.

13. The U-Diagnose Program would run on equipment with limited memory and no special video adaptors.

14. Software would be generic, allowing for its use in other disciplines.

During the process of development, the computerized diagnostic reasoning evaluation system was granted a United States Patent (Arnold, Greenhalgh, & Rutgers, The State University, 1990). The outcome was a generic software program consisting of two disks: a test disk and scoring disk. The test disk is used for data entry and the scoring disk is used for grading the respondents' choices.

Using a U-Diagnose Nursing Situation Test

A U-Diagnose Situation Test can run on an IBM or IBM compatible microcomputer requiring minimum memory (128K).

When the program is started, a welcome screen is displayed. The software begins with a request for the user's name and unique identification number. Then the user is presented with a brief description of the testing process. Next, the problem identification answering sheet appears with function key choices at the bottom of the screen. The function keys allow the user to access the situation and lists of problems, objectives, criteria, actions and rationale. The narrative scenario, varying in length from one to several screens, begins with directions for the problem identification section and definition of terms. The user moves back and forth from the scenario to the problem listing to complete the problem identification section. Figure 33.3 illustrates the problem identification answer sheet and a sample problem listing. The left side of the screen is used for displaying information, and the right side of the screen is used for entering data. There is no limit on the number of problem choices. Supporting data are phrases within the scenario that are relevant to a specific problem.

The planning section requires the user to refer to the problem listing a second time to identify the major problems for the situation (diagnoses). A listing of objectives, criteria, actions, and rationale is provided for the user to make choices and enter them by number. Figure 33.4 illustrates the action plan answer sheet and sample action choices.

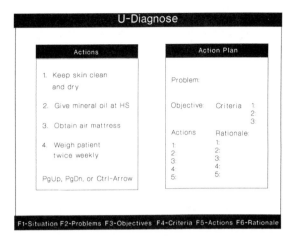

Figure 33.4 U-Diagnose actions and action plan. (Source: *U-Diagnose Program* by J. M. Arnold & W. H. Greenhalgh, 1989, Newark, NJ: Rutgers, The State University. Copyright © 1990, by J. M. Arnold, W. H. Greenhalgh, & Rutgers, The State University. Reprinted by permission.)

Scoring the Test

Although the scoring system required extensive testing, it does work with a variety of

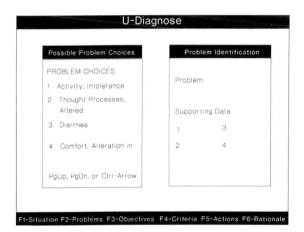

Figure 33.3 U-Diagnose problem choices and problem identification answer sheet. (Source: *U-Diagnose Program* by J. M. Arnold & W. H. Greenhalgh, 1989, Newark, NJ: Rutgers, The State University. Copyright © 1990, by J. M. Arnold, W. H. Greenhalgh, & Rutgers, The State University. Reprinted by permission.)

simulations as desired originally. The scoring disk is used in conjunction with the test disk. An answer key can be created on a word processor and entered as a text file. The answer key must differentiate between major and minor problem choices and include only correct problems, objectives, criteria, action, and rationale. The scoring disk can be used to grade one or several subjects simultaneously. The scoring process terminates with a detailed printout which is an individual profile of each user's diagnostic reasoning for the given situation. The U-Diagnose Program yields an objective score for each of the two sections and a total score. The computer printout reveals the learner's problem choices and indicates if supporting data are correct. Each action plan is delineated indicating if choices made are correct or incorrect. General classifications of ratings for assessment, hypotheses, actions, and rationale are "valid," "some validity," and "without validity." If responses are mostly correct, a valid response is obtained; if responses are a mixture of correct and incorrect, a rating of some validity is given. If the responses are more incorrect than correct, a rating of irrelevant validity or without validity is given. Scoring is determined by comparing the user's responses with answer key. Figure 33.5 is a partial U-Diagnose printout. Interpretation sheets are provided for users.

The scoring disk has been used in-house and is not available for distribution at the present time. Instead, U-Diagnose Situation Tests are being marketed as situations with the scoring service available from the developers (Arnold & Greenhalgh, 1991). The U-Diagnose Situation Tests can be purchased in paper or disk versions. The decision to sell the tests and not the scoring disk was made due to the specialized needs of outside users for a modification of the scoring system. One user group requested scoring only of the assessment section as a measure of teaching strategies for nursing diagnosis; another user in social work requested scoring of assessment, major problems, and actions; a nursing service department desired use of problems, actions, and rationale to evaluate competencies of practicing nurses.

TESTING OF U-DIAGNOSE SITUATION TESTS

The development and testing process for a U-Diagnose Situation Test has been described elsewhere (Arnold, 1990). Written versions of the simulations were used initially and then modified for microcomputer use. The inclusion of the scenario on the test disk resulted in shortening of the situations. Too much information on the screen interfered with the diagnostic reasoning pro-

---

U-Diagnose Situation Test Printout: Miss G.
Student Number: 0102034 PROBLEM IDENTIFICATION SECTION

Problem number: 1 Diversional Activity Deficit

Data Phrases: 4 True
              5 True
              7 False
            15 False

Problem ID Rating: Assessment with some validity

Section Score: 23 out of 40

ACTION SECTION

Problem number: Diversional Activity Deficit

Objective: 8 Correct

Criteria 1: 7 Correct
Criteria 2: 5 Incorrect
Criteria 3: 4 Correct
Action: 10 Correct   Action: 15 Correct
Rationale: 27 Incorrect   Rationale: 25 Incorrect
Action Rating: Correct Intervention
Rationale Rating: Mixed Rationale

Figure 33.5 U-Diagnose situation test printout. (Source: *U-Diagnose Program* by J. M. Arnold & W. H. Greenhalgh, 1989, Newark, NJ: Rutgers, The State University. Copyright © 1990, by J. M. Arnold, W. H. Greenhalgh, & Rutgers, The State University. Reprinted by permission.)

cesses. The problem component of a North American Nursing Diagnosis Association (NANDA) nursing diagnosis has been used in problem listings for nursing situations. The writing of uniform objectives, criteria, actions, and rationale was more difficult because a taxonomy of these components is not available in nursing. The structure for these diagnostic reasoning protocols is based on the format used in written nursing care plans. A verb was used to describe actions of the nurse. An example of the format for actions is illustrated in Figure 33.4. U-Diagnose situations have been used to test baccalaureate nursing students' diagnostic reasoning about acute and chronic care at two schools. The nursing management U-Diagnose Situation Test has been used to compare expert and novice nurses' ability to manage care.

OUTCOMES

The formation of a database of nursing diagnoses with related objectives, criteria, actions, and rationale was an outcome of the writing of six gerontological nursing situations. The use of a custom item analysis interface with a U-Diagnose Situation Test resulted in detailed descriptions of a group's responses (Arnold, 1991). Results of these studies indicate that U-Diagnose Situation Tests measure different behaviors than other written and performance tests of decision making (Arnold, 1991). U-Diagnose is a microcomputer program that will score situations in a uniform manner and measure diagnostic reasoning across disciplines. The diagnostic reasoning model can be used to teach novices how to relate data to problems and develop action plans. U-Diagnose Situation Tests can be used as summative evaluation measures within educational programs as well as preparation for licensing and cer-

tification examinations in nursing. The challenge is to develop more tests of this nature. Future applications of this software will include its interface with intelligent tutoring systems.

REFERENCES

Arnold, J. M. (1988). Diagnostic reasoning protocols for clinical simulations in nursing. In O. L. Strickland, & C. F. Waltz (Eds.), *Measurement of nursing outcomes: Measuring nursing performance: Practice, education and research* (Vol. 2, pp. 53–75). New York: Springer.

Arnold, J. M. (1990). Development and testing of a diagnostic reasoning simulation. In C. F. Waltz, & O. L. Strickland (Eds.), *Measurement of nursing outcomes: Measuring clinical skills and professional development in education and practice* (Vol. 3, pp. 85–101). New York: Springer.

Arnold, J. M. (1991). Custom item analysis interface with a U-diagnose gerontological nursing simulation. In E. J. S. Hovenga, K. J. Hannah, K. A. McCormick, & J. S. Ronald (Eds.), *Lecture notes in medical informatics: Nursing informatics '91* (pp. 541–544). New York: Springer-Verlag.

Arnold, J. M., & Greenhalgh, W. H. (1989). *U-Diagnose* [Computer program]. Newark: Rutgers, The State University.

Arnold, J. M., & Greenhalgh, W. H. (1991). Miss G. U-Diagnose situation test: Acute gerontological nursing care, Mr. Rex U-diagnose situation test: Community gerontological nursing care & Mrs. Luxo U-diagnose situation test: Community gerontological nursing care. In C. Bolwell (Ed.), *Directory of educational software for nursing* (4th ed.) (pp. 424–430). New York: National League for Nursing and Athens, Ohio: Fuld Institute for Technology in Nursing Education.

Arnold, J. M., Greenhalgh, W. H., & Rutgers, The State University. (1990). Patent number: 4,895,518 Computerized diagnostic reasoning evaluation system. *Official Gazette of U.S. Patent & Trademark Office: Patents, 1,110* (4), 1803.

Barrows, H. S., & Tamblyn, R. M. (1976). An evaluation of problem-based learning in small groups utilizing simulated patient. *Journal of Medical Education, 51*, 52–54.

Tanner, C. A., & McGuire, C. (1983). Research on clinical judgment. In W. L. Holozemer (Ed.), *Review of research in nursing education* (pp. 2–32). Thorofare, NJ: Slack.

Verhonick, P. (1968). I came, I saw, I responded: Nursing observation and action survey. *Nursing Research,* 17 (1), 38–44.

Yura, H., & Walsh, M. B. (1978). *The nursing process: assessing, planning, implementation, evaluating* (3rd ed.). New York: Appleton-Century-Crofts.

Note: The U-Diagnose® trademark was designated in February, 1992, as book was going to press. See trademark list.

Section Seven
Nursing Research about
Computer Applications

This section presents research about computer applications in nursing education with implications for nursing practice. An innovative use of an application database and computer assisted simulations with nursing students to teach and evaluate documentation of nursing process is presented by Krumme.

Jacobs and dela Cruz share the development process of their informatics survey instrument and the results of its use with graduate nursing students. The findings illustrate the need for integrating informatics in graduate education.

Mikan and Aiken compiled self-reports of more than 500 undergraduate nursing programs of instructional and non-instructional use of computers. These findings are important to know due to their similarity to other regional surveys during the same time period.

Thiele and Holloway describe the creation of their taxonomy for classifying decision making attributes of computer-based simulations. The taxonomy helps the nurse educator choose low-level as well as high-level decision making simulations and thereby increases the learner's ability to problem solve.

Arnold concludes the text by sharing her student software evaluation form. The instrument's use with one class of students to evaluate eight computer assisted instructional programs is described.

34

Computer Learning Experiences to Develop and Measure Nursing Process Competencies

Ursel Krumme

INTRODUCTION

Nurse educators are continually challenged to develop and measure nursing process outcomes (American Association of Colleges of Nursing, 1986; Strickland & Waltz, 1988; Waltz & Neuman, 1988; Waltz & Strickland, 1990). New technologies in clinical practice, particularly the increasing use of computerized care plans, add another dimension to this challenge (Summers, Ratliff, Becker, & Resler, 1989). Higher acuity levels also heighten the need for better preparation of students in nursing process skills. The purpose of this chapter is to provide the nurse educator with teaching–learning strategies involving the use of computers to enhance the development and measurement of nursing process outcomes of students. The author presents two alternative approaches which have been used during the past five years in a baccalaureate program: a learning experience using computerized care plans with peer assessment health appraisal data and computer patient simulations.

REVIEW OF THE LITERATURE

Nursing Process Competencies: Expected Behaviors for Practice

Nursing process competence continues to be an essential educational outcome of baccalaureate programs, as reaffirmed by the most recent national study conducted by the American Association of Colleges of Nursing (1986): "every program preparing nurses for the first professional degree should include educational experiences for each of the essentials" (p. 1). In another recent study comparing the use of clinical evaluation tools between hospitals and affiliated baccalaureate programs, Grabbe (1988) reported that nursing process competencies tended to be assessed in both environments; the inclusion of these behaviors "points to shared emphasis on these behaviors in schools and hospitals" (p. 396).

Given this emphasis, there is then also a continuing need to explore educational experiences which promote such competencies. Most nursing service administrators

The author gratefully acknowledges the support of a Seattle University Summer Fellowship.

"strongly agree" that the following behaviors were among those which were expected, but not evidenced in nursing practice of baccalaureate degree graduates: selects and organizes relevant data in a systematic manner, records data, formulates a plan of care with client and health care professionals, specifies nursing actions necessary to assist client to goal achievement, initiates actions designated by plan of care, and maintains the "Standards of Practice" of the American Nurses' Association (Joyce-Nagata, Reeb, & Burch, 1989). The same authors conclude that "a predominant deficit seemed to be . . . in the application of the nursing process" and recommend "further study of nursing curriculum in relation to activities and experiences that facilitate and enable students to meet competencies" (p. 321).

The Use of Computer Care Plans for Documenting Nursing Process

In the early 1980s, computer documentation of nursing care was considered to be among the emerging health care technologies (U.S. Department of Health and Human Survey, Office of Health Research, Statistics, and Technology, 1981). One writer, in referring to this report, asks, "As we approach our challenges for the technological future, what necessary educational adaptations will prepare nurses for the changing health care environment . . . of documenting nursing practice?" (McCormick, 1984, p. 381). Perlich (1986), in delineating the issues of health care economics from both the service and education perspectives, identifies "the need for faculty to change the nursing school curriculum to more accurately reflect the realities of health care today" and cites one of the issues for curricular change to "include communication/coordination strategies: use of the computer" (p. 6). Such calls were accompanied by findings that computerized care plans in the clinical area were available to the students of only 21 percent of (generic)

baccalaureate programs surveyed, while 59 percent indicated that none or only a few recent graduates were prepared to apply computer technology in nursing practice (National League for Nursing, 1986).

Documenting nursing practice is now cited as a recommended informatics competency identified for the practicing nurse (Peterson & Gerdin-Jelner, 1988). A related resolution for nursing informatics was passed at the National League for Nursing 1991 Convention: "That nurse . . . educators identify ways in which the learning needs of nurses and nursing students for nursing informatics can be met" (National League for Nursing, 1991). Sinclair (1989), in addressing this educational task, posits that "conveying content related to computer applications for nursing presents unusual challenges to an instructor" and advocates "hands-on experiences which will enhance comprehension of the concepts . . . if time and resources permit" (p. 82).

INTRODUCTION OF COMPUTER EXPERIENCES IN CARE PLANNING IN A BACCALAUREATE PROGRAM

In 1986, the introduction of computerized care plans at a Seattle medical center, with plans under way at other affiliated clinical agencies, underscored the urgency of providing appropriate learning experiences in Seattle University's baccalaureate nursing curriculum. University funding of a School of Nursing proposal ($6,000) made implementation possible. Criteria for computer care plan program selection were: (1) microcomputer compatibility (IBM); (2) compatibility with the nursing diagnosis approach; (3) free text data-entry capability; and (4) cost within funded budget. Software chosen by the faculty was the RNact Corporation (1989) *Nursing Careplan Generator* (1984). All junior-level students participated as part of the requirements for a 5-credit

Health Appraisal course. A one-hour orientation to the RNact software program was provided. Instructions were posted in the computer laboratory to provide cues for recall of software commands.

Computer Care Plan Experience in Health Appraisal Laboratory (Lab)

Three classes were required to submit a printed standardized nursing care plan as well as an individualized nursing care plan weekly. Data for nursing care plans were based on health appraisals of students elicited from peer partners. Students individualized the RNact standard nursing care plan for the components nursing diagnoses, related interventions, and patient objectives and then highlighted these changes with a yellow marker for easier review and comparison by faculty. Figures 34.1 and 34.2 illustrate selected items from health appraisals on a peer and an individualized care plan: "Non-Compliance R/T Failure to Participate in Monthly Breast Self-Exam (BSE)."

Examiner: _____

Client's Initials: _____

LAB RESPONSE SHEET FOR ASSESSMENT OF BREASTS AND AXILLAE

I. Interview Data:

   Sex: F   Age: 25   Race/Ethnic Background: Caucasian   L.M.P.: 9/18/88

   A. Review the results of the "Breast Cancer Risk Scale"

      1. Score: 85

      2. Meaning of score: Practice BSE q. month and have breast examination by an M.D. or nurse practitioner q. 3 yrs. Client does not practice BSE.

   B. Symptomatic complaints: Tenderness approx. 1 week prior to the start of menstrual cycle.

II. Objective Data (sample of one area addressed):

   A. Inspection:

      1. Breasts:

         a. Size: bilaterally equal with left slightly > right; chest diameter 36"; states wears a B-cup bra

         b. Symmetry: has no marked asymmetry; states she has had no unilateral increase in size

         c. Contour: bilaterally smooth, convex, even contour without dimpling retractions, fixation

         d. Skin color/texture: silver-toned striae bilaterally; light pink breasts with darker pink areola; no erythema

         e. Venous pattern: bilaterally even venous patterns

         f. Nevi/moles: generalized nevi bilaterally on upper inner quadrants and on sternum; client reports no tenderness nor recent changes in nevi

Figure 34.1 Nursing database: selected items from Health Appraisals on Peer. (Underlined material = Peer data.)

MEDICAL I-Z LIBRARY REFERENCE: NON-COMPLIANCE*

NURSING DIAGNOSIS: Noncompliance r/t failure to participate in monthly breast self-exam (BSE)

RELATED INTERVENTIONS:
1. Assess client's attitude towards BSE and possible reasons for lack of performance (such as cultural values or just lack of time)
2. Assess previous knowledge regarding BSE technique and breast disease
3. Assess client's willingness and readiness to learn or relearn BSE

PATIENT OBJECTIVES:
1. Client able to perform BSE on return demonstration
2. Client will see a benefit in performing BSE monthly and carry technique learned into lifestyle
3. Client will be able to relate signs of breast disease and cancer

*RNact Corporation (1984)

Figure 34.2 Individualized nursing care plan: selected items from Health Appraisals on Peer.

Student Response to Computer Care Plan Experience in Health Appraisal Lab

Three classes of junior-year baccalaureate students subsequently participated in the computerized care plan learning experience. The majority of these students reported use of computers prior to this learning experience (see Table 34.1); almost all of the respondents (98%) felt that computer skills were necessary or would be necessary for work as a nurse in clinical settings. Most students were female; exceptions were: class of 1988, one of 54; class of 1989, twelve of 58; and class of 1990, three of 54. Mean age of respondents ranged from 25 to 27 for the three classes.

Data were collected for measuring students' affective responses to these learning experiences using a semantic differential five-step scale with bipolar adjectives for the variables of computer use: interesting, simple, friendly and comfort level (ratings: 1 = lowest; 5 = highest). Means on the semantic differential of students' affective responses about computers prior and after their use in Health Appraisal for total group, those with and those without prior computer experience are presented in Table 34.2. It was hypothesized that there would be a significant change in the affective responses (in the positive direction) following the learning experiences of writing computerized care plans in the Health Appraisal course. Using one-tail t-tests of significance, these hypotheses were supported for total student group. The exception was for the variable "boring-interesting" for those with prior computer experience in the class of 1988 (see Table 34.2). These findings lend support to those reported by Jacobson, Holder and Dearner (1989) that computer education and experience are associated with decreased anxiety.

Data on students' self-timed care plan

Table 34.1 Three Classes' Use of RNact Program By Percentage (Number): 1988–1990

	Group with Prior Computer Experience	Group with No Prior Computer Experience	Total Sample
Class of 1988	67 (36)	33 (18)	100 (54)
Class of 1989	53 (31)	47 (27)	100 (58)
Class of 1990	57 (31)	43 (23)	100 (54)

Table 34.2   Means on Semantic Differential Before and After Computer Experiences in Care Planning: Class of 1988, 1989, and 1990

	Group with Prior Computer Experience		Group with No Prior Computer Experience		Total Sample	
	Before	**After**	**Before**	**After**	**Before**	**After**
Class of 1988:						
Boring-Interesting	3.97	4.11	3.22	4.78*	3.72	4.33*
Complex-Simple	2.89	3.92*	2.00	4.33*	2.59	4.06*
Unfriendly-Friendly	3.44	4.00*	2.17	4.50*	3.02	4.17*
Uncomfortable-Comfortable	3.25	4.22*	2.06	4.61*	2.85	4.35*
Class of 1989:						
Boring-Interesting	3.65	4.23†	2.63	4.11*	3.17	4.17*
Complex-Simple	2.97	4.39*	1.74	4.07*	2.40	4.24*
Unfriendly-Friendly	3.19	4.29*	2.15	4.07*	2.71	4.19*
Uncomfortable-Comfortable	3.32	4.35*	1.89	4.07*	2.66	4.22*
Class of 1990:						
Boring-Interesting	3.61	4.00†	3.00	3.83*	3.35	3.93*
Complex-Simple	3.35	4.13*	2.52	4.00*	3.00	4.07*
Unfriendly-Friendly	3.39	3.94*	2.87	4.04*	3.17	3.98*
Uncomfortable-Comfortable	3.65	4.13*	2.87	4.17*	3.31	4.15*

(Ratings: 1 = lowest; 5 = highest)
* $p < .01$
† $p < .05$

transactions for all three classes also revealed a significant decrease: whereas average times of 32, 27, and 25 minutes were needed to print a standardized care plan the first two weeks, it only took 12 or 13 minutes thereafter; likewise, whereas it took 39, 43 or 44 minutes to print an individualized care plan the first two weeks, it took only 22 or 23 minutes the remainder of the quarter (see Table 34.3; mean number of edited lines ranged from 13–15 the first two weeks and 16–20 the remainder of the quarter). These data come close to the 15 minutes needed on average by staff nurses for initiating a computerized diagnoses-based care plan as reported by Mehmert (1987).

Students also responded positively to the opportunity to write weekly computerized care plans in the Health Appraisal course: mean rating for overall value of learning experience for all three classes ranged from 4.4 to 4.5 out of a maximum of 5. Ninety-two percent of the class of 1988, 94 percent of the class of 1989, and 85 percent of the class of 1990 also stated they *enjoyed* writing computerized care plans, an unexpected but welcome finding! Over 90 percent of all three classes also stated they would support the retention of the computer care plan writing experience as part of the course grade. The majority of students (84–85%) felt they received the needed assistance. Such positive responses by students to this computer learning experience are comparable with those cited by Schwirian, Malone, Stone, Nunley and Francisco (1989): "students' attitudes toward computer use in nursing were positive, and the more computer experience students had, the more positive their attitudes" (p. 168). Most recently, care planning as a computer application was identified as one of the two most preferred

Table 34.3 Mean Minutes Used for Printing Standardized and Individualized Care Plan Weeks 1 & 2 and Remainder of Quarter: Class of 1988, 1989, and 1990

	Group with Prior Computer Experience		Group with No Prior Computer Experience		Total Sample	
	Weeks 1 & 2	Remainder of Qtr.	Weeks 1 & 2	Remainder of Qtr.	Weeks 1 & 2	Remainder of Qtr.
Class of 1988:						
Standardized Plan	24	12*	51	14*	32	13*
Individualized Plan	40	20*	54	23*	43	22*
Class of 1989:						
Standardized Plan	24	10*	31	16*	27	13*
Individualized Plan	36	20*	49	23*	44	22*
Class of 1990:						
Standardized Plan	18	10*	35	14*	25	12*
Individualized Plan	35	22*	45	27*	39	23*

* $p < .01$

learning activities students would like to see used in their nursing curricula (Van Dover & Boblin, 1991, p. 78).

CURRICULAR FOLLOW-UP WITH COMPUTER PATIENT SIMULATIONS

In Fall 1989, new university "Core" requirements and a new nursing curriculum were instituted that encouraged faculty to search for creative teaching and learning approaches which actively involve students (Bean, 1991; Seattle University, 1990). They also emphasized writing skills across the curriculum and thereby served as an impetus to look for other computer learning experiences that could, at the same time, enhance the development and measurement of students' nursing process skills. Grant application and subsequent external funding (by the Helene Fuld Foundation) made additional computer teaching–learning experiences possible for course implementation.

Computer patient simulation was one strategy faculty felt could assist students in

applying nursing process knowledge in their first Nursing Care of Ill Adults theory course. The literature on the use of simulations as a teaching–learning strategy for clinical decision-making has already been described by Arnold in Chapter 19. Other studies suggest that computer simulations can also serve as a more "realistic" approach for students' introduction to essential nursing care activities (Sparks, 1989). The new curriculum also specified that students' nursing process skills would be assessed against the profession's standards of practice. In a survey of National League for Nursing-accredited BSN programs, Gaines and McFarland (1984) had earlier reported that the majority of such programs hold students accountable for nursing process competencies according to the profession's standards of practice.

"Impaired physical mobility" was the nursing diagnosis selected for the learning experience with computer care plans. This diagnosis was ranked among the ten most frequently encountered in patient care settings (Gordon, 1987). Students also were assigned, concurrently, to inpatient hospitals on orthopedic units to make use of opportunities to apply theory to practice. Criteria for computer patient simulation program selection were: (1) compatibility with selected nursing diagnosis; (2) appropriate student educational level; (3) provision of immediate feedback with rationales for choices; (4) inclusion of graphics and visuals for enhanced learning; and (5) availability of screen printing option. The software program *Simulated patient encounters in medical–surgical nursing: Patients who need help with mobility* (Gomez, 1988) was chosen by faculty. Large computer screen projection using a newly purchased liquid crystal display (LCD) unit provided an interactive instruction mode encouraging students' *active* involvement in the classroom. Students could debate the underlying rationales for their selections of nursing process activities from a list of options. After the instructor's feedback, a final choice of action was made.

Computer Care Plan Experience Using Computer Patient Simulations

Fall 1989 and 1990, students were asked to submit a printed care plan which applied the *Orthopedic nursing practice: Process and outcome criteria for selected diagnosis* (American Nurses Association and National Association of Orthopedic Nurses, 1986) for the diagnosis "Impaired physical mobility." Students could select one of three simulated patient encounters: Mr. Flint, A Gentleman with a Fractured Tibia; Mrs. Misty, A Lady with a Fractured Femur; or Mrs. Peppy, A Lady with a Hip Replacement. Individualization of the standard nursing care plan occurred in the components of nursing diagnoses, related interventions, and patient objectives and were highlighted (again using a yellow marker) by students. All students submitted a printed standardized and individualized care plan using the RNact Corporation (1989) *Nursing Careplan Generator program.*

Student Response to Computer Care Plan Experience Using Computer Patient Simulations

With the National League for Nursing's curricular accreditation process increasingly focusing on measurement of student outcomes (Waltz & Neuman, 1988), collection of learning data for this computer care plan writing experience consisted of (1) scores on test items which accompanied the selected software programs and (2) analyses of students' nursing process performance on items for simulated patients with "Impaired physical mobility" (adapted from the *Orthopedic Nursing Practice Process and Outcome Criteria* using methodology described by Krumme (1988); validity and interrater reliability testing for items retained for the simulations were accomplished Fall 1989).

Analysis of scores on test items accompanying the selected software programs revealed that 88 percent of students attained the mastery level (designated at 80%) for the three identified patient encounters in Fall 1989 and 83 percent for Fall 1990. Results from item analyses of 61 students' nursing process performance for the nursing diagnosis "Impaired physical mobility" Fall 1990 showed that a large number of the expected behaviors were also met (see Table 34.4). For example, more than 80 percent stated that the nurse assesses a client's ability to transfer/walk, functional range of motion, and muscle strength; more than 80 percent also incorporated positioning, range of motion, and muscle strengthening exercises for maintaining limb function. Nevertheless, findings also revealed that several expected nursing process behaviors were not attained at the desired 80 percent level, for example, providing pain relief measures prior to and during activity and collaboration with other health professionals. Such findings allow for a systematic evaluation of students' learning outcomes for nursing pro-

Table 34.4 Item Difficulty Summary of Students' Nursing Process Competencies by Percentage (Number) for Simulated Patients with Impaired Physical Mobility, Fall 1990

	Mr. Flint: Fx. Tibia & Cast	Mrs. Misty: Fx. Femur & Traction	Mrs. Peppy: Total Hip Replacement	All Three Simulated Patients
	a	b	c	d
A. States etiology: Impaired physical mobility "related to" client's:				
1. Imposed activity-mechanical restriction/ decreased range of motion-muscle strength and/or pain	92 (11)	100 (13)	86 (31)	90 (55)
B. Describes assessment parameters: Nurse assesses client's:				
1. Ability to turn/bed mobility skills (0-4 scale)	58 (7)	54 (7)	75 (27)	67 (41)
2. Ability to transfer/walk (0-4 scale)	75 (9)	NA (NA)	83 (30)	81 (39)
3. Functional range of joint motion (0-1800)	83 (10)	62 (8)	86 (31)	80 (49)
4. Muscle strength (0-5 assessment scale)	83 (10)	92 (12)	81 (29)	84 (51)
5. Coordination/gait pattern	75 (9)	NA (NA)	83 (30)	81 (39)
6. Comfort level (0-10 intensity scale)	83 (10)	92 (12)	92 (33)	90 (55)
C. Incorporates process criteria: Nurse assists client in maintaining function of limbs by:				
1. Encouraging bed mobility/use of trapeze	50 (6)	92 (12)	89 (32)	82 (50)
2. Positioning the individual in alignment	67 (8)	92 (12)	86 (31)	84 (51)
3. Joint range of motion exercises: upper/lower	92 (11)	92 (12)	81 (29)	85 (52)
4. Muscle strengthening exercises: upper/lower	75 (9)	85 (11)	92 (33)	87 (53)
5. Using ambulation devices: walker/ crutches	67 (8)	NA (NA)	86 (31)	81 (39)
6. Providing pain relief measures prior to/ during activity	83 (10)	77 (10)	58 (21)	67 (41)
7. Collaboration with other health professionals	67 (8)	31 (4)	50 (18)	49 (30)
D. Integrates outcome criteria: Nurse assesses client's limb function/safe movement within imposed limitations by:				
1. Participation in bed mobility activities	50 (6)	69 (9)	58 (21)	59 (36)
2. Body limbs positioned in alignment: upper/lower	42 (5)	92 (12)	83 (30)	77 (47)
3. Full range of motion of joints: upper/lower	92 (11)	100 (13)	69 (25)	80 (49)
4. 5 + Muscle Strength: upper/lower body	83 (10)	92 (12)	64 (23)	74 (45)
5. Safe use of ambulation devices in environment	92 (11)	NA (NA)	89 (32)	90 (43)
6. Comfort level for performing mobility activities	42 (5)	62 (8)	56 (20)	54 (33)

a N = 12 for all items
b N = 13 for all items
c N = 36 for all items
d N = 61 for all items except B2, B5, C5, D5 (N = 48)

cess and can serve as guides for further teaching–learning activities.

SUMMARY AND CONCLUSIONS

Learning experiences with computer care plans can assist faculty in developing and measuring student outcomes in nursing process. They allow students to practice their nursing process skills, provide opportunities for faculty to evaluate their behaviors against the profession's standards of practice, and also can be a vehicle for preparing that computer literate nurse so increasingly demanded in practice. Learning experiences with computer care plans also address the new curricular goal for nursing informatics in the curriculum (National League for Nursing, 1991). Baccalaureate programs that include health assessment courses with lab sessions may be able to implement the writing of computerized care plans as one (even enjoyable!) way to integrate computers in the curriculum. Integration of computer patient simulations for computer care planning may be yet another, perhaps even more realistic, way to develop and evaluate students' nursing process skills in a nursing theory course. Such learning experiences may even improve the preparation of students for computerized National Council Licensing Examination (NCLEX) RN examinations slated for implementation in 1993. More importantly, inclusion of such interactive, "hands-on" computer experiences described in this chapter may well provide that "missing ingredient" which is not usually included in course content (Skiba, 1985).

A word of caution, however, needs to be addressed to nurse educators contemplating learning experiences in computerized care plan writing: do *not* consider only the costs involved in initial hardware and software acquisition; be prepared for increased fac-

ulty time spent on solving initial glitches that inevitably arise; down-time of computers (encourage students to plan for sufficient lead time); loss of text by pressing the wrong key to print out plan (have students write their changes on hard copy and save the program on their own disks); failure of liquid crystal display unit for large classroom projection (instructor needs backup presentation or extraordinary extemporaneous speaking skills); incompatibility of care plan program with hospital system (instructor needs to stress hospital hardware constraints and transfer of learning principles); and so forth. In conclusion, one may ask: Does the value of implementing computer nursing care plan learning experiences in a curriculum outweigh the problems encountered? For this nurse educator, the answer is a resounding "Yes!" For better preparation of students to function in current and future clinical practice, there does not seem to be any other alternative.

REFERENCES

American Association of Colleges of Nursing. (1986). *Essentials of college and university education for professional nursing*. Washington, DC: Author.

American Nurses Association and National Association of Orthopedic Nurses. (1986). *Orthopedic nursing practice: Process and outcome criteria for selected diagnoses*. Kansas City, MO: Authors.

Bean, J. C. (1991). *Expecting excellence: A faculty guide to writing and active learning in the core curriculum at Seattle University*. Seattle: Seattle University.

Gaines, B. C., & McFarland, M. B. (1984). Nursing diagnosis: Its relationship and use in nursing education. *Topics in Clinical nursing, 5* (4), 39–49.

Gomez, S. P. (1988). *Simulated patient en-*

counters in medical-surgical nursing: Patients who need help with mobility [Computer program]. Philadelphia, PA: J. B. Lippincott.

Gordon, M. (1987). *Nursing diagnosis: Process and application* (2nd ed.). New York: McGraw-Hill.

Grabbe, L. L. (1988). A comparison of clinical evaluation tools in hospitals and baccalaureate nursing programs. *Journal of Nursing Education, 27* (9), 394–398.

Jacobson, S. F., Holder, M. E., & Dearner, J. F. (1989). Computer anxiety among students, educators, staff, and administrators. *Computers in Nursing, 7* (6), 266–272.

Joyce-Nagata, B., Reeb, R., & Burch, S. (1989). Comparison of expected and evidenced baccalaureate degree competencies. *Journal of Nursing Education, 28* (7), 314–321.

Krumme, U. (1988). Measuring baccalaureate students' nursing process competencies: A nursing diagnosis framework. In O. Strickland & C. Waltz (Eds.), *Measurement of nursing outcomes: Measuring nursing performance: Practice, education and research* (Vol. 2, pp. 252–293). New York: Springer.

McCormick, K. A. (1984). Preparing nurses for the technologic future. *Nursing & Health Care, 5* (7), 379–382.

Mehmert, P. A. (1987). A nursing information system: The outcome of implementing nursing diagnoses. *Nursing Clinics of North America, 22* (4), 943–953.

National League for Nursing. (1986). *Nursing data review: 1986.* New York: Author.

National League for Nursing. (1991). Resolutions accepted at 1991 convention. *Nursing & Health Care, 12* (7), 358.

Perlich, L. J. M. (1986). Catalyzing educational change. *Journal of Nursing Administration, 16* (1), 6.

Peterson, H. E., & Gerdin-Jelger, U. (Eds.). (1988). *Preparing nurses for using informa-tion systems: Recommended informatics competencies.* New York: National League for Nursing.

RNact Corporation. (1984). *The nursing care-plan generator* [Computer program]. LaGrange, IL.

Schwirian, P., Malone, J., Stone, V., Nunley, B., & Francisco, T. (1989). Computers in nursing practice: A comparison of the attitudes of nurses and nursing students. *Computers in Nursing, 7* (4), 168–177.

Seattle University School of Nursing. (1990). *Self-study report for the National League for Nursing.* Seattle: Seattle University.

Sinclair, V. G. (1989). Addressing challenges in nursing informatics instruction. *Journal of Nursing Education, 28* (2), 82–84.

Skiba, D. J. (1985). Interactive computer experiences: The missing ingredient. *Nursing Clinics of North America, 20* (3), 577–584.

Sparks, S. M. (1989). *Computer-based education in nursing.* Bethesda, MD: U.S. Dept. of Health and Human Services, National Institutes of Health.

Strickland, O., & Waltz, C. F. (Eds.). (1988). *Measurement of nursing outcomes: Measuring nursing performance: Practice, education and research* (Vol. 2). New York: Springer.

Summers, S., Ratliff, C., Becker, A., & Resler, M. (1989). Computerized nursing diagnosis and documentation of nursing care in inpatient health care agencies. In R. M. Carroll-Johnson (Ed.), *Proceeding of the Eighth Conference of the North American Nursing Diagnosis Association: Classification of nursing diagnoses* (pp. 270–274). Philadelphia: J. B. Lippincott.

U.S. Department of Health and Human Services, Office of Health Research, Statistics, and Technology. (1981). *1980–1981 List of emerging health care technologies.* Washington, DC: The National Center for Health Care Technology.

Van Dover, L., & Boblin, S. (1991). Student

nurse computer experience and preferences for learning. *Computers in Nursing, 9* (2), 75–79.

Waltz, C. F., & Neuman, L. H. (Eds.). (1988). *Educational outcomes: Assessment of quality* (Vol. 1–4). New York: National League for Nursing.

Waltz, C. F., & Strickland, O. (Eds.). (1990). *Measurement of nursing outcomes: Measuring clinical skills and professional development in education and practice* (Vol. 3). New York: Springer.

35

The Informatics Education Needs
of Graduate Nursing Students

Angeline M. Jacobs
Felicitas A. dela Cruz

INTRODUCTION

This chapter describes a study that determined the informatics curriculum needs of graduate nursing students at Azusa Pacific University (APU). Informatics is defined as "the field that concerns itself with the cognitive, information processing, and communication tasks of . . . practice, education, and research, including the information science and the technology to support these tasks" (Greenes & Shortliffe, 1990, p. 1114). The survey developed for this study assessed computer and information-seeking skills required for both education and advanced nursing practice, with special emphasis on retrieval of information from large databases. The immediate use of the study's findings will be to modify the curriculum for a federally funded graduate clinical specialization program in high-risk home health nursing at Azusa Pacific University. Although findings in a single institution are not necessarily generalizable to other settings, the survey instrument, with its proven reliability and content validity, could be adapted for use by other graduate nursing programs.

REVIEW OF THE LITERATURE

The need to incorporate informatics in nursing education, research, and practice has been well documented in the literature, particularly since the late 1980s (Newbern, 1985; Parks, Damrosch, Heller, & Romano,

This project was funded by a grant from the Division of Nursing, Advanced Nurse Education, U.S. Department of Health and Human Services (Grant #5 D23 NU 00820). The authors acknowledge with gratitude the contributions of the project assistant, Constance Collins, RN, who did the data entry and statistical analyses; and two nursing student assistants, Grace Mandani and Tami Mackley, who assisted with the literature search.

1986; Saba, 1982; Schwirian, Malone, Stone, Nunley, & Francisco, 1989). The review of the literature was conducted to inform and guide the development of the survey instrument.

Nurses are being challenged to develop ways of using computer technology in caring for their patients, because of spiraling technological advances (Andreoli & Musser, 1985). Indeed, while a major use of computers in the health care field is administrative, with the proliferation of large, centralized hospital information systems (Mikan, 1984), computers are used in every aspect of nursing, including practice, administration, research, and education (Armstrong, 1989). In their daily care of clients, nurses enter data and retrieve information about clients, monitor clients, diagnose nursing problems, plan care, and document care by means of computers. Saba summarized the advancement of computerized management information systems in community health nursing—systems that manage the "flow of information in the proper time frame and thus, assist in the decision-making process" (Saba, 1982, p. 510). Saba urged nurses to concentrate on research and development in the use of computers, especially on the promotion of computer applications and understanding of systems theory concepts in nursing education.

In addition to practice applications, computers abound in nursing educational and research arenas, as well. Computer literacy is becoming a necessity in nursing education, for both students and faculty (American Nurses Association, 1977). Nurse faculty need to understand computers, to be aware of their uses and potential, to become adept and comfortable in their use, and to transmit this comfort and skill to their students (Newbern, 1985). On the other hand, achieving computer competency in faculty and students is not an easy task. Newbern (1985) lists some barriers to integrating informatics

in nursing curricula: motivation, resources, control, the interface with practice, and the paucity of software. She urges sharing of scarce resources and overcoming geographical constraints in order to achieve the enormous potential of the new age of computer technology.

The need for implementation of computer technology courses in nursing curricula on a national basis is recognized by the National League for Nursing (NLN). According to the NLN, only 13.2 percent of all nursing programs and 31.3 percent of graduate nursing programs require computer courses (National League for Nursing, 1988). Following a 1987 NLN resolution promoting computer technology and its publication of the *Guidelines for basic computer education in nursing* (Ronald & Skiba, 1987), the NLN Council on Nursing Informatics requested that the Committee on Accreditation "examine the issue of technology in nursing informatics education and make recommendations about its inclusion in nursing curricula . . ." (National League for Nursing, 1989, p. 12).

The need for computer technology instruction in graduate nursing programs has been supported by a number of nursing leaders (Andreoli & Musser, 1985; Armstrong, 1989; Gothler, 1985; Romano, Damrosch, Heller, & Parks, 1989; Mikan, 1988; Newbern, 1985; Sparks, 1989). Indeed, Sparks urges not only the incorporation of informatics courses in undergraduate and graduate curricula, but also the development of graduate nursing programs to prepare nurse computer and information scientists, similar to programs in medical informatics (Sparks, 1989). Three such programs exist—at the University of Maryland, the University of Utah, and the State University of New York at Buffalo.

Two additional areas of need for the integration of informatics into graduate nursing education curricula are decision making and information seeking (Mikan, 1988). Decision analysis programs patterned after expert systems existing in medicine and other professions are beginning to emerge in nursing. These programs allow the nurse to modify the knowledge base with the addition of new information, thus increasing the nurse's clinical effectiveness (Badger, 1988). Gaston (1988) believes that the increased use of computer-model simulations in clinical teaching will result in a greater aptitude in decision-making skills and will stimulate information seeking in nursing students.

In spite of the obvious need for computer education in graduate nursing programs, there is a dearth of existing programs (Armstrong, 1989). Although the 1988 NLN report indicates that 31.3 percent of the graduate programs require computer courses, and 17.4 percent report that computer courses are available as electives, more than one-third (39.1%) do not even have computer courses available (Sparks, 1989).

Among those graduate programs that have integrated computer instruction into graduate curricula, some exemplary programs involve innovative strategies. At the University of Kansas, graduate students may enroll in a two-credit elective entitled *Computers in Nursing* (Summers, Penny, Fortin-Boyer, Loutzenhiser, & Arnold-Biogoli, 1990). This course enables "first-time computer users" to integrate and creatively link microcomputer hardware and software capabilities to solve nursing practice problems of their choice. Researchers at the University of Maryland (Romano et al., 1989) have proposed a three-level model for computer education in professional nursing: (1) basic skills for undergraduate students; (2) foundational skills for graduate nursing students preparing for advanced roles as educators, clinicians, or administrators; and (3) skills for graduate nursing students preparing for specialized roles in nursing informatics, as managers of technological innovations, systems analysts, and systems evaluators. Based on their success with the graduate foundational

course, these investigators recommend informatics education as an "essential" component of graduate nursing curricula.

PROJECT DESCRIPTION AND METHODOLOGY

The impetus for considering integration of nursing informatics into the APU graduate nursing curriculum came from a federally funded grant—the High Risk Home Health Clinical Specialty Program. In the process of developing the clinical specialization curriculum, the need for informatics skills in home health care nursing became increasingly evident. In addition to the practice applications of informatics, there was a crucial need for skills to help clinical nurse specialists cope with the explosion of information and research. To fully realize their roles as expert clinicians, consultants, educators, and researchers, the clinical specialists will have to know how to access and analyze important new knowledge as it becomes available. These information-seeking skills are especially crucial in home health care, where traditional library services are generally unavailable.

With the exception of statistical analysis, instruction in informatics is not provided within the graduate nursing courses at APU. Incorporating additional informatics content in the home health curriculum necessitates examination of the entire graduate curriculum, because home health care students take 21 of their 43 required units in common with students in other graduate nursing tracks. Thus it was necessary to survey all the graduate students to determine what might be their specific informatics needs.

Although the literature contains many survey and attitude assessment studies, none of them were especially suited to the requirements of the study. Therefore, the authors decided to develop a questionnaire specifically for the APU population. Standard instrument development procedure was used, including review of the literature, drafting of the instrument by a team of content and curriculum experts, content validation, and reliability assessment.

Questionnaire Development

The project staff, with input from an informatics expert, prepared a draft of the questionnaire. The content of the questionnaire included: (1) demographic and experiential characteristics of the students, (2) extent of use of computers, (3) types of computers and systems used by the student, (4) self-reported skill in 16 computer applications in practice and education settings, (5) types of word processing and spreadsheet software used, (6) specific questions about competency in conducting literature searches and using computerized databases, (7) an overall self-rating of extent of computer skills possessed, and (8) an open-ended comment section. A sample of the self-rating section of the questionnaire is shown in Figure 35.1.

The first draft was reviewed and revised by the graduate committee of the School of Nursing. Two undergraduate students critiqued the clarity of the questionnaire. Following revisions, the completed questionnaire was mailed to the homes of the 90 students in January 1991 as an enclosure with a newsletter from the director of the graduate nursing program. The students were urged to respond to the questionnaire and to voice their opinions in order to assist the faculty's curriculum decision-making process. The questionnaires were coded to facilitate sending reminder letters and to protect student anonymity. At no point in the data processing or analysis was any student's name associated with the data. One reminder letter was sent, two weeks after the first mailing, with a fresh copy of the questionnaire. All returns (n = 67) received came in within one month of the first mailing. A content validity analysis was conducted concurrent with the fielding of the survey to the students. Four weeks later, a test/retest reliability assessment was completed. The results of these efforts are described below.

Content Validity

Eight experts assessed the content validity of the questionnaire. Four are professors in local graduate schools of nursing; one is a nationally known nurse–researcher; one is employed in an informatics capacity by a private firm; one owns a publishing and information services company and has considerable expertise in computerized databases; and the last directs an innovative informatics program at a school of nursing in the western United States. Each expert rated the validity of each questionnaire item on a four-point scale, from 1 (not valid) to 4 (valid), in terms of whether the item tapped some aspect of computer/informatics skill or experience. All eight experts responded. A content validity index of .92 was derived, using Popham's method of average congruency (Popham, 1978). This method involves assessing the proportion of all the items rated valid by each rater and deriving the mean of the proportions for all the raters. Table 35.1 shows the number and percentages of items rated either 3 or 4 by each rater.

Reliability

The test/retest reliability was conducted on a subsample of the study population. Of the 67 respondents to the survey, 34 names were randomly selected and a letter of re-

Listed below are some uses and applications of computers. Please circle, in the first column, whether you personally have ever used a computer in the way indicated by each statement (Y = yes, N = no).

In the second column, circle the number that reflects the extent of your competence in the stated activity, using the following scale:

> 1 = Beginning knowledge, competence or experience
> 2 = Advanced knowledge, competence or experience
> 3 = Expert knowledge, competence or experience

Activities	Column 1 Do you use a computer in this way?		Column 2 Extent of Competence		
Word Processing. If yes, what type of software do you use?_____ _____	Y	N	1	2	3
Spread sheets. If yes, what type of software do you use?_____ _____	Y	N	1	2	3
Patient accounts/billing/insurance. etc.	Y	N	1	2	3
Monitoring patients' vital signs and status	Y	N	1	2	3
Retrieving information about the patient, for example medications, orders, assessment data	Y	N	1	2	3
Planning patient care	Y	N	1	2	3
Documenting care	Y	N	1	2	3
Decision analysis	Y	N	1	2	3
Using learning modules	Y	N	1	2	3
Doing statistical analyses	Y	N	1	2	3

Figure 35.1 Sample items from questionnaire on informatics education needs of graduate students.

quest was sent to them with a fresh copy of the same questionnaire. The timing of the retest was one month after final returns were received from the original survey. This amount of time is sufficient to negate the effects of memory and is short enough to obviate most learning effects or the effects of additional experience. The students were offered an honorarium of $10 for completing the second questionnaire. In a two-week period, 23 (68%) of the 34 questionnaires were returned. Following reminder calls, seven more questionnaires were received, for a total of 30 questionnaires (88%). The test/retest reliability was .86, which was the mean of the agreement scores on each of the questionnaire items when the responses of the test and retest administrations were compared.

Sample

As described in the questionnaire development section above, the questionnaire was mailed to all 90 students enrolled in the

Table 35.1 Rating of Items by Eight Content Experts

Rater	Number of Items Rated "Valid"	Proportion of Total Items with Ratings of 3 or 4 (n = 26)
1	26	1.00
2	26	1.00
3	23	.88
4	23	.88
5	23	.88
6	25	.96
7	22	.85
8	23	.88
		7.33

Content validity*: Mean = 7.33 ÷ 8 = .92

* Popham's method of average congruency (Popham, 1978).

graduate nursing program. It was completed by 67 students, with a response rate of 74 percent. The demographic characteristics of the respondents closely approximated those of the graduate nursing student population as a whole. These characteristics included length of experience in the program, focus of program of studies, enrollment in the BS/MS-articulated program for nurses with non-nursing baccalaureate degrees, and self-reported skill in 16 computer skills or applications. The demographic and experiential characteristics of the 67 respondents are summarized in Table 35.2.

Most of the respondents (51%) are enrolled in clinical specialty options and are in the regular BSN to MS track. The majority of these respondents (46%) are in clinical positions. More than one-half of the respondents (60%) have completed less than one-half of the units required for graduation. This is consistent with the fact that the graduate program is fairly new and almost all of the students are employed full time; most of them enroll in six units each semester. Eighty percent of the students are over thirty

years of age and 33 percent are over 40. They are experienced nurses; 78 percent have worked in nursing for six or more years, and 63 percent for 11 or more years.

Statistical Procedures

Descriptive statistics were used—frequencies, percentages, and measures of central tendency. Cross-tabulations and Chi Square were used to determine whether there was any difference in the responses based on:

- the respondent's experience in the program as defined by the number of units completed (more experienced respondents completed 23 units or more)
- prerequisite degree (whether the respondent was in the regular master's track or in the BS/MS articulated program for nurses with non-nursing baccalaureate degrees)
- the respondent's position (clinical positions versus all others)
- the respondent's program option (clinical versus all others)

Narrative responses were content analyzed and summarized for discussion with the graduate committee.

FINDINGS

Respondents rated their skill in specific computer applications ranging from word processing to literature searching. In addition they indicated the extent of their use of computers.

Skill in Computer Applications

While 82 percent of the respondents had word processing experience, about one-half

Table 35.2   Graduate Nursing Students: Demographic and Experiential Characteristics (n = 67)

Characteristics		Frequency and Percentage of Respondents	
Graduate Program Option			
Education track		16	(24%)
Administration track		17	(25%)
Clinical Specialty track		34	(51%)
	TOTAL	67	(100%)
Experience in Program			
Completed 23 or more units		27	(40%)
Completed less than 23 units		40	(60%)
	TOTAL	67	(100%)
Enrollment in Graduate Nursing Track			
RN with non-nursing BS/MS track		16	(24%)
RN with BSN/MS track		51	(76%)
	TOTAL	67	(100%)
Age			
22–29 years		13	(20%)
30–39 years		31	(47%)
40 or more years		22	(33%)
	TOTAL	66	(100%)
Years of Nursing Experience			
1–2 years		4	(6%)
3–5 years		11	(16%)
6–10 years		10	(15%)
11 or more years		42	(63%)
	TOTAL	67	(100%)
Current Position			
Clinical		31	(46%)
Educational		16	(24%)
Administration		13	(20%)
Other		7	(10%)
	TOTAL	67	(100%)

of those respondents had only beginning skills (see Table 35.3). Only 24 percent had some experience using spreadsheets; 21 percent had used learning modules; three percent had used computers in decision analysis applications; and 33 percent had performed statistical analyses. The percentage of respondents with skill in nursing practice applications ranged from 10 percent for patient

accounts to 58 percent for retrieving patient information from records.

Almost 50 percent of the 55 students who reported skill in word processing used Word-Perfect. Other software programs used, in order of frequency, were: Microsoft Word, MultiMate, WordStar, Word, Volkswriter, Easy Works, Microsoft Works, Symphony, First Choice, and Apple Works.

Table 35.3 Graduate Nursing Students: Self-reported Skill in Computer Use

Skills/Application	Number of Respondents	Frequency and Percentage of Respondents			
		Beginning Skill	Advanced Skill	Total Having Some Skill	No Skill
• Word processing	67	27 (40%)	28 (42%)	55 (82%)	12 (18%)**
• Spreadsheets	66	12 (18%)	4 (6%)	16 (24%)	50 (76%)*
• Learning modules	66	8 (12%)	6 (9%)	14 (21%)	52 (79%)
• Decision analysis	65	1 (1.5%)	1 (1.5%)	2 (3%)	63 (97%)
• Statistical analysis	66	15 (23%)	7 (10%)	22 (33%)	44 (67%)***
• Practice applications					
Patient accounts	63	3 (5%)	3 (5%)	6 (10%)	57 (90%)
Patient monitoring	66	7 (10.5%)	7 (10.5%)	14 (21%)	52 (79%)
Patient information	66	19 (29%)	19 (29%)	38 (58%)	28 (42%)
Med. information	66	8 (12%)	6 (9%)	14 (21%)	52 (79%)
Med. calculation	66	5 (8%)	6 (9%)	11 (17%)	55 (83%)
Care planning	66	4 (6%)	8 (12%)	12 (18%)	54 (82%)*
Documenting	66	7 (11%)	8 (12%)	15 (23%)	51 (77%)
• Literature search					
Do own search	67	12 (18%)	8 (12%)	20 (30%)	47 (70%)
Ask others to do	59	22 (37%)	21 (36%)	43 (73%)	16 (27%)**
Choose search words	57	18 (32%)	23 (40%)	41 (72%)	16 (28%)
• Use of DOS	65	—	—	29 (45%)	36 (55%)**
• Use of IBM PC	66	—	—	43 (65%)	23 (35%)**
• Use of Macintosh	64	—	—	18 (28%)	46 (72%)

Chi Square between more experienced and less experienced students.
* p < .05
** p < .01
*** p < .001

Most of the 16 respondents who reported using spread sheets used Lotus 1-2-3. Other software used, in order of frequency, included: Microsoft Excel, Symphony, Microsoft Works, Harvard Graphics, Crunch, Paradox 3, First Choice, and Apple 2E.

Literature Search Skills

While 73 percent of the respondents had asked a librarian to do a search for them, only 30 percent had ever done one themselves (see Table 35.3). These students accessed MEDLINE, CINAHL, and ERIC using DIALOGUE or CD-ROM. Forty-one students (72%) had chosen their own descriptor words for the search. In response to a question about their competence in choosing the search words, 26 students (64%) had little or no difficulty, but most of these "competent" students were in the "more experienced" group (p of Chi Square < .01). Twenty-seven percent of the respondents had never used a computerized database. Of those who had (43 respondents), 13 were familiar *only* with MEDLINE; an additional seven were familiar only with CINAHL; and nine had used both MEDLINE and CINAHL. Only eight of the respondents (12% of the entire sample) had experience with three or more databases. The databases that were reported, in order of frequency, were: MEDLINE, CINAHL, ERIC, BIOETHICS LINE, HEALTH, SOCIAL SCISEARCH, MED ETHX, and MICRO MEDIX.

Extent of Computer Use

Fifty-three of the 67 respondents (79%) reported that they are required to use a computer at work, school situations, or at home, and 64 (95%) have access to a computer, either at home, at work, or at school. As indicated in Table 35.3, more students use IBM or IBM compatible systems (65%) than Macintosh (28%). Less than one-half of all the respondents have some skill in using Disk Operating System (DOS). Those students who have been in the program longer more often reported skill in using IBM microcomputers and DOS.

Self-rating of Informatics Competency

Seventy-eight percent of the students felt they needed to develop computer skills for either home, work, or school situations; 19 percent would like some advanced skills; and 3 percent felt they have good computer skills. The more experienced students indicated that they needed advanced skills more often than did the less experienced students, who more often indicated that they needed beginning skills. The specific areas of advanced skills desired were: report presentation, manuscript preparation, literature searching, statistical analysis, graphics, spreadsheets, designing forms, research, and business applications.

General Comments

Seventeen students wrote comments that were supportive of integrating informatics into the graduate curriculum. More than one-half of these respondents said they needed training and would welcome a course in computers. One student commented that a prerequisite computer course for the required course in quantitative research would have been helpful because there was not enough time in the research course to assimilate the computer knowledge. Two students criticized the editing program for SPSS in the student computer lab (which has since been changed). Many of the students indicated that owning or having access to a computer was very useful and even fun, but that they needed to learn more. The dilemma for these students is captured in one comment, as follows: "I never felt I needed a computer until after I had one. Now I don't know how I got along for so long without one. I only wish I knew more about them. All my knowledge has been self-taught and there are definite gaps in what I am able to do."

SUMMARY

The major finding was that graduate students required education in almost all the computer applications addressed. The need is strongly related to experience in the program, as defined by the number of units completed toward the master's degree. In Table 35.3, significance levels are indicated for the Chi Square determinations between students with more experience and those with less experience, as defined by number of units earned. Students who had completed more than one-half of the units toward the degree more often reported skills than did those with fewer units.

The need is unrelated to the prerequisite degree held by the student (i.e., BSN or BS in a non-nursing field). Nevertheless, when responses were cross-tabulated by the respondent's focus of specialization (as defined by specialization area and employment position) there was a predictable positive relationship—although not always statistically significant (Table 35.4). Those respondents with a clinical specialization focus or in clinical positions more often reported skills in clinical applications than did those in other specializations or positions. The re-

Table 35.4 Graduate Nursing Students: Self-reported Skill by Specialization Area and Employment Position

Skills	Specialization Area		Employment Position	
	Respondents[1] Indicating Skill	Significance of χ^2	Respondents[2] Indicating Skill	Significance of χ^2
Word processing				
Clinical	30 (86%)	.35	34 (81%)	.42
Other	25 (88%)		21 (84%)	
Spreadsheets				
Clinical	7 (21%)	.11	7 (17%)	.03*
Other	10 (31%)		10 (40%)	
Patient accounts				
Clinical	4 (11%)	.25	4 (9%)	.42
Other	2 (6%)		2 (8%)	
Patient monitoring				
Clinical	10 (29%)	.07	12 (29%)	.03*
Other	4 (13%)		2 (8%)	
Using patient information				
Clinical	21 (60%)	.47	28 (67%)	.05*
Other	17 (53%)		10 (40%)	
Obtaining med. information				
Clinical	7 (20%)	.28	9 (21%)	.29
Other	6 (19%)		4 (16%)	
Calculating med. dosage				
Clinical	5 (14%)	.44	8 (19%)	.10
Other	6 (19%)		3 (12%)	
Patient care planning				
Clinical	8 (23%)	.12	8 (19%)	.19
Other	4 (13%)		4 (16%)	
Documenting care				
Clinical	11 (31%)	.05*	10 (24%)	.20
Other	4 (13%)		5 (20%)	
Decision analysis				
Clinical	1 (3%)	.48	1 (2%)	.46
Other	1 (3%)		1 (4%)	
Using learning modules				
Clinical	7 (20%)	.43	9 (21%)	.47
Other	7 (22%)		5 (20%)	
Statistical analysis				
Clinical	12 (34%)	.14	12 (29%)	.48
Other	10 (31%)		10 (40%)	

[1] There were 35 students in clinical tracks and 32 in all other graduate program tracks.
[2] There were 42 students in clinical positions and 25 in all other positions.
* $p < .05$

verse was true for the use of word processing or spread sheet applications, in which clinically oriented students less often reported skills than did the other students. In decision analysis and the use of learning modules there was virtually no difference.

For statistical analysis applications, the results were mixed—more students in the clinical specialization option, but fewer in clinical positions, reported skill in this application.

The findings support the need for integrating informatics into the curriculum. Areas of need include: computer literacy and grasp of basic skills, especially the use of DOS, word processing, spreadsheets, learning modules; statistical analysis; decision analysis applications; nursing practice applications; information searching; and the use of large computerized databases. Still, many questions need to be answered. Given the strong relationship between student experience in the program and level of skill, there is a need to determine how and where these students obtain experience in informatics. Some of it is probably through program courses, either directly, as in the quantitative research course (where students learn to use SPSS), or indirectly because certain skills are required by the demands of the course (e.g., literature searching). Other questions are: What is the best placement of informatics content in the curriculum? Should it be in one course or should parts of it be integrated into many courses? Are there other resources in the community through which students can acquire the skills they need in a time frame and at a cost they can afford? As curriculum changes are planned, successful models in place at other graduate nursing programs, such as at the University of Maryland, will be examined. In this information age, there is no longer a choice regarding involvement with computers. It is now nursing education's charge to be as responsive as possible to student needs and to provide them with the informatics knowledge and experiences that will help them fully realize their professional growth potential.

REFERENCES

American Nurses Association. (1977). *Computers in nursing education.* Kansas City, MO: American Nurses Association.

Andreoli, K., & Musser, L. A. (1985). Computers in nursing care: The state of the art. *Nursing Outlook, 33* (1), 16–21.

Armstrong, M. L. (1989). Computer competencies identified for nursing staff development educators. *Journal of Nursing Staff Development, 5* (4), 187–191.

Badger, L. (1988). A nurse's view of technology. *Computers in Healthcare, 9* (2), 31–32.

Gaston, S. (1988). Knowledge, retention, and attitude effects of computer-assisted instruction. *Journal of Nursing Education, 27* (1), 30–34.

Gothler, A. (1985). Nursing education update: Computer technology. *Nursing and Healthcare, 6,* 509–10.

Greenes, R. A., & Shortliffe, E. H. (1990). Medical informatics an emerging academic discipline and institutional priority. *Journal of the American Medical Association, 263* (8), 1114–1120.

Mikan, K. J. (1984). Computer integration: A challenge for nursing education. *Nursing Outlook, 32* (1), 6–8.

Mikan, K. J. (1988). Curriculum planning for instructional use of computers. In *Impact of DRG's on nursing: Report of the Southern Regional Education Board* (pp. 13–28). Rockville, MD: Division of Nursing. (NTIS No. HRP-0907181).

National League for Nursing. (1988). *Nursing data review 1987* (Publication No. 19-2213). New York: National League for Nursing.

National League for Nursing. (1989, December/January). NLN forum on computers in health care and nursing. *Nursing Educators Microworld,* p. 12.

Newbern, V. B. (1985). Computer literacy in nursing education: An overview. *Nursing Clinics of North America, 20* (3), 549–556.

Parks, P. L., Damrosch, S. P., Heller, B. R., & Romano, C. A. (1986). Faculty and student perceptions of computer applications in nursing. *Journal of Professional Nursing, 2* (2), 104–113.

Popham, W. J. (1978). *Criterion-referenced*

measurement. Englewood Cliffs, NJ: Prentice-Hall.

Romano, C. A., Damrosch, S. P., Heller, B. R., & Parks, P. L. (1989). Levels of computer education for professional nursing: Development of a prototype graduate course. *Computers in Nursing, 7* (1), 21–28.

Ronald, J. S., & Skiba, D. J. (1987). *Guidelines for basic computer education in nursing.* New York: National League for Nursing.

Saba, J. K. (1982). The computer in public health: Today and tomorrow. *Nursing Outlook, 30* (9), 510–514.

Schwirian, P., Malone, J. A., Stone, V. J., Nunley, B., & Francisco, T. (1989). Computers in nursing practice. *Computers in Nursing, 7* (4), 168–177.

Sparks, S. M. (1989). *Computer-based education in nursing.* Bethesda, MD: U.S. Department of Health and Human Services, National Institutes of Health, National Library of Medicine.

Summers, S., Penny, S., Fortin-Boyer, J., Loutzenhister, J., Arnold-Biogioli, B. (1990). Creative use of microcomputer software by graduate students. *Computers in Nursing, 8* (5), 198–200.

36

Computer Use in Undergraduate Nursing Education Programs

Kathleen J. Mikan
Eula Aiken

INTRODUCTION

The purposes of this descriptive study of 513 undergraduate nursing education programs in 1989 were to document the use of microcomputers as instructional or non-instructional tools and to compare their use in programs located in 15 southern states with those in states outside the South. Few of the studies, conducted prior to 1985, included information about the use of microcomputers in associate and baccalaureate degree nursing programs. The early studies in nursing education focused on accessibility (Hales & Rothenberg, 1982), administrative uses (Johnson, 1984), and use in baccalaureate and higher degree programs (Thomas, 1985). In 1983, Spector conducted a survey of the collegiate nursing programs in the South to determine the extent of faculty interest in computer use and continuing education activities. The findings of the 1983 survey indicated a high level of faculty interest and documented the need for continuing education activities aimed to help faculty become competent computer users (Spector, 1983).

The increasing availability of microcomputers in academe and the concurrent rapid expansion of the use of computers in health care agencies in the mid-1980s contributed to a need for nurse educators to address the use of microcomputers as instructional tools in nursing education. Faculty preparation was a key factor in the process of incorporating computers within the nursing curricula. Recognizing the need for faculty development in the area of computer technology, the Southern Council on Collegiate Education for Nursing, in affiliation with the Southern Regional Education Board (SREB), sought funds to support a regional project.

In 1985, the Division of Nursing, Bureau of Health Professions, Health Resources and Services Administration, U.S. Department of Health and Human Services, awarded a three-year Nursing Special Project grant (D10NU24198) to the Southern Regional Education Board. This grant provided funds to support a series of computer-related workshops and conferences for nurse educators in 15 southern states (Alabama, Arkansas, Florida, Georgia, Kentucky, Louisiana, Maryland, Mississippi, North Carolina, Oklahoma, South Carolina, Tennessee, Texas, Virginia, West Virginia). The major focus of the continuing education activities was the use of the computer as an instructional tool at the undergraduate level in nursing programs. Throughout the project period, data on computer use were collected from the college-based nursing programs in the South. In 1987, data collection was expanded to include all college-based nursing programs in the nation (Aiken, 1988, 1989, 1990).

METHODOLOGY

The tool used for data collection, a questionnaire, was mailed in August 1989 to the administrators of the nursing programs (dean, director, chair, head of department) at 1,311 institutions in the United States. The 55 items on the questionnaire were based on the actual and potential uses of microcomputers in education in general, and in nursing education in particular, that were described in the literature. Before the initial administration of the instrument in 1985, an expert panel of nurse educators reviewed the instrument for content validity and clarity. The panelists, directors of learning resource centers and located outside of the South, were engaged in computer-related activities in nursing education.

RESULTS

Findings

The overall national response rate was 39 percent, with returns from 49 states; the response rate for the 15 southern states was 48 percent. The majority of the 513 institutions, representing all parts of the United States,

were public. The administrators of the nursing programs completed the majority of the forms. A summary of the findings, structured according to the five major questions related to computer use, follows.

Do the Undergraduate Nursing Majors Receive Any of Their Pre-nursing or Non-nursing Instruction with Computers? Over one-half of the returns indicated that nursing majors used microcomputers in the pre-nursing or non-nursing education courses. A majority of the nursing programs used microcomputers in the nursing portion of the curriculum while a low percent indicated undergraduate nursing students used terminals connected to the mainframe computer in their nursing courses. The percent of programs in the 15 southern states that used a mainframe computer in nursing courses was lower than the percent of programs in other states. On the other hand, the use of microcomputers in pre-nursing and nursing courses was similar across the nation.

Does the Nursing Program Have Microcomputers Available for Noninstructional Uses? The top five noninstructional uses of computers were word processing, student records, test construction, grade calculation, and test scoring. Word processing was the most frequently reported noninstructional purpose. Of the top five noninstructional uses there was little difference in percentage of responses from institutions located in the 15 southern states and those in other states.

What Are the Major Instructional Purposes for which Microcomputers Are Being Used within Nursing Courses? The major instructional uses of microcomputers at the undergraduate level in nursing programs were identified from a list of possible uses, for example, enrichment, remedial, testing, self-help, diagnostic. Enrichment and remedial activities were used by a majority of the nursing programs. Less than one-third of the undergraduate nursing programs used microcomputers for instructional testing, evaluation, self-help, or diagnosis of learning needs. Comparison of undergraduate nursing programs in the South with those in other states indicated higher use for southern programs. The category with the highest percent difference was diagnosing student learning needs. The percentage of programs in the South that used computers for diagnostic purposes was seven percent higher than those in other states. Nevertheless, the overall percentage of programs across the nation was low.

Microcomputers were used for two major instructional purposes: to supplement classroom and clinical learning. A higher percentage of the programs used microcomputers to enrich classroom learning experiences (72%) than clinical learning experiences (53%). Few nursing programs used microcomputers to replace or substitute for classroom or clinical learning experiences. Less than 10 percent used the microcomputer to replace clinical learning experiences. The percentage of nursing programs in the South that used computers to enrich classroom learning, supplement classroom learning, or enrich clinical learning experiences was higher than those in other states. On the other hand, a higher percentage of nursing programs in other states used microcomputers as a substitute for clinical learning, a supplement to clinical learning, and a replacement for clinical learning. Moreover, the percent difference between responses of programs in the South and other states was less than seven percent.

Identify All Types of Learning Activities Currently Provided by Microcomputers in Undergraduate Nursing Courses. Of 11 types of computer-related learning activities, the top five in this study were simulations, tutorials, drill and practice, word processing, and testing. There was little difference in any of the categories (less than 6%) between programs in the South and other states.

Name All Content Areas (Nursing-related) Taught, in Whole or Part, by Microcomputers. A majority of the nursing programs—in the South and in other states—reportedly used microcomputers to teach in the following top five nursing-related content areas: calculations (drugs and solutions), adult nursing, clinical case studies, clinical decision making, and maternity nursing. The percent difference in responses elicited from nursing programs in southern and other states was low (Table 36.1).

Discussion

This study was limited to the self-reports about computer use at 513 institutions with undergraduate nursing programs. No attempt was made to validate the extent of use or to contact administrators of nursing programs who did not return the questionnaire. Despite these limitations, the findings provide important information for nurse educators. The historical significance of the study cannot be ignored since it was conducted during the period when availability of microcomputers for instructional purposes in nursing education was in its infancy.

There was little difference in responses elicited from the 210 undergraduate nursing programs in 15 southern states and the 303 in the remaining states—a percent difference of seven or less. Cost, access, and availability of nursing-related software were important variables that influenced computer use. The availability and cost of commercially prepared software for specific nursing-related content areas probably influenced computer use in many settings. The reason for greater use in nursing (77 %) than

Table 36.1 Nursing-related Content Areas Taught with Microcomputers by Percentage and Frequency (N = 393)

	South N = 157		Other N = 236		Total N = 393	
	Percent	Frequency	Percent	Frequency	Percent	Frequency
Calculations	75	118	69	163	72	281
Adult nursing	65	102	65	153	65	255
Clinical case studies	61	95	59	139	60	234
Clinical decision-making	54	85	51	120	52	125
Maternity nursing	52	80	51	120	51	200
Basic mathematics	51	80	47	111	49	191
Clinical topics	48	75	39	92	42	167
Nursing leadership	48	75	39	92	42	167
Mental health	45	71	43	101	44	172
Nursing process	44	69	44	104	44	173
Medical terminology	16	25	19	44	18	69
Nutrition	24	38	27	64	26	102
Psychomotor skills	18	28	20	47	19	75
Research	22	34	26	61	24	95
Anatomy/physiology	8	12	10	24	9	36
Pathology	2	3	6	14	4	17
Pharmacology	36	57	36	85	36	142
Community health	11	17	15	35	13	52
Literature searches	3	42	28	67	28	109
Nursing management	1	13	13	30	11	43
Statistics/data analysis	22	35	19	45	20	80
Computer literacy	41	65	40	95	41	160

Note. Based on "Yes" responses to Question: Do undergradute nursing majors receive any of their nursing instruction with microcomputers?

in pre-nursing (55 %) courses is unknown. A lack of awareness of use in pre-nursing courses may be a contributing factor in these responses. Greater use of microcomputers than terminals connected to mainframe computers was consistent with the trend in society toward increased use of microcomputers for undergraduate educational purposes.

In sum, the findings indicated that microcomputers were used (1) in pre-nursing and nursing courses, (2) more frequently for noninstructional than for instructional purposes, and (3) to supplement and enrich classroom and clinical learning experiences. Few nurse educators used the microcomputer to replace either classroom or clinical learning experiences. Microcomputers were used primarily for word processing, simulations, tutorials, drill and practice, and testing and most frequently in nursing-related content areas to teach calculations, adult nursing, clinical case studies, clinical decision making, and maternity nursing.

The findings of the 1989 study were consistent with the results of other regional surveys that were conducted during the project period. The top five noninstructional and instructional uses, as well as nursing-related content areas, remained constant throughout this period. Additional research is needed at the regional and national levels to address issues related to the extent of use, cost effectiveness, and cost benefits of computer use in nursing education.

REFERENCES

Aiken, E. (1988). *Computer use in undergraduate nursing education programs: A study of 550 programs.* Atlanta: Southern Regional Education Board.

Aiken, E. (1989). *Computer use in 513 undergraduate nursing programs.* Atlanta: Southern Regional Education Board.

Aiken, E. (1990). *Continuing nursing education in computer technology: A regional experience.* Atlanta: Southern Regional Education Board.

Hales, G., & Rothenberg, L. (Eds.). (1982, May-June). Preliminary analysis of survey. *Computers in Nursing*, 1, 3. (Available from School of Nursing, The University of Texas at Austin.)

Johnson, B. M. (1984). Improving decision-making in the dean's office. In G. S. Cohen (Ed.), *Proceedings of the Eighth Annual Symposium on Computer Applications in Medical Care*, 8, 610–613.

Spector, A. F. (Ed.). (1983). *Survey of microcomputer use in southern nursing education: Report of findings.* Atlanta: Southern Council on Collegiate Education for Nursing.

Thomas, B. S. (1985). A survey study of computers in nursing education. *Computers in Nursing*, 3, 173–179.

37

Development of a Taxonomy of Decision-Making Properties of Computerized Clinical Simulations

Joan E. Thiele
Janet R. Holloway

INTRODUCTION

Today's complex health care knowledge and technology demand accurate clinical decision-making skills of all nurses. Proficiency in clinical decision making is acquired through practice with feedback. Concern for the health and safety of patients requires the use of simulated experiences for a large portion of the decision-making practice of students. In nursing education today, computerized simulations offer realistic situations for learning and practice purposes without the attendant risks to patients found in the clinical arena.

Currently, the decision-making processes and level of skill in decision making attained through use of computerized simulations is unknown. Development of a taxonomy of interactive computerized simulations is needed for production and selection of software appropriate to student learning needs. A taxonomy is also needed for the identification of levels of clinical decision making resulting from practice of decision making. Nevertheless, the literature identifying characteristics and categories of computer-assisted instructional materials is limited.

PURPOSE OF STUDY

The purpose of this study was to develop a taxonomy for identification and classification of levels of cognitive processing pre-

Funding for this project was provided by the National League for Nursing, Council for the Society for Research in Nursing Education. Additional support was obtained from Washington State University, Intercollegiate Center for Nursing Education.

This study was presented at the Ninth Annual Conference of the Council for Research in Nursing Education, National League for Nursing, San Francisco, CA, February 6–8, 1991.

sented in computer-assisted simulations. The taxonomy was designed to serve as an indicator of the level of decision making presented in a variety of computer-assisted instructional simulations. The taxonomy may be used to identify decision-making complexity contained within simulations that purport to teach or measure decision-making processes.

BACKGROUND OF STUDY

A body of literature is available supporting the use of computer assisted instruction (CAI) for teaching decision making. CAI in nursing began in the late 1960s, more than 30 years ago (Sweeney, 1985). Study of the effectiveness of CAI established that learning time could be reduced to as much as one-third for traditional instruction by lecture and reading of textbooks (Bitzer, 1970). CAI is equally as effective as other instructional strategies and far more efficient (Ball & Hannah, 1984).

In a 1988 nursing education survey, the major learning activities presented via CAI were simulations, drill and practice, tutorials, testing and evaluation, and word processing (Southern Regional Education Board, 1988). In a review of research on the effectiveness of CAI Roblyer (1988) reported that "computer applications in science areas [using] primarily simulations yield higher effects than in any other area. Science results are followed by mathematics and cognitive skills" (p. 86).

Effective use of computer simulations requires identification of learning outcomes. As Glenn and Rakow (1985) noted, "simulations can be effective learning experiences, as students can learn in an environment designed to allow for error and discovery" (p. 59). To date, efforts to categorize CAI have

produced evaluation tools for assessing the technical merit of CAI software (Underwood, 1988), identifying job performance (Harmon, 1985), and specifying types of simulations (Gredler, 1986). Development of a tool for evaluating decision-making skills for nursing practice resulting from use of computer simulations has not been reported in the literature.

Pilot work reported by Thiele (1989) indicated that simulations for teaching clinical decision making can be categorized according to cognitive complexity. Levels of clinical performance have been categorized as novice, advanced beginner, competent, proficient, and expert (Benner, 1984). Characteristics of clinical performance levels provide a base for identification of decision making as practiced in simulations. As shown in Figure 37.1, CAI offers clinical decision-making practice consistent with novice to proficient performance.

Determination of clinical judgment levels from simulations requires identification and classification of the cognitive components, task complexity, and nursing focus required to formulate a judgment (Tanner, 1983). Categories for the proposed taxonomy were developed from the literature and subjected to pilot testing. Fifteen commercially available CAIs were analyzed to identify descriptors of performance consistent with novice to proficient levels of practice (Benner, 1984). The category of expert was not included, as the principal investigator (Thiele, 1989) had concluded, from an earlier pilot study, that existing computer simulations were not ca-

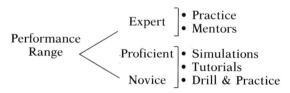

Figure 37.1 Sources of decision-making practice.

pable of requiring the cognitive processing consistent with expert performance. The next step was to define how the concepts were used in relation to CAI.

Review of the 1989 *Directory of Educational Software* (Bolwell, 1989) revealed a list of 201 CAI software items that were IBM compatible, developed in 1987 or later, and had a rating of 2.7 or higher on a four-point scale. The numerical ratings were those assigned by reviewers who judged each program in relation to ease of use, microcomputer attributes, general interest, and overall impression. The rating of 2.7 was arbitrarily chosen to represent programs that had above average and higher ratings. Of the 201 software programs identified, 29 were described as "drill and practice," 76 were "tutorials," and 96 were listed as "simulations." The terms "drill and practice," "tutorial," and "simulation" were used to reflect the classification of the CAI as identified by the reviewer (Bolwell, 1989).

Our goal was to review all of the tutorials and simulations that were rated 2.7 or higher and produced in 1987 or later. After eliminating duplicate entries, those CAIs listed as both tutorial and simulation and the ones we had previously reviewed, 30 CAIs were identified for review. Viewing these 30 software programs provided the basis for further refinement of the taxonomy. The most consistent findings produced by this review were:

1. the majority of programs described as tutorial or simulations required non-complex decision making, identified as Level II, or advanced beginner

2. the focus of tutorials or simulations was on presentation of factual information, rather than application of facts

3. the taxonomy was very helpful in determining the nature and level of decision-making components in software, al-though some degree of overlapping was present

4. variations in instructional design, particularly the extent of interaction with the learner required in different software programs, contributed to differences in identified level of decision making.

The review also pointed out that CAIs are becoming increasingly sophisticated. In fact, a number of newer CAIs presented materials that contained different degrees of complexity; learners could select their own performance levels at the start of the program. The learner who does not perform at a satisfactory level is told to read a particular book, review other materials, or do something other than continue in the program.

After reviewing the 30 programs, the first draft of the taxonomy was generated. Commonalities that served to differentiate levels of nursing practice in CAIs were identified. Grouping of common elements provided sets of descriptors of CAI format and instructional components that formed the crux of the taxonomic classifications. These instructional components were then matched with descriptions of human performance characteristics (Benner, 1984). CAI characteristics and related peformance levels are displayed in the model depicted in Figure 37.2.

VALIDATION OF DESCRIPTORS

Construct validity of the taxonomy was established by asking 11 individuals to compare the CAI with human performance descriptors and to match one with the other. One hundred percent agreement between the two sets of descriptors was obtained from these experts. At this point, the principal investigator decided that validity between the

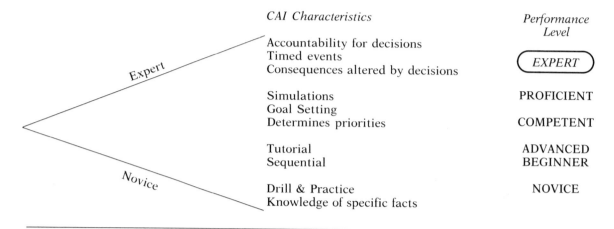

Figure 37.2   Model of decision-making from CAI.

sets of descriptors was present. The next step was to ask various individuals to review selected CAI programs and identify the level of decision making in each by using the Thiele-Holloway CAI Decision-Making Taxonomy (shown in Appendix A). To facilitate the process of using the taxonomy, a checklist format was developed.

A list of 12 CAIs that represented all levels of the taxonomy was generated. Reviews of each of these 12 programs were obtained from faculty and graduate students. The percentage of agreement between these reviews was calculated to establish reliability and provide information for further refinement of the taxonomy. Agreement was obtained among 95 percent of the ratings.

RELIABILITY OF THE TAXONOMY

To determine reliability of the taxonomy, individuals were asked to evaluate the decision-making characteristics of 12 different software programs. The CAI had been previously evaluated by the investigators and was selected to represent different decision-making levels and a variety of content areas. Most of the individuals who agreed to assist with evaluating the taxonomy viewed only one or two pieces of software. Of 39 reviews, only two disagreements between rankings of programs occurred. Interrater reliability was determined by dividing the total number of agreements by the total number of agreements plus disagreements. To obtain the percent of agreement, this sum was multiplied by 100.

$$\frac{\text{number of agreements}}{\substack{\text{number of} \\ \text{agreements} + \text{number of} \\ \text{disagreements}}} \times 100$$

Use of this formula produced a 95% interrater reliability.

$$\frac{37}{37 + 2} \times 100 = 95\%$$

The multiple reviews of CAI established reliability of the taxonomy across performance levels. In addition, many comments were received that assisted in revising the taxonomy.

By recording the critical determiners that were most often used to identify decision-making levels, a subset of factors that increase in complexity across levels was identified. These factors are: (1) decision making required of the learner, (2) the complexity of the situation, (3) interaction and feedback to the learner, (4) format, and (5) scoring method. The Thiele-Holloway Taxonomy displayed in Appendix A combines these specific determiners with general characteristics that apply to all levels of simulations. Regardless of the level of performance achieved by the user, computer-assisted simulations share common characteristics. That is, simulations typically begin with a brief scenario, then involve the learner in a variety of decision-making activities. Often, the CAI is designed to inform learners of the accuracy of their choices and the potential consequences of incorrect decisions. Simulations are structured so as to offer learners more than question and answer sequences. These characteristics differentiate simulations from other types of teaching materials. The general characteristics of simulations provided guides for categorization of instructional materials. The categories are summative in nature; overlapping of characteristics from one category to the next higher level occurs. Classification of CAI was based upon a determination of the taxonomic level that the software *most closely* represented.

CHARACTERISTICS OF CAI AT LEVEL I—NOVICE

As you might expect, CAI at the novice level consists primarily of drill and practice or tutorial programs. The CAI typically includes extensive feedback in a variety of forms; feedback is provided regardless of whether an answer is right or wrong. Instructive feedback is provided to reinforce learning. The learner can receive help both in running the software and with the content of the course. Usually, the learner cannot proceed after providing an incorrect answer; the correct choice must be selected (or, is provided to the learner) before advancing to the next portion of the program. Software written as decision-making Level I (novice) assumes that the learner has acquired the rudiments of the content, but needs additional factual information to increase understanding.

CHARACTERISTICS OF CAI AT LEVEL II—ADVANCED BEGINNER

In addition to the general characteristics of Level I simulations, the complexity of the performance required of the learner increases in Level II materials. Tutorials and situation-based events are noted. Multiple facts or pieces of information are required to interpret and correctly respond to the simulations. Feedback is provided, but more often when incorrect answers are given.

CHARACTERISTICS OF CAI AT LEVEL III—COMPETENT

A change in both the computer-assisted simulation materials and performance demands on the learner was noted in Level III. This change was seen as a shift to requiring priority setting in complex situations. Typically, materials request the learner to identify *the most appropriate* action(s) or interpret events. The learner must select between answers that are correct, but not equal in priority.

CHARACTERISTICS OF CAI AT LEVEL IV—PROFICIENT

Simulations requiring a proficient level of performance typically increase in complexity of the events. Accompanying the increased complexity is a greater focus upon accountability for decisions. In some instances, the first decision the learner had to make was the pathway or branch of the program that they wished to follow. Forced choices must be made by the learner; decisions, whether right or wrong, are used as the basis for subsequent events in the simulation. Additional data relating to the simulation is often available to the learner, but must be specifically requested. The consequences of the decisions are emphasized to the learner. Often, a timed event is included; not only must the learner make complex decisions, the decisions must also be made in a timely fashion.

SPECIFIC RESULTS OF STUDY

This study produced a useful taxonomy, presented in Appendix A, that provides a means of classifying decision-making performance provided in CAI. Rating CAI according to decision-making characteristics may be of value to educators in selecting curricular experiences for students and authors in planning quality software. It was interesting to note that of the 39 reviews, seven were rated as level I (novice); almost one-half, or 19, were rated as level II (advanced beginner); seven were rated for level III (competent practitioners); and six were rated as level IV (proficient). Of the 13 rated level III or IV, each included multiple pathways or branching modes as an instructional design strategy. In these CAIs, the learner identified his or her skill level on a range

from genius to beginner prior to actually beginning the program.

The resulting taxonomy provides a means for differentiating performance requirements of CAI. Identification of the descriptive domain of decision making from CAI yielded a measure that can be interpreted according to established performance indicators (Glaser, 1972). As additional refinement occurs and specific performance standards are established, a criterion-referenced measure or taxonomy may emerge (Waltz, Strickland, & Lenz, 1984).

SUMMARY

The effort to develop a taxonomy of decision making as found in computerized simulations was a fascinating study. At this time, a useful taxonomy has emerged. We suggest that educators review the level of decisions required in the CAI assigned to students. Perhaps some of the criticism of lack of decision-making ability of students and graduates is a reflection of lack of increase in complexity of the decisions required in the common source of practice simulations, computer-assisted instruction. Obviously, to move students beyond the level of an advanced beginner, teaching materials must demand higher performance levels of the learner. Multiple level CAI allows for greater usefulness of the software. Learners at various levels, advanced beginners to employees being oriented to new positions, may find such materials useful.

Both educators and authors of CAI need to be cognizant of the decision-making ability of students. Use of a taxonomy for identification of cognitive complexity in CAI software may promote identification of decision-making abilities of learners. A taxonomy of decision-making levels of simulations may contribute to more effective use of computerized instructional materials.

REFERENCES

Ball, M. J., & Hannah, K. J. (1984). *Using computers in nursing*. Reston, VA: Reston.

Benner, P. (1984). *From novice to expert: Excellence and power in clinical nursing practice*. Menlo Park, CA: Addison-Wesley.

Bitzer, M. A. (1970). Nursing in the decade ahead. *American Journal of Nursing, 70*, 2117–2118.

Bolwell, C. (Ed.). (1989). *Directory of educational software*. New York: National League for Nursing.

Glaser, R. A. (1971). A criterion-referenced test. In W. J. Popham (Ed.), *Criterion-referenced measurement* (pp. 41–51). Englewood Cliffs, NJ: Educational Technology Publications.

Glenn, A. D., & Rakow, S. J. (1985). Computer simulations: Effective teaching strategies. *The Computing Teacher, 12* (5), 58–59.

Gredler, M. B. (1988). A taxonomy of computer simulations. *Educational Technology, 26* (4), 7–12.

Harmon, P. (1985). Instructional software: A basic taxonomy. *Performance and Instruction Journal, 24* (5), 9–11.

Roblyer, M. D. (1988). The effectiveness of microcomputers in education: A review of the research from 1980–1987. *Technological Horizons in Education Journal, 16* (2), 85–89.

Southern Regional Education Board, 1988. *Computer use in undergraduate nursing education programs: A study of 550 programs*. Atlanta, GA: Author.

Sweeney, M. A., 1985. *The nurse's guide to computers*. New York: Macmillan.

Tanner, C. A. (1986). Research on clinical judgment. In W. L. Holzemer (Ed.), *Review of research in nursing education, 1,* 3–40. New York, National League for Nursing.

Thiele, J. E. (1989). *Decision-making properties of clinical simulations*. In *Simulation Design for Teaching and/or Measuring Clinical Decision-making*. Symposium conducted at the annual meeting of the Society for Research in Nursing Education, San Francisco, January 11–13, 1989.

Underwood, S. M. (1988). Measuring the validity of computer assisted instructional media. In O. L. Strickland, & C. F. Waltz (Eds.), *Measurement of nursing outcomes* (pp. 294–307). New York: Springer.

Waltz, C. F., Strickland, O. L., & Lenz, E. R. (1984). *Measurement in nursing research*. Philadelphia: F. A. Davis.

APPENDIX A: THIELE-HOLLOWAY TAXONOMY

Decision-Making Characteristics of Computer-Assisted Instruction Directions for Use and Taxonomy

Directions for Use. The following pages enumerate decision-making characteristics *common* to four levels of computer-assisted instruction (CAI). As you review CAI software, place a check mark in the column that best describes the software in relation to: (1) decision making required of the learner, (2) complexity of the situation(s), (3) interaction and feedback, (4) format, and (5) scoring method. As you review software, use the Thiele-Holloway CAI Taxonomy to identify the decision-making level presented. While overlapping of categories will occur, each CAI will "best fit" a single category. Rate the CAI according to the highest level of decision making that the majority of the program addresses. Complete the rating below after reviewing the software.

Evaluation Summary

Title of CAI _____

Date Produced _____ Source of CAI _____

Overall Rating of CAI:

Level I—Novice _____

Level II—Advanced Beginner _____

Level III—Competent _____

Level IV—Proficient _____

Overall Impression:

Additional Comments:

Level One—Novice

General Description. Primarily drill and practice (i.e., a series of problems to solve). Characterized by extensive feedback; multiple forms or modes of feedback provided. Help is readily available. Typically, the learner cannot proceed on an incorrect answer; must select the right choice before proceeding. Feedback is given frequently; often, regardless of whether an answer is right or wrong. Instructive feedback provided to reinforce learning. The learner is expected to have acquired the rudiments of the content.

Decision-making characteristics of computer-assisted instruction. Level One.

Characteristics of CAI	Present?	Comments
A. Decision making required of learner Recall of facts/information Rote memory		
B. Complexity of situation Usually not based on situations Rule guided Answers to questions do not build on previous items Drill and practice format		
C. Interaction and feedback Extensive feedback Cues and prompts used Multiple reinforcers used Correct answer provided after each item Help readily available		
D. Format One pathway; all learners follow same sequence of materials Answers provided on a list or menu from which learner selects Question/answer sequence—primarily Stand-alone questions		
E. Scoring Method Count of right/wrong responses		

NOTE: Use the back of the form for additional comments.

Level Two—Advanced Beginner

General Description. Level II CAI increases in complexity. Tutorials, situation-based events presented in a question, answer, feedback sequence are noted. Multiple events and/or multiple facts are required to interpret and respond to the simulations.

Decision-making characteristics of computer-assisted instruction. Level Two.

Characteristics of CAI	Present?	Comments
A. Decision making required of learner Some (limited) application of facts to new situation Base of knowledge (of events) assumed		
B. Complexity of situation Situation-based presentation(s) Answers to questions begin to build on previous items Complexity increased (no longer drill and practice) Exceptions to rules provided in situation		
C. Interaction and feedback Feedback provided frequently Cues and prompts used Must select a correct answer to advance to the next item Often given more than one opportunity to select correct answer May be given a chance to change answer; additional information may be provided Help readily available		
D. Format Tutorial—situation presented with some degree of instruction accompanying One pathway; all learners follow same sequence of materials Answers provided on a list or menu from which learner selects		
E. Scoring Method Count of right/wrong responses		

Level Three—Competent

General Description. Changes in both the computer-assisted simulation materials and performance demands on the learner are noted at Level III. These changes are: greater focus upon priority setting, interpretation of multiple concurrent events in situations of increased complexity, decreased feedback, and a change in scoring methods. Simulations are used to approximate real-world experiences.

Decision-making characteristics of computer-assisted instruction. Level Three.

Characteristics of CAI	Present?	Comments
A. Decision making required of learner Increased focus on planning Priority setting expected		
B. Complexity of situation Multiple simultaneous events presented Identification of priorities expected Case study presentation(s)		
C. Interaction and feedback Feedback accompanied by supporting rationale Frequency of feedback decreased; often provided at the end of a related sequence of information		
D. Format Pathway may be partially determined by the learner's responses Sequence not the same for each learner		
E. Scoring Method Scored by content area(s); decision making, priority or goal setting part of scoring		

Level Four—Proficient

Characteristics. Level IV materials are noted by presentation of dynamic situations. Accompanying the complexity is a greater focus upon accountability for decisions. Forced choices are presented to the learner. The decisions made must be retained throughout the simulation.

Decision-making characteristics of computer-assisted instruction. Level Four.

Characteristics of CAI	Present?	Comments
A. Decision making required of learner Priority setting demanded Learner held accountable for decisions made in situation		
B. Complexity of situation Priority setting demanded Learner held accountable for decisions made in situation Multiple complex events/situations presented Evaluation of multiple circumstances/events required Rapid response often required (timed responses)		
C. Interaction and feedback Minimal corrective feedback offered Frequency of feedback decreased; often provided at the end of a related sequence of information Learner often must provide own responses Decisions of learner alter sequence of events; once made, responses cannot be changed		
D. Format Pathway determined by the learner selects performance level; held accountable for level Sequence not the same for each learner Multiple difficulty levels may be found in a single program Additional information may be available to learner, but only when requested and correctly identified Learner must often provide own response		
E. Scoring Method Scored by analytical attributes of simulation Decision making/goal setting part of scoring		

38

Development and Testing of a Student Software Evaluation Form for Computer-Assisted Instruction

Jean M. Arnold

INTRODUCTION

Computer-assisted instruction (CAI) is a means to individualize instruction. CAI is the use of a computer to provide instruction in the form of drill and practice, tutorials, and simulations (Chambers & Sprecher, 1983, p. 3). The instructional design of CAI simulations is a portrayal of a realistic situation. With the advent of the personal computer CAI has become more readily available to the nurse educator. Nevertheless, the literature related to the use of CAI contains little or no evaluation information or data (Schwirian, 1987, p. 128; C. Bolwell, personal comunication, August 1991). Measurement capabilities of instruments such as reliability and validity were not addressed (Schwirian, 1987). Instead there was an emphasis on software selection. These tools assist the faculty to examine hardware and software requirements, content, instructional design, documentation, and motivation (Skiba, 1986; Smith, 1985). Although these instruments were helpful in examining software features, they could not be used to examine

learning. Recommendations for items to consider when evaluating learning included learner satisfaction, joy of learning, effects of feedback (Smith, 1985; Schwirian, 1987).

These recommendations influenced the writer to develop items for a student software evaluation tool. Three items were developed to address the instructional design of computer-assisted instruction (CAI): self-pacing, feedback, and comparison to other strategies. Self-pacing and feedback were selected, due to their inclusion in all the CAI software used with this baccalaureate student population. Since simulations were used to facilitate the transition between classroom and clinical practice, subjects were queried regarding simulation usefulness in preparing for actual client care.

The writer also thought there should be an item comparing CAI to other instructional strategies. Ease of use was added to determine if the respondents preferred the programming features of CAI. This instructional design of providing information, asking a question, and requiring a response with feedback is thought to facilitate learning. Enjoy-

363

ment of learning was addressed to determine learner's feelings about CAI.

Computer-assisted instruction was provided to one class of baccalaureate nursing students during both junior and senior years of their baccalaureate nursing program. Funding for the purchase and use of software was made possible by the New Jersey Department of Education. Evaluation of the use of software was a critical component of the project.

Objectives

1. To develop a student software evaluation form for use with CAI.
2. To test the Student Software Evaluation Form with the same population of baccalaureate nursing students over a two-year period.
3. To evaluate use of eight CAI programs by a class of baccalaureate nursing students.
4. To determine time requirements for using each of the eight software programs.

Because the project was initially funded for one year, a decision was made to develop a short tool that could be used with a variety of software programs and also assess the usefulness of CAI software. It was also decided not to focus on the subject matter of the software. Rather, the faculty or project director would make the match of the software with course content. Thus, the features, not the subject matter of computer-assisted instruction were used as criteria. These objectives were expanded as funding for the project increased.

The first two objectives were established for the first-year grant which provided hardware and software purchases for use at one

location. The goal of second-year funding was to expand integration and evaluation of CAI within the curriculum. Additional software was purchased and used with both new and ongoing students.

Since it was anticipated that the software evaluation form would be used each time a student used software, the questionnaire was restricted to five items.

A Likert scale was used to elicit a range of responses from the learner as opposed to dichotomous "yes" or "no" responses. A four point scale indicating degree of agreement was established including "strongly agree," "somewhat agree," "somewhat disagree," and "strongly disagree."

Faculty did not reduce class time to allow learners additional time to complete computer-assisted instruction. Their rationale was, "we do not give students reduced class time to view audiovisuals." The students did complain about the additional assignment of computer-assisted instruction. How much viewing time was actually required for CAI was unknown. Thus, time frames were added to the software evaluation data. The time frames selected were 0–15 minutes, 16–30 minutes, 31–45 minutes, 46–60 minutes, and 61 minutes or more. The software evaluation tool is illustrated in Figure 38.1. The Likert scale is used with five items and time requirement is designated via the five options described above. A comment section provides opportunity for open-ended responses.

METHODOLOGY

A nursing faculty member with expertise in measurement and evaluation reviewed the software evaluation tool. The faculty member recommended the use of a Likert Scale. Content validity was established through review of literature and discussion of items with nursing experts using CAI.

DIRECTIONS: Choose from accompanying list title(s) of computer software.

Software Title: _____

EVALUATION OF CAI

	Strongly Agree	Somewhat Agree	Somewhat Disagree	Strongly Disagree
Found self-pacing useful in learning the material				
Found client simulations useful in preparing for real client care situations				
Was able to learn the material easier than non-CAI learning approaches				
Found CAI enjoyable to use				
Found immediate feedback useful in learning the material				

Amount of minutes spent	0–15	16–30	31–45	over 61
on each CAI program:	_____	_____	_____	_____

Be sure to complete this evaluation form for each software program used.

COMMENTS: Please focus your feedback on how well this software facilitated learning of course content.

Figure 38.1 Student software evaluation form.

The next step was to select software. The writer, as project director, made software selections by using the following criteria:

1. Description of software available within *Computers in Nursing Software Exchange* (*Computers in Nursing,* Annual March/April issue).

2. Review of software, either written or via personal communication with colleagues

3. Content match with a selected nursing course

4. Preview of software on site by project director

Descriptions and reviews of software assisted in the decision whether to request preview copies of software from the publishers. These materials determined if there was compatibility of the software program with hardware and course content. Previews of software were difficult to obtain, but vendor negotiation was usually successful.

Several software titles were selected using these criteria, but only a few were required for all students. The software programs included three tutorials and five simulations. The software selected is presented in Table 38.1 by title, type, and use in level of program.

Hardly any faculty and student input was used due to their lack of both interest and familiarity with computer-assisted instruction. Nevertheless, the project director did review the software and read reviews whenever possible. A match with curriculum content was one major goal, and faculty did assist in this manner. The project director was familiar with the software evaluation process and had conducted workshops with faculty regarding CAI.

Three one-year grants to integrate CAI within undergraduate nursing programs were obtained in succession from the New Jersey Department of Education. These funds provided the opportunity for software evaluation within the same population of students during their junior and senior years of study for a baccalaureate degree. Repeated use of the software evaluation tool was made possible by these grants as well.

The most difficult component of this project was that of obtaining evaluation data. Both faculty and computer laboratory staff felt it was not their responsibility. One may wonder why faculty were not interested in this information since evaluation of instruction is an integral component of teaching. To overcome this obstacle, students were required to sign out software, and the software evaluation forms were to be distributed with the software. Nevertheless, laboratory personnel simply placed the software on a table in the laboratory away from the sign-in counter. Thus, it was necessary to hire a part-time staff person to distribute and collect software evaluation forms. The number of students who completed each software program varied, however, the sample was drawn from the same class of students. The software evaluation tool illustrated in Figure 38.1 was used with each software title as a repeated measurement design. The reliability measure, Cronbach Alpha Statistic was calculated for each software program.

FINDINGS

Reliability Results

The reliability results by type and level are illustrated in Table 38.2. The sample size ranged from 30 to 49. The unstandardized reliability results ranged from 0.753 to 0.882. These findings indicate that the Student Software Evaluation Form consistently measured students' appraisal of software at a moderate to high level. The outcome of a

Table 38.1 Software Titles by Type and Level

Title	Type	Level
Thorax and Lungs	Tutorial	I
ABGee!	Tutorial	II
Unconscious Patient	Simulation	II
Suicidal Adolescent	Simulation	II
Elliott: Seizures	Simulation	III
Jason: Meningitis	Simulation	III
Roy: SCI	Simulation	III
Managing to the Top	Tutorial	IV

Table 38.2 Reliability Results for Software Evaluations

Software by Title	n	Alpha
Thorax and Lungs	37	0.787
ABGee!	36	0.808
Managing to the Top	30	0.882
Unconscious Patient	32	0.833
Suicidal Adolescent	46	0.753
Elliott: Seizures	49	0.846
Jason: Meningitis	32	0.778
Roy: SCI	41	0.823

Items = 5

reliability analysis of the scale using 300 cases was an unstandardized reliability co-efficient of 0.797. It is unusual that a scale with only five items generated positive results each time it was used.

Time Requirements

The students were also requested to record the amount of minutes spent using each CAI program. The five time periods were collapsed into three to portray findings in bar graphs that were easier to read. The three time periods included 0–30 minutes, 31–60 minutes, and over 61 minutes. The software time requirements are illustrated in Figure 38.2. The tutorial program *Thorax and Lungs* time requirement varied from 16 minutes to over one hour with the majority of the respondents (n = 35) finishing the program within one hour. The *ABGee! The arterial blood gas learning program* (Thompson, 1988) software program required an average of 31–60 minutes (n = 39). The *Clinical simulations in nursing: Medical surgical series: Unconscious Patient* (Neil, 1987) simulation had a variation in time requirement from 16 to over 60 minutes with average time requirement of 31–60 minutes (n = 30). The time requirement for the psychiatric simulation, *Clinical simulations in nursing: Psychiatric*

Series: A suicidal adolescent, (Dibner, 1985) varied considerably ranging from under 15 minutes to over one hour (n = 32). Nearly one-half of the respondents (n = 46) completed the simulation *University of Washington neurological series: Elliott: Seizures,* (Ozuna, 1988) in less than one-half of an hour and the remainder required one hour. The time requirement for the *University of Washington neurological series: Jason: Meningitis* (McCarthy, 1988) simulation varied from 16 minutes to over one hour with the majority completing this software within 45 minutes (n = 50). Most of the subjects completed the third simulation, *University of Washington neurological series: Roy: SCI,* (Konikow, 1987) within 31 to 60 minutes (n = 34). The respondents (n = 42) varied considerably in time required for completion of the tutorial *Managing to the Top* (Career Development Software, Inc., 1985) ranging across all time periods. The majority of the subjects required one hour to finish this program although some respondents completed the software within one-half of an hour. In summary, the time period most selected by the respondents for all eight titles was one-half of an hour to one hour.

The number of subjects who recorded this information varied from one program to another; yet, the information has been helpful to other students and faculty who have been concerned about the time involved in using CAI. One reason why the number of respondents completing the software varied was the manner in which faculty assigned the software. Some stated the assignment was required and monitored its usage. Others stated it was required and designated its point value within the course grade.

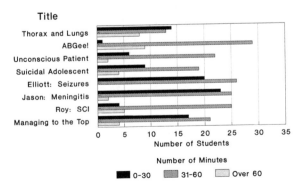

Figure 38.2 Software time requirements.

Students' Evaluation of the Software

Responses to the five items listed in the Student Software Evaluation Tool are illustrated in Figures 38.3 to 38.7. The bar graph in Figure 38.3 displays the subjects' evaluations of the self-pacing feature of CAI by title. The sample size for each of the programs is presented with the first item of the instrument, self-pacing. The same number of respondents is represented in the discussion of the other four items of the Student Software Evaluation Form for CAI.

Most of the respondents rated the *Thorax and Lungs* program positively but two chose the item "somewhat disagree" (n = 40). The "strongly agree" item was the dominant choice used for the *ABGee!* software (n = 40). The subjects varied in their evaluation of the *Unconscious Patient* program (n = 30) and *Suicidal Adolescent* (n = 32) using three of the four choices, with most subjects agreeing that self-pacing was useful. The softwares *Elliott* (n = 46) and *Jason* (n = 49) were the only two programs in which the respondents chose the "somewhat agree" item predominantly. The subjects rated the self-pacing of *Roy* program (n = 32) and *Managing to the Top* program (n = 42) positively. In general, self-pacing was rated highly by most of the respondents across the eight software titles used in this study.

The responses to the clinical preparation item is illustrated in Figure 38.4. The "somewhat agree" choice was dominant in six of the software programs used by this class of

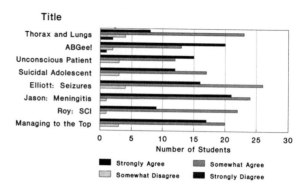

Figure 38.4   Clinical preparation.

baccalaureate students. The respondents used the four points on the Likert Scale for two of the three tutorial programs (*ABGee!* and *Thorax and Lungs*). This finding is not surprising because tutorials generally focus more on presenting information than applying it to situations. It was anticipated that the respondents would rate the simulation as more useful in preparing them for the clinical area. Figure 38.4 illustrates that the simulation *Unconscious Patient* was rated the highest by the respondents; that is, the "strongly agree" item was the dominant choice for this program. The subjects chose the "somewhat agree" Likert point predominantly for the other four simulations (*Suicidal Adolescent, Elliott, Jason* and *Roy*). The *Managing to the Top* tutorial was evaluated as useful in preparing for clinical practice due to its content focus on administering care to clients. The positive points were used more often than the negative points of the Likert scale across all software used by this sample of baccalaureate students.

Item three of the Student Software Evaluation Form addressed the ease of learning with computer assisted instruction. Figure 38.5 is a bar graph of the sample's evaluation of this feature of CAI. *ABGee!* software was rated the highest for ease of learning by these baccalaureate students. The four points of

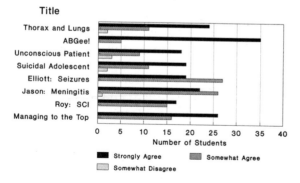

Figure 38.3   Self-pacing.

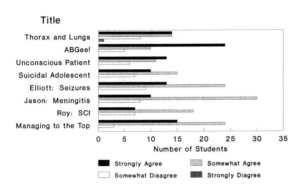

Figure 38.5 Ease of learning.

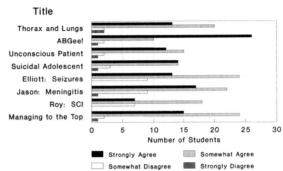

Figure 38.6 Enjoyment.

the Likert scale were only used with the *Thorax and Lungs Program.* The "somewhat disagree" Likert item was used by the respondents for each of the eight programs. Nevertheless, the respondents rated all of the eight programs as easier to learn than non-CAI approaches. This class of students did not have previous experience with CAI, a factor which may have accounted in the variation of responses across the programs. Also the content differences within the software programs may have affected the ratings by the respondents.

"Is CAI enjoyable to use?" This question was addressed in item four of the Student Software Evaluation Form and the findings are illustrated in Figure 38.6. It appears that the respondents enjoyed some software more than others. *ABGee!* was rated the highest for enjoyment, yet some respondents did not enjoy using it. Most of the respondents enjoyed CAI. The "somewhat agree" point on the Likert scale was selected most often by these respondents. The type and content of the software did not seem to affect this variable. Most of the respondents enjoyed CAI with a minority indicating they did not. Six of the software programs were not enjoyed by some respondents. These findings were shared with faculty along with the invitation to select additional software for purchase.

The usefulness of immediate feedback in CAI was measured in the fifth item of the Student Software Evaluation Form (see Figure 38.7). The "strongly agree" point of the Likert scale was the dominant choice used by the respondents for seven of the eight software titles. Feedback was rated more highly for the tutorial programs than simulation programs although more of this sample rated feedback positively than each of the other four items of the scale.

In summary, CAI was a satisfactory and enjoyable learning experience for this group of baccalaureate nursing students. The bar graphs for the five items of the student software evaluation form reveal a consistent pattern of positive ratings for the software programs used.

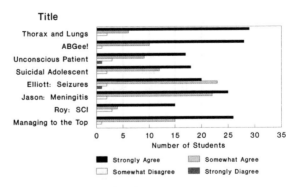

Figure 38.7 Feedback.

RECOMMENDATIONS

The following recommendations are made to assist others concerned with involving learners in software evaluation.

1. Require the learner to use software. Learners need explicit direction regarding learning activities. When making a computer assignment, inform the learner of the assignment's relationship to course requirements.

2. Use a software evaluation form; students like to offer their opinions about learning experiences. Also students may prefer software that you least expect, as illustrated by responses to *Managing to the Top*. Sometimes faculty consider software as simplistic and too easy. Yet students may disagree and become involved with the content through discussion with others.

3. Whenever possible, use a computer-based evaluation form instead of a paper form. It is preferable to have the computer track learners' responses as opposed to collecting forms and compiling data. Many hours of time were required to collect and organize the data for this project. In this study the student software evaluation form was added to the computer work stations. Nevertheless, because it was not part of the commercial software, the student was able to bypass it.

4. Allow the user time to use the software. Determine if some class time could be used for this purpose. If students are asked to view more software, nurse educators should consider the additional time burden for the learners.

Evaluation is a critical component in nursing education. Why not involve the student in the process? The development and use of the Student Software Evaluation Form was presented here to encourage its use in other nursing programs. CAI is an alternative teaching strategy that was highly acceptable to this sample. Student evaluation forms are outcomes measures of teaching effectiveness. Why not use CAI more and evaluate it further using reliable instruments? What other option is there to individualize instruction?

REFERENCES

Career Development Software, Inc. (1985). *Managing to the Top* [Computer program]. Vancouver, WA: Author.

Chambers, J. A., & Sprecher, J. (1983). *Computer-assisted instruction: Its use in the classroom.* Englewood Cliffs: Prentice-Hall.

Dibner, L. A. (1985). *Clinical simulations in nursing, Psychiatric Nursing Simulations I: A Suicidal Adolescent* [Computer program]. New York: Medical Examination Publishing Company.

Konikow, N. (1987). *University of Washington neurological series: Roy: SCI.* [Computer program]. Philadelphia: Saunders.

March, G., & Price, B. J. (1987). *A Software guide to physical assessment: Thorax and lungs* [Computer program].

McCarthy, A. M. (1988). *University of Washington neurological series: Jason: Meningitis* [Computer program]. Philadelphia: Saunders.

Neil, R. M. (1987). *Clinical simulations in nursing: Medical surgical series: Unconscious patient* [Computer program]. New York: Medical Examination Publishing Company.

Ozuna, J. (1988). *University of Washington neurological series: Elliott: Seizures* [Computer program]. Philadelphia: Saunders.

Schwirian, P. M. (1987). Evaluation research in computer-based instruction. *Computers in Nursing, 5* (4), 128–131.

Skiba, D. J. (1985). Evaluation of computer-assisted instruction courseware. *Computers in Life Science Education, 2* (2), 11–14.

Smith, J. M. (1985). Courseware evaluation: A Guide for nursing educators. *Computers in Nursing. 3* (3), 117–121.

Thompson, D. A. (1988). *ABGee! The arterial blood gas learning program* [Computer program]. Chapel Hill: Health Sciences Consortium.

Acronyms

AAAI—American Association for Artificial Intelligence
AACN—American Association of Colleges of Nursing
ACM—Association for Computing Machinery
ADCIS—Association for the Development of Computer-based Instructional Systems
ADL—Activities of Daily Living
ADT—Admission-Discharge-Transfer
AFIPS—American Federation of Information Processing Societies
ALA—American Library Association
AMIA—American Medical Informatics Association
AMRA—American Medical Record Association
ANOCOVA—Analysis of Covariance (Statistical procedure)
ANOVA—Analysis of Variance (Statistical procedure)
AONE—American Organization of Nurse Executives
ASCII—American Standard Code for Information Interchange
ASIS—American Society for Information Science

BCF—Basic Conditioning Factors

CAI—Computer-Assisted Instruction
CBVI—Computer-based Video Instruction
CBX—Computer-based examinations
CCP—Comprehensive Care Plan
CD-ROM—Compact Disc-Read Only Memory
CINAHL—Cumulative Index to Nursing and Allied Health Literature
CIS—Capacity Information System
CIPP—Context-Input-Process-Product
CNIS—Computerized Nursing Information System
CPU—Computer Processing Unit
CUSSN—Computer Use in Social Service Network

DHHS—Department of Health and Human Services
DRG—Diagnostic Related Groups
DSCR—Developmental Self-Care Requisites

EDUCOM—Educational Communication
ERIC—Educational Resources Information Center

FTE—Full-Time Equivalents

HCFA—Health Care Financing Administration
HDSCR—Health Deviation Self-Care Requisites
HeSCA—Health Science Communications Association
HIMSS—Healthcare Information and Management System Society
HIS—Hospital Information System
HISSG—Healthcare Information Systems Sharing Group
HL7—Health Level Seven
HRF—Health Related Facility

IDR—Item Discrimination Ratio
IEEE—Institute of Electrical & Electronic Engineers
IVD—Interactive Videodisc

JCAHO—Joint Commission on Accreditation of Healthcare Organizations

LAN—Local Area Network

MBTI—Myers-Briggs Type Indicator
MDS—Minimum Data Set
MEDINFO—Medical Informatics
MIB—Medical Information Bus

NANDA—North American Nursing Diagnosis Association
NCLEX—National Council Licensing Examination
NIRA—Nursing Incentives Reimbursement Award
NYQAS—New York Quality Assurance Standards

PBCC—Point biserial correlation coefficient
PCS—Patient Care System
PNUT—Portable Nursing Unit Terminal
PRI—Patient Review Instrument

RAPS—Resident Assessment Protocols
RUG II—Resource Utilization Groups II

SBIR—Small Business Innovative Research
SCAMC—Symposium on Computer Applications in Medical Care
SCDMS—Society for Clinical Data Management Systems
SCDNT—Self-Care Deficit Nursing Theory
SIG—Special Interest Group
SNF—Skilled Nursing Facility

USCR—Universal Self-Care Requisites

Trademarks

ABGee!®
Allen Electric and Communications Company®
Alpha Three® (Alpha Software Inc.)
Apple Computer, Inc.®
Apple®
Asymetrix®
AppleWorks®

Borland International, Inc.®

CliniCare®
CliniCom Incorporated®
CliniPac®
CliniView®
CLINSTAR®
CompuServe™
Crosstalk®
Crunch®

Data General®
dBASE III® (by Ashton Tate)
dBASE III PLUS®
dBMAN®
Dataflex®
DIALOG®

EasyNet®
Epson®
The Examiner® (software system)
ExamSYSTEM®
ERIC® (Educational Resource Information Center)—database
Elliott® (software program)

First Choice®

Harvard Graphics®
Hewlett-Packard® Corporation
HyperCard™
HEALTH® (database)
HealthQuest℠/HBO & Company

IBM®
IBM InfoWindow®
IBM Micro Channel®
IBM Presentation Manager™

JASON® (program title)

LaserJet Series®
Lotus 1-2-3®

Macintosh®
MediPac™
MEDLINE®
MicroPro International Corporation®
Microsoft Corporation®
MicroPac®
Microsoft Windows®
MicroTEST®
MicroTim®
MS-DOS®
MultiMate®
MUMPS® (Massachusetts General Hospital Utility Multi-Programming System)
MYSTAT®

NASDAQ® (North American Security Dealers Automated Quotations)
NCS® (National Computer Systems)

Opscan®

Paradox® (Borland International, Inc.)
Paragon®
PARSystem®
PROCOMM Plus®
Pioneer®
PC Paintbrush®
PsycINFO®
PsycLIT®

Quantum℠
QuestNet® (Healthcare Enterprise Information Network)

RNact®
Reflex® (Borland International Inc.)

SprintNet (formerly Telenet®)
SPSS® (SPSS Software, Inc.)
ScanTools™
Symphony®
SYSTAT®

ToolBook®
TRENDSTAR®

U-Diagnose®
UNIX®

VAX® (computer system)
Volkswriter® (software)

White Knight®
WordPerfect®
Word®
WordStar®

Zenith®

INDEX

Italicized page numbers represent figures and tables.